# A Handbook of Neurological Investigations in Children

T0260992

# A Handbook of Neurological Investigations in Children

## Mary D King and John BP Stephenson

2009
Mac Keith Press
Distributed by Wiley–Blackwell

© 2009 Mac Keith Press

Editor: Hilary M Hart
Managing Director, Mac Keith Press: Caroline Black
Indexer: Dr Laurence Errington

The front cover illustration includes part of an original painting by
Margaret Stephenson of Harrogate, North Yorkshire, UK

First published in this edition 2009 by
Mac Keith Press, 2nd Floor, Rankin Building, 139-143 Bermondsey Street, London SE1 3UW, UK

Reprinted with update 2014, 2018, 2019
British Library Cataloguing-in-Publication Data
A catalogue record of this book is available from the British Library

ISBN: 978-1-898683-69-8

Printed by The Lavenham Press Ltd, Water Street, Lavenham, Suffolk

# Contents

Authors viii

Acknowledgements ix

Foreword xi
*Rob Rust*

Abbreviations xiii

**Introduction** 1

**Part 1**

1.1 **History Highlights** 7

1.2 **Examination Essentials** 11

**Part 2. Investigations**

2.1 **Video with Audio** 14

2.2 **Electroencephalography** 22

2.3 **Electromyography and Nerve Conduction Studies** 40

2.4 **Evoked Potentials** 49

2.5 **Structural Imaging** 55

| 2.6 | Functional Imaging | 85 |
| 2.7 | Cerebrospinal Fluid | 93 |
| 2.8 | Cardiac Tests and Autonomic Function | 105 |
| 2.9 | Microscopic Examinations: Cells and Biopsies | 112 |
| 2.10 | Microbiology | 123 |
| 2.11 | Haematology | 129 |
| 2.12 | Immunology | 134 |
| 2.13 | Genetic Investigations | 144 |
| 2.14 | Biochemistry | 151 |
| 2.15 | Antiepileptic Drug Monitoring | 198 |
| 2.16 | Diagnosis by Clinical Trial | 201 |

Part 3. Clinical Settings

| 3.1 | Neonatal Seizures | 208 |
| 3.2 | Abnormal Neonatal Neurology | 214 |
| 3.3 | Delayed Development | 223 |
| 3.4 | Floppy Infant | 228 |
| 3.5 | Abnormal Head Size | 235 |
| 3.6 | Wobbly-eyed Baby | 240 |
| 3.7 | 'Cerebral Palsy' | 243 |
| 3.8 | Peculiar Gait | 251 |
| 3.9 | Learning Disability/Mental Retardation | 259 |
| 3.10 | Speech and Language Disorders | 265 |
| 3.11 | 'Psychiatric' Disorders | 271 |

3.12    Epileptic Seizures and Epilepsy                              275

3.13    Febrile Seizures                                             294

3.14    Paroxysmal Non-epileptic Disorders                          297

3.15    Epileptic and Non-epileptic Disorders Together              305

3.16    Acquired Neurological Deficits                              310

3.17    Acute Encephalopathy                                        318

3.18    Headache                                                    327

3.19    Weakness and Fatigue                                        330

3.20    Ataxia                                                      333

3.21    Movement Disorders                                          337

3.22    Progressive Loss of Skills and Dementia                     344

3.23    Rare Treatable Disorders                                    355

Appendix 1. Predictive Value of Investigation Results               364

Appendix 2. Some Normal Values                                      368

Appendix 3. List of Clinical Vignettes                              371

Index                                                               373

# Authors

**Professor Mary D King**, Consultant Paediatric Neurologist, Children's University Hospital, Rotunda Hospital and Beaumont Hospital, Dublin; *and* Associate Professor in Paediatric Neurology, University College Dublin School of Medicine and Medical Science, Dublin, Ireland

**Professor John BP Stephenson**, Hon. Professor in Paediatric Neurology and Senior Research Fellow, Division of Developmental Medicine, Faculty of Medicine, University of Glasgow; *and* Consultant in Paediatric Neurology Emeritus, Fraser of Allander Neurosciences Unit, Royal Hospital for Sick Children, Glasgow, Scotland

# Acknowledgements

We would first like to say thank you to Rob Rust of the University of Virginia not only for agreeing to write the Foreword but for making detailed constructive comments on the whole book.

We are extremely grateful to the following who have helped us greatly in many ways, with writing, editing, criticizing and revising, although of course any remaining errors or omissions are our own. So very special thanks to: Stephanie Ryan, Robert McWilliam, Vijeya Ganesan, John Tolmie, Amre Shahwan, Stephanie Robb, Michael Farrell, Francesco Muntoni, Peter Clayton, Jo Poulton, Mary Cafferky, David Coman and Sameer Zuberi.

Most of the Clinical Vignettes come from our own experience, but we are especially thankful to those doctors who have provided information about other children under their care, in alphabetical order of given name: Alla Nechay (Ukraine), Adnan Manzur (UK), Bryan Lynch (Ireland), Christopher Rittey (UK), Daniel Tibussek (Germany), Edward Wong (Hong Kong, PRC), Enrst Christensen (Denmark), John Heckmatt (UK), Lieven Lagae (Belgium), Rachel Kneen (UK), V Ramesh (UK), Robert McWilliam (UK), Russell Dale (Australia), Sameer Zuberi (UK), Wendy Mitchell (USA). We would also like to thank the family of the late Stuart Green, the families of the many children included, and in particular the family of Malcolm, who is in the first vignette.

Some details of the children in several of the vignettes have appeared in various medical journals and we thank them for permission to publish.

We are indebted to Bernie Larkin and Andrew Patton for assistance with the preparation of the manuscript and to Jean Hyslop for additional images.

Hilary Hart, Caroline Black and Udoka Ohuonu of Mac Keith Press have been very patient and greatly supportive.

To

Rory and Philippa

# Foreword

In days not so long ago when there were few tests excepting biopsy or postmortem against which the surmises of history and clinical examination could be tested, great neurological textbooks were nonetheless written by the likes of Kinnier Wilson, Frank Ford, Ray Adams and others. A remarkable and important quality of such texts was their capacity to teach us how to select historical details and observe clinical findings that guided us toward a correct formulation. Such texts manifested analytical honesty, practicality, and exceptional judgment, each having a particular 'personality'. The reader of such texts thus acquired sufficient confidence and authority to allay appropriately the uncertainty and anxiety of patients and their families, and they placed generations of readers in a position to refine the classification of diagnoses, accuracy of tests, and efficacy of treatments. In doing so they acquired facility in dealing with the uncertainties not only of the precise nature of neurological disease, but also those concerning the validity of tests, since in most there is a degree of imprecision and potential false-positivity. Errors in the selection or omission of appropriate confirmatory tests carried the risk of missing the point entirely, for which the consequences included inappropriate prognostication, a lack of genetic counselling, and inappropriate or untried treatments.

Upon this foundation a quite remarkable edifice of clinical and scientific sophistication has been constructed. If so much less was known, those intellectual ancestors were observant, experienced, critical thinkers who took great pride and satisfaction in acquiring exceptional skill at dealing with what they knew within the context of what was not yet known. The past three decades have, with astonishing and rapidly accelerating speed, filled in so many details and brought forward concepts and mechanisms that have made memorization of detail less burdensome, so improving the power of both our questions and our observations. With this great wealth of information, few general neurological texts are now the product of one or a few authors. There are exceptions: those of Aicardi (with a few remarkable associates) and Volpe are among the very small group that retain the particular virtue of the older texts, a personality that retains the integrity of method and point of view that can be so instructive, upon which one may model a durable and practical approach to the uncertainties of diagnosis that will prove both satisfying and productive.

In their Introduction to this handbook, Professors King and Stephenson raise themselves the question as to what possible use there might be for this work, since there is now such a plethora of information concerning the neurological diseases of children, their manifestations, pathogenesis, treatment, and outcome. Their excuse is to provide "a paper compendium of guidance on principle" together with a "philosophy of tests." This is a very modest description of this very remarkable handbook. What Professors King and Stephenson have done is to enrich and enable the success with which those who approach children with neurological diseases will utilize this wealth of information. They have provided an element that may be lost in the midst of so much information – the kind of judgment that only extensive experience and the tendency to ask difficult questions are able to generate. They organize our desire to confirm our formulations around the principle that we must first have formulated well and that our tests must be specifically selected to affirm or discredit that formulation. Armed with exceptionally sophisticated knowledge of clinical child neurology they have taken on a glittering array of tests in order to help us organize our approach to them.

This handbook is well organized, and the well-selected references are remarkably current. The principles of test selection are highly enriched with diagnostic tips, and the approach is illustrated with an instructive array of clinical vignettes. For busy academics, the vignettes themselves will provide an excellent aid to teaching our successors how to become judicious physicians. For scientists, this handbook is a reminder that their chances of identifying pertinent genes and elucidating disease mechanisms are far greater if they adhere to the valuable principles of formulation advocated in this book. Professors King and Stephenson obviously savor the ever richer opportunities for diagnostic testing but are evidently keenly aware of Aicardi's prediction, now nearly twenty years old, that "spectacular future progress in imaging ... neurophysiological or other laboratory examinations ... will remain of little value when applied indiscriminately without a previous careful [clinical] analysis." They are aware that the concept that "screening tests" for neurological disease might soon replace the adept clinician is a very dangerous one. They are just the sort of exceptionally adept clinicians and thinkers as are qualified to show us how to make the best use of what has become available to us to answer the questions posed so anxiously by children with neurological dysfunction and their families.

Robert S Rust, MA, MD
Thomas E Worrall Professor of Epileptology and Neurology
Professor of Pediatrics
Director of Child Neurology
The University of Virginia
USA

# Abbreviations

α–AASA – alpha-aminoadipic semialdehyde

AADC – aromatic L-amino acid decarboxylase

ABCD1 – ATP-binding cassette, subfamily D, member

AChR – acetylcholine receptor

ACTH – adrenocorticotrophic hormone

AD – autosomal dominant

ADC – apparent diffusion coefficients (map)

ADEM – acute disseminated encephalomyelitis

ADNFLE – autosomal dominant frontal lobe epilepsy

*ADSL* – adenylosuccinate lyase gene

AED – antiepileptic drug

aEEG – amplitude-integrated EEG

AES – anoxic–epileptic seizure(s)

AGAT – L-arginine:glycine amidinotransferase

AGS – Aicardi–Goutières syndrome

AIS – arterial ischaemic stroke

alb – albumin

ALD – adrenoleukodystrophy

*ALDH7A1* – aldehyde dehydrogenase 7 family, member A1 (antiquitin) gene

ALT – alanine transaminase

ANE – acute necrotizing encephalopathy

ANF – antinuclear factor

anti-DNAase B – antideoxyribonuclease B

anti-GQ1b IgG – an antibody to a specific ganglioside, but not an acronym

anti-Hu, -La -Ri, -Ro – various autoantibodies, meaning of abbreviation not important

anti-RNP – anti-ribonucleoprotein

AOA1/2 – ataxia with oculomotor apraxia 1/2

*AQP4* – aquaporin 4 gene

AQP4-IgG – antibody to AQP4 (same as NMO-IgG)

AR – autosomal recessive

AR-GCH1 – autosomal recessive GCH1 (deficiency)

ARSA – arylsulphatase A

*ARX* – Aristaless gene (ARX also used for conditions caused by mutations)

ASO – antistreptolysin O

AST – aspartate transaminase

ATM – ataxia telangiectasia mutated gene

ATP – adenosine triphosphate

*ATP1A3* – ATPase, Na⁺/K⁺ transporting, alpha 3 polypeptide gene

*ATP7A* – ATPase, copper transporting, alpha polypeptide gene

*ATP7B* – ATPase, copper transporting, beta polypeptide gene

ATRX – alpha-thalassaemia–mental retardation syndrome, X-linked (gene is *ATRX*)

BAEP – brainstem auditory evoked potential(s)

BECTS – benign epilepsy with centrotemporal spikes (same as BRE)

BG – basal ganglia

$BH_4$ – tetrahyrobiopterin

BNSM – benign neonatal sleep myoclonus

BOLD – blood-oxygen-level dependent (as in fMRI)

BRE – benign rolandic epilepsy (same as BECTS)

BSN – bilateral striatal necrosis

CACH – childhood-onset ataxia with CNS hypomyelination (old term for eIF2B-related disorders, same as VWM disease)

CACNA1A – calcium channel, voltage-dependent, P/Q type, alpha 1A subunit

CAE – childhood absence epilepsy

CAG – see G A T C below: codes for glutamine, hence polyglutamine repeats

CCA – catheter cerebral angiography

CDG (1a) – congenital defect of glycosylation (type 1a)

*CDKL5* – cyclin-dependent kinase-like 5 gene (also called *STK9*)

CGH – comparative genomic hybridization (as in array CGH)

CHAT – choline acetyltransferase or ChAT

*CHRNE* – cholinergic receptor, nicotinic, epsilon gene

CIS – clinically isolated syndrome

CK – creatine kinase

*CLN1, CLN3* – see INCL, JNCL

CMAP – compound muscle action potential

CMD – congenital muscular dystrophy

CMS – congenital myasthenic syndrome(s)

CMT – Charcot–Marie–Tooth

CMV – cytomegalovirus

CNS – central nervous system

COL4A1 – collagen type IV, alpha-1

*COLQ* – collagen-like tail subunit (single strand of homotrimer) of asymmetric acetylcholinesterase

CoQ(10) – ubiquinone

COX – cytochrome c oxidase

CP – cerebral palsy

CPP – cerebral perfusion pressure

CPT – carnitine palmitoyl transferase

CRMCC – cerebroretinal microangiopathy with calcifications and cysts

CSF – cerebrospinal fluid

*CSTB* – cystatin B gene

CSWS – continuous spike–wave in sleep (same as ESES)

CT – computerized tomography

CVST – cerebral venous sinus thrombosis

*DARS2* – mitochondrial aspartyl-tRNA synthetase gene

DBP – D-bifunctional protein

DEND – delay epilepsy neonatal diabetes mellitus

DESC – devastating encephalopathy in school-age children (same as FIRES)

DHAP-AT – dihydroxyacetone phosphate acyltransferase

DHPR – dihydropteridine reductase

DNA – deoxyribonucleic acid

*DOK7* – docking protein 7 gene (acronym: downstream of kinase 7)

DRD – dopa-responsive dystonia (Segawa disease)

dsDNA – double-stranded DNA (as in anti-dsDNA)

DTP – diphtheria, tetanus and pertussis vaccine

DWI – diffusion-weighted imaging

DYT1 – dystonia 1 = early-onset primary dystonia (torsion dystonia)

DYT5 – dystonia 5 = DRD

DYT11 – dystonia 11 = myoclonus–dystonia

DYT12 – dystonia 12 = rapid onset dystonia parkinsonism

DYT16 – dystonia 16 = dystonia parkinsonism not rapid onset

EA1 – episodic ataxia type 1

EA2 – episodic ataxia type 2 (other numbers exist)

ECG – electrocardiogram

EEG – electroencephalogram

*EGR2* – early growth response 2 gene

eIF2B – eukaryotic translation initiation factor 2B

*EIF2B1–5* – genes for the 5 subunits of eIF2B

EMG – electromyogram

*EPM2A, B* – epilepsy, progressive myoclonus type 2A, 2B

ERG – electroretinogram

ESES – electrical status epilepticus in sleep (same as CSWS)

ETF – electron transfer flavoprotein

ETF-DH – ETF dehydrogenase

F-wave – the second CMAP after supramaximal nerve stimulation – via cord neurons

FAB-MS – fast atom bombardment mass spectrometry

*FAM126A* – family with sequence similarity 126, member A gene

FDG – fluorodeoxyglucose, as in FDG-PET

FIRES – febrile infection responsive epileptic encephalopathies of school age (same as DESC)

FISH – fluorescent in situ hybridization

FLAIR – fluid-attenuated inversion recovery

fMRI – functional MRI

FT3 – free T3 (metabolically active T3)

FT4 – free T4 (metabolically active T4)

FXN – frataxin

GA 1, 2 – glutaric aciduria (type 1, type 2)

GAA – guanidinoacetate

*GAA* – alpha glucosidase gene

GABA – gamma-aminobutyric acid

GAG – glycosaminoglycan(s)

GAMT – guanidinoacetate methyltransferase

G A T C – guanine, adenine, thymine, cytosine: the bases of DNA and RNA that are combined in trinucleotide repeats as GAA, CGG, CTG, etc., and as CAG in the 'polyglutamine repeats'

GCH1 – GTP cyclohydrolase 1 (gene is *GCH1*)

GC-MS – gas chromatography mass spectroscopy

GEFS+ – genetic (previously generalized) epilepsy with febrile seizures plus

*GJA12* – gap junction protein, gamma 2 gene

GLRA1 – strychnine-sensitive α-subunit of glycine receptor (gene is *GLRA1*)

GluR3 – glutamate receptor 3 (as in anti-GluR3)

GLUT1 – glucose transporter 1

GlyT2 – glycine transporter 2 (gene is *SLC6A5*)

GM1, 2 – monosialic gangliosides with N-acetylneuraminic acid

GROD – granular osmiophilic deposits (on electronmicroscopy)

GTP – guanosine triphosphate

GTP-CH – GTP-cyclohydrolase

HABC – hypomyelination and atrophy of the basal ganglia and cerebellum

HARP – hypoprebetalipoproteinaemia, acanthocytosis, retinitis pigmentosa and pallidal degeneration

HCU – homocystinuria syndrome

*HEXB* – hexosaminidase B gene

HGPRT – hypoxanthine phosphoribosyltransferase 1

HHH – hyperornithinaemia–hyperammonaemia–homocitrullinaemia

HHV6, 7 – human herpes virus 6, 7

HIAA – 5-hydroxyindole acetic acid

HIE – hypoxic–ischaemic encephalopathy

HIV – human immunodeficiency virus

HLA – human leukocyte antigen

HMMA – 4-hydroxy-methoxymandelic acid (same as VMA)

HMPAO – $^{99m}$Tc hexamethyl propylene amine oxime

H-MRS – $^1$HMRS, proton magnetic resonance spectroscopy

HMSN – hereditary motor and sensory neuropathy

*HPRT1* – hypoxanthine phosphoribosyltransferase 1

HSAS – hydrocephalus due to congenital stenosis of aqueduct of Sylvius

*HSD17B4* – hydroxysteroid (17-beta) dehydrogenase 4 gene (codes for D-bifunctional protein)

HSP – hereditary spastic paraplegia

HSV – herpes simplex virus

HVA – homovanillic acid

ICP – intracranial pressure

IEF – isoelectric focusing

IFN-α – interferon-alpha (IFN-alpha)

IgG, M – immunoglobulin G, M

INAD – infantile neuroaxonal dystrophy

INCL – infantile neuronal ceroid lipofuscinosis (*CLN1*)

JME – juvenile myoclonic epilepsy

JNCL – juvenile neuronal ceroid lipofuscinosis (*CLN3* or *CLN1*)

*KCNA1* – potassium voltage-gated channel, shaker-related subfamily, member 1 gene

*KCNJ11* – potassium channel, inwardly rectifying, subfamily j, member 11

*KCNQ2* – potassium voltage-gated channel, KQT-like subfamily, member 2 gene

LCMV – lymphocytic choriomeningitis virus

*LICAM* – encodes L1 cell adhesion molecule (mutated in HSAS and MASA)

*L2HGDH* – L-hydroxyglutarate dehydrogenase gene (also called *DURANIN*)

LHON – Leber hereditary optic neuropathy

LINCL – late infantile neuronal ceroid lipofuscinosis (*CLN2*)

LQT – long-QT (syndrome 1, 2, 3, etc.)

LR+ – positive likelihood ratio (likelihood ratio of disease given a positive test)

LR– – negative likelihood ratio (likelihood ratio of disease given a negative test)

MADD – multiple acyl-CoA dehydrogenase deficiency (same as GA2)

MAE – myoclonic–astatic epilepsy

MASA – mental retardation, aphasia, shuffling gait and adducted thumbs

MCAD – medium-chain acyl coenzyme A dehydrogenase (deficiency)

MCT8 – monocarboxylate transporter 8 (gene is *MCT8* or *SLC16A2*)

MECP2 – methyl CpG binding protein 2 (gene is *MECP2*)

MELAS – mitochondrial myopathy, encephalopathy, lactic acidosis and stroke-like episodes

MERRF – myoclonic epilepsy with ragged red fibres

MIBG – meta-iodobenzylguanidine (technetium 99m tagged)

MICS – microcephaly intracranial calcification syndrome

MLD – metachromatic leukodystrophy

MLPA – multiplex ligation-dependent probe amplification

MNGIE – mitochondrial neurogastrointestinal encephalomyopathy

MPS – mucopolysaccharidosis

*MPZ* – myelin protein zero gene

MRA – magnetic resonance angiography

MRI – magnetic resonance imaging

MRS – magnetic resonance spectroscopy (usually proton – see H-MRS)

MRV – magnetic resonance venography

MSUD – maple syrup urine disease

5-MTHF – 5-methyltetrahydrofolate

MTHFR – 5,10-methylenetetrahydrofolate reductase

MTLE – mesial temporal lobe epilepsy with hippocampal seizures

*MTMR2* – myotubularin-related protein 2 gene

MuSK – muscle-specific receptor tyrosine kinase

NAA – N-acetyl aspartate

NAITP – neonatal alloimmune thrombocytopenic purpura

NCL – neuronal ceroid lipofuscinosis

NCV – nerve conduction velocity

NF1 – neurofibromatosis type 1

NKH – nonketotic hyperglycinaemia (glycine encephalopathy)

NM – neuromyelitis (optic neuritis not obligatory)

NMDA – N-methyl-D-aspartic acid

NMO – neuromyelitis optica

NMO-IgG – antibody to NMO = AQP4 protein (same as AQP4-IgG)

Nup62 – nucleoporin-62 kilodaltons (nuclear pore component)

OCB – oligoclonal bands (qualitative IgG)

*OCRL1* – gene for oculocerebrorenal syndrome of Lowe

OTC – ornithine transcarbamylase

PANDAS – paediatric autoimmune neuropsychiatric disorder associated with streptococcal infection

*PANK2* – pantothenate kinase 2 gene

*PCDH19* – protocadherin 19 gene

PCR – polymerase chain reaction

PDE – pyridoxine-dependent epilepsy

PDH – pyruvate dehydrogenase

PET – positron emission tomography

*PEX1* – peroxisome biogenesis factor 1 gene

pFN – false negative proportion

pFP – false positive proportion

*PHOX2b* – paired-like homeobox 2b gene

PIND – Progressive Intellectual and Neurological Deterioration (study)

PiZZ, PiSZ – α1-antitrypsin alleles (Pi = protein inhibitor)

PKAN – pantothenate kinase-associated neurodegeneration

PKD – paroxysmal kinesigenic dyskinesia

PKU – phenylketonuria

PLA1 – phospholipase 1 (also as in anti-PLA1)

*PLA2G6* – phospholipase A2, group VI (cytosolic, calcium-independent) gene

PLAN – PLA2G6-associated neurodegeneration

PLP – proteolipid protein 1 (gene)

PLP – pyridoxal-5′-phosphate

PMD – Pelizaeus–Merzbacher disease

PMLD – Pelizaeus–Merzbacher-like disease

*PMP22* – peripheral myelin protein 22 gene

(31)PMRS – phosphorus magnetic resonance spectroscopy

PNP – purine nucleoside phosphorylase

PNPO – pyridox(am)ine 5′-phosphate oxidase

PNS – peripheral nervous system

*POLG1* – mitochondrial polymerase gamma 1 gene

*POMT1* – protein-O-mannosyltransferase 1 gene

PPT – protein palmitoyl thioesterase

*PRKRA* – protein kinase, interferon-inducible double-stranded RNA dependent activator gene

PSAT1 – phosphoserine aminotransferase 1

PT – prothrombin time

pTN – true negative proportion

pTP – true positive proportion

PTPS – 6-pyruvoyl-tetrahydropterin synthase

PV+ – positive predictive value

PV– – negative predictive value

PVL – periventricular leukomalacia

$Q$ – quotient (as in $Q_{alb}$ and $Q_{IgG}$)

QTc – corrected QT interval

RANBP2 – ran-binding protein 2 (nuclear pore component)

*RAPSN* – receptor-associated protein of the synapse gene

RBC – red blood cells

RHADS – rhythmic high-amplitude delta with superimposed (poly)spikes

RNA – ribonucleic acid

*RNASEH2(B)* – ribonuclease H2 (subunit B) gene

ROC – receiver operating characteristic

SAMHD1 – SAM domain and HD domain-containing protein 1 (5th gene for AGS)

*SCN1A* – sodium channel alpha-1 subunit gene

*SCN2A* – sodium channel alpha-2 subunit gene

*SCN9A* – sodium channel alpha-9 subunit gene

SE – status epilepticus

SFEMG – single-fibre EMG (see also stimSFEMG)

*SGCE* – sarcoglycan gene

*SLC2A1* – solute carrier family 2 (facilitated glucose transporter), member 1 gene (codes for GLUT1)

*SLC6A5* – solute carrier family 6 (glycine transporter) member 5 gene (codes for GlyT2)

*SLC6A8* – solute carrier family 6 (creatine transporter) member 8 gene

*SLC9A6* – solute carrier family 9 (sodium/hydrogen exchanger), isoform 6 gene

*SLC16A2* –solute carrier family 16 (monocarboxylic acid transporter), member 2 gene (codes for MCT8)

*SLC19A3* – solute carrier number 19 (folate transporter), member 3 gene

*SLC25A22* – solute carrier family 25 (mitochondrial carrier: glutamate), member 22 gene

SLE – systemic lupus erythematosus

SMA – spinal muscular atrophy

SMARD1 – spinal muscular atrophy with respiratory distress 1

SMEI – severe myoclonic epilepsy in infancy (Dravet syndrome)

*SMN* – survival motor neuron (1 telomeric, 2 centromeric)

*SPAST* – current name for *SPG4*: codes for spastin

SPECT – single photon emission computerized tomography

*SPG4* – spastic paraplegia 4 gene (old name for *SPAST* gene)

*SPG11* – spastic paraplegia 11 gene (autosomal recessive)

SSADH – succinic semialdehyde dehydrogenase (deficiency)

SSEP – somatosensory evoked potential

SSPE – subacute sclerosing panencephalitis

stimSFEMG – stimulation single-fibre EMG

*STXBP1* – syntaxin binding protein 1 gene

SUDEP – sudden unexpected (unexplained) death in epilepsy (or in 'epilepsy')

*SURF1* – surfeit 1 gene

S/W – spike and wave

T3 – triiodothyronine (see also FT3)

T4 – thyroxine (see also FT4)

*TCF4* – transcription factor 4 gene

TE – echo time

TITF1 – thyroid transcription factor 1

TLR – toll-like receptor

TORCH(S) – toxoplasma, rubella, CMV, HSV (syphilis)

TPO – thyroperoxidase (as in anti-TPO)

*TREX1* – three prime repair exonuclease 1

tRNA – transfer RNA

TSC – tuberous sclerosis (complex)

TSH – thyroid stimulating hormone

*TTPA* – tocopherol (alpha) transfer protein gene

*UBE3A* – ubiquitin protein ligase E3A gene

VEP – visual evoked potential

VGKC-Ab – voltage-gated potassium channel antibodies

VLCFA – very long chain fatty acid

VMA – vanillylmandelic acid (same as HMMA)

VWM – vanishing white matter (subtype of eIF2B-related disorder)

WBC – white blood cells


We don't like abbreviations either, but we can't do without them!

MDK, JBPS

# Introduction

This handbook aims to help all those involved in the diagnosis of children with suspected neurological disorders. The authors are paediatric neurologists but we hope to reach out to a wider range of disciplines. Neonatologists, general paediatricians, child psychiatrists, intensivists, metabolic physicians, clinical geneticists and indeed neurologists who deal with adults may all be involved in trying to answer the question, "Why did this disorder happen?"

With the explosion of electronic information such as is found on PubMed and the availability of freely accessible diagnostic software such as SimulConsult (www.simulconsult.com) one might ask what possible use there is for a handbook like this. We think that even in this age of accelerating knowledge many will still wish for a paper compendium of guidance on principle. In particular we are keen to emphasize the philosophy of tests, which we discuss in the next section.

The handbook is divided into three parts. In the first part we provide extremely short outlines of what we believe to be the essence of clinical history and examination.

Part two deals with the investigations themselves. Because the question the clinician asks is "How do I investigate such and such a neurological disorder?" we have included two types of investigations. Firstly there are investigations which are more or less primarily concerned with the function and structure of the nervous system. Secondly we consider tests which may be necessary to explain what is wrong. Thus we have not only to give guidance within the disciplines of neurophysiology and neuroradiology but also to venture into the subtleties of biochemistry and other disciplines.

In part three we adopt a problem-oriented approach, and discuss the most appropriate choice of investigations in selected clinical settings. We hope that overlap and repetition between and within these last two parts will illuminate rather than irritate.

1

At the end of each chapter in parts one and two we include one or more illustrative clinical vignettes. We do this because it is through case histories that clinicians learn. The first vignette below is chosen because it embraces most of the principles of neurological investigation discussed in this book and illustrates the importance of never giving up the quest for a diagnosis.

This is neither a textbook of child neurology nor a practical manual, and it is certainly not intended to be a cookbook.

### Philosophy of tests

Jean Aicardi in his Hower Award Lecture of 1986 wrote: "Clinical medicine is basically an intellectual process whereby data from all sources, whether strictly clinical (in the restricted sense) or from the laboratory and other technical tools, is integrated and shaped into a meaningful profile." It is worth giving some thought as to how this is done.

It is important to undertake investigations with a specific question in mind. For example, if the history is of an intelligent 8-year-old boy with episodes of waking at night with contraction of one side of the face, salivation and inability to speak then the question is does he have benign rolandic epilepsy? Frequent centrotemporal spikes on the electroencephalogram (EEG) will confirm this diagnosis. On the other hand, to do an EEG on a child with loss of consciousness and stiffening during a swimming race risks not only finding irrelevant spike discharges but also missing a cardiac conduction disorder that could be revealed by electrocardiogram (ECG) (long-QT syndrome type 1).

In neurology it is important to understand the meaning of terms and concepts however apparently simple they seem. It is easy to assume that ataxia should point to investigation of the cerebellum, whereas it might be sensory ataxia (or even visuomotor ataxia) with completely different investigational priorities.

Screening tests or bundles of investigations are increasingly popular. If as we suggest a specific diagnostic question is being posed, it is important to ensure that the 'screening tests' will be able to answer it. If the 'metabolic screen' in a floppy infant or a young child with mixed epilepsy does not include simultaneous fasting blood and cerebrospinal fluid (CSF) glucose then the treatable disorder GLUT1 (glucose transporter type 1) deficiency will be missed.

It is worth devoting some attention to the diagnostic power of positive and negative investigations and what to do when an unexpected normal or abnormal result is received. We discuss the simple mathematics of this conundrum in Appendix 1.

### Geographical and financial constraints

A word is in order about the economics of neurological investigations. There may be difficulties not only as one might expect in underdeveloped countries but also in those in which political and insurance company regulations prohibit clinically appropriate investigations. We hope our approach of targeting investigations on the basis of clinical analysis may foster the best use of scarce resources.

## Clinical vignette

### Introduction.1 *Neurological investigations in a child*
We realize that those handy with the retrospectoscope (not an investigation in the index of this Handbook) will have less difficulty than we did puzzling over this boy's problems 30 years ago. Nonetheless, we think that the detail of one of our most difficult and interesting patients still holds lessons today.

PRESENTATION
An 8-month-old Scottish infant was referred to hospital in December 1976 because he had been unwell since his second triple vaccine (diphtheria, tetanus and pertussis – DTP) five days before. From the day after the immunization he had been irritable and 'dopey' with vomiting and loss of appetite (off his food).

His mother said that since birth he had passed large soft stools and he had not gained the expected weight. Moreover, he had been slower in his general development than his healthy sister and still could not sit unsupported.

On examination he was afebrile but was described as ill, and he showed *tache cérébrale* (the fiery red line left after stroking the abdominal skin that Trousseau first described, thought to be a feature of tuberculous meningitis, albeit nonspecific). He lay still and cried quietly at times, occasionally arching his back and neck, moving his right lower limb up and down on the bed but not his left. He tended to keep his thumbs in his palms.

INVESTIGATIONS (1)
(We refer to investigations here, as in later vignettes in this Handbook, in the order of the chapters in which they are discussed: EEG was not the first investigation undertaken!)

*EEG* – Theta dominated, within normal limits.

*CSF* – Pale yellow, white blood cells (WBC) 2–10/mm$^3$, red blood cells (RBC) 230/mm$^3$, protein 5.1g/L (510mg/dL), glucose 2.8mmol/L. Repeat CSF showed no appreciable change.

*Microbiology* – Tuberculous meningitis was ruled out.

*Haematology* – Haemoglobin 12.3g/100mL, film (smear) normal.

*Biochemistry* – Plasma albumin 37–42g/L, aspartate transaminase (AST) 336IU/L, alanine transaminase (ALT) 732IU/L.

COURSE (1)

A provisional diagnosis of mild cerebral palsy was made by the general paediatricians, the high CSF protein being attributed to 'bloody tap' (traumatic lumbar puncture).

By the age of 14 months his failure to thrive was more obvious, with little weight gain and head circumference falling to just below the 2nd centile. His mother said that after his immunization at age 8 months he lost interest and "there was no smile out of him" for 3 weeks. However, she said he never regressed apart from during illnesses. On examination he behaved as if he was aged 10 months, and the striking neurological finding was that tendon reflexes could not be elicited on meticulous examination. Plantar responses were inconsistent.

Poor growth and weight gain, a low serum iron and blood folate and continued loose (and sometimes foul smelling) stools prompted jejunal biopsy at 18 months. This was normal, and neurological investigations resumed.

INVESTIGATIONS (2)

*EEG* – Prominent theta but within normal limits.

*Nerve conduction* – Lateral popliteal velocity 32m/s, distal latency 8.5ms, no sensory response in sural, H reflex absent.

*CSF protein* = 8.5g/L.

*Sural nerve biopsy* – Normal.

*Muscle biopsy* – Gastrocnemius: probably not abnormal but some unusual profiles and possible abnormality of distribution of mitochondria in most of the fibres.

*Biochemistry* – Plasma lactate 1.7mmol/L, pyruvate 94mmol/L (lactate/pyruvate ratio 20), leukocyte arylsulphatase normal.

COURSE (2)

He continued to have bouts of lethargy, unsteadiness and vomiting. He made intellectual progress but he had evidence of increasing cerebellar ataxia and cerebellar dysarthria. Rombergism was demonstrated unequivocally on one occasion.

INVESTIGATIONS (3)

*Serial photography* was undertaken, showing *no* ptosis aged 17 months but unequivocal ptosis aged 8 years. Video of progress was recorded.

*EEGs* were not repeated after earlier normal recordings.

*Nerve conduction* – Velocities fluctuated but showed clear evidence of both conduction slowing and very small evoked potentials, indicating combined axonal and demyelinating neuropathy.

*Structural imaging* – Brain computerized tomography (CT) showed no abnormality (advanced imaging was not yet available).

*CSF protein* ranged up to 10.7g/L with CSF:serum albumin ratio ~150 (normal <9).

*Biopsies* – Further nerve and muscle biopsies did not clarify, showing only demyelinating neuropathy without specific abnormality in muscle and no visible mitochondrial abnormality.

*Biochemistry* – CSF and venous plasma lactates occasionally rose to 3.8mmol/L and lactate/pyruvate ratio was sometimes as high as 20–30, but some later values were normal.

Detailed studies of all respiratory chain activities in fresh muscle were carried out and no abnormalities were detected.

Several of these investigations were repeated in another national unit and the opinion was "probably not mitochondrial".

COURSE (3)
He remained a thin boy who was interactive between bouts of vomiting and lethargy and irritability. Lower limb distal weakness and wasting became more pronounced. When aged 9 years twitching of his right eyelid and right face and right limbs began and developed into epilepsia partialis continua. At the same time he had rapid onset of external ophthalmoplegia and pigmentary retinopathy with narrow retinal vessels, optic atrophy and loss of vision. Right-sided twitching persisted but he could still ask with his scanning dysarthria, "How is my EEG?"

INVESTIGATIONS (4)
EEG showed left 1Hz or slower (1/1.5s) occipital spike or sharp complexes. There were two and sometimes three sharp waves within each complex, superimposed on the slow wave.

COURSE (4)
He remained at a school for children with physical impairment, continuing to have intermittent right clonic epileptic seizures. He had a further bout of vomiting when he was aged nearly 11 years and then was found moribund, dying shortly afterwards. His devoted mother suggested post-mortem examination before it was requested.

INVESTIGATIONS (5)
*Liver and muscle pathology* were not contributory.

*Brain pathology* showed extensive loss of neurons in the cerebellum and olives, together with a leukodystrophy involving deep central white matter and certain spinal tracts, there being an extensive abnormality of myelinated axons in the dorsal columns and in the lateral columns but not in the pyramidal tracts.

COURSE (5)
In discussion with his parents it was decided never to abandon his diagnosis.

INVESTIGATIONS (6)
When methods became available for detecting deletions and duplications within the mitochondrial genome these were examined and excluded.

Course (6)
His diagnosis was reconsidered as a part of preparing this Handbook.

Investigations (7)
Screening for common mutations in the nuclear mitochondrial polymerase gamma gene (*POLG1*) was normal, but on further analysis he was found to be a compound heterozygote for pathogenic mutations in *POLG1*, one of which was novel.

Comment
This was a story of neurological investigations in a boy whose illness was difficult to diagnose in part because of the limitations of scientific advances at the time. We now know that *POLG1* mutations are relatively common, and associated with an expanding phenotypic spectrum of neurological disorders. The parents of a child affected by a neurological disorder wish for a cure, but failing that they may not want investigations to stop until a diagnosis is made, however late. The parents of this particular boy have asked if we could publish his name: his name was Malcolm.

## Further reading

Aicardi J. (1987) The future of clinical child neurology. *J Child Neurol* 2: 152–159.

Donnai D, Read AP. (2003) How clinicians add to knowledge of development. *Lancet* 362: 477–484.

Grimes, DA, Schulz KF. (2002) Uses and abuses of screening tests. *Lancet* 359: 881–884.

Guyatt G, Drummond M, Feeny D, et al. (1986) Guidelines for the clinical and economic evaluation of health care technologies. *Soc Sci Med* 22: 393–408.

Hudson G, Chinnery PF. (2006) Mitochondrial DNA polymerase-gamma and human disease. *Hum Mol Genet* 15: R244–R252.

Pagon RA. (2006) GeneTests: an online genetic information resource for health care providers. *J Med Libr Assoc* 94: 343–348.

Segal M. (2007) How doctors think, and how software can help avoid cognitive errors in diagnosis. *Acta Paediatr* 96: 1720–1722.

## Addendum

Since the first printing of this handbook at the end of 2009 there have been many advances. Because most of these may be found without much difficulty through searching PubMed we have not thought it worth listing them here. Rather, we reiterate our view that recent technology is compatible with what we have called the philosophy of tests. In particular we still maintain that homing in on a single diagnosis or diagnostic category – solely on the basis of the clinical history and examination - is fully compatible with the use of panels of diagnostic possibilities.

At the same time we would caution against reliance on a single investigation. Rather we would support what we have called "diagnostic greed". By this we mean what in law would be called corroboration. So that in making the diagnosis of Glut1 deficiency (one of the most common and important of the rare treatable disorders) we would suggest both seeking a mutation in SLC2A1 and measuring fasting blood and CSF glucose levels (and lactate).

Mary D King & John BP Stephenson, June 2014

# Chapter 1.1
## History Highlights

Although this book is about neurological investigations, the best pointer to the appropriate tests and the correct diagnosis is the clinical history. The historian is the person taking the history, and this may take longer than the time allowed by many health systems.

A crucial aspect of the elicited biography is the situation, setting, state, stimulus and provocation. Like other aspects of the clinical history such details may need to be elicited in the sense of being squeezed out from the memory of the informants. Sometimes the existence of triggers may be denied, but if one allows undirected talk then a significant pointer may emerge. Although prolonged interrogation is often required, sometimes the simplest association gives the diagnostic clue. If an infant deteriorates shortly after DTP vaccine, then this is likely to be the start of Dravet syndrome with a mutation in the *SCN1A* gene or a mitochondrial disorder or occasionally a metabolic decompensation, as in glutaric aciduria type 1 (GA1).

In the case of paroxysmal disorders it has been said that the "diagnosis is as good as the history" and this is true provided that the history is taken meticulously from the witness or witnesses to the event and from the child if sufficiently old. "The objective is to elicit a sequence which, replayed in the mind's eye, is as good as or better than video recording with full polygraphy" (Stephenson 1990). Nonetheless, home video, with accompanying audio, may add to this moving picture, and even more so if such recordings are made with a specific question in mind (Chapter 2.1).

In subsequent chapters we include examples of specific approaches to history taking. As a very simple example, if the problem is delayed motor development, the first questions will focus on the style of developmental trajectory: is there a crawling sequence as is usual, or a bottom shuffling one (Chapters 3.3, 3.4, 3.7)? When the consultation relates to recently recognized learning difficulties (Chapter 3.9) the question is more difficult and one must dissect the skills history to ensure that there has been no loss of abilities (Chapter 3.22) or even a rare treatable disorder (Chapter 3.23).

In several neurological disorders the family history may be difficult to elicit or completely denied. Although this might seem particularly common in certain paroxysmal disorders and channelopathies, it is a widespread problem. It may be necessary to interview other members of the family, particularly the oldest living female relative (the 'matriarch'), to elicit the true state of affairs, and in several situations such as genetic epilepsy with febrile seizures plus (GEFS+) (Chapters 3.12, 3.13) this is essential.

If a diagnostic problem has not been solved by the sequence history → examination → targeted investigation(s), then one returns to the history and begins this process again.

We sometimes regard the Guthrie test (neonatal blood spot analysis) as an extension of the clinical history: although it was introduced to detect inborn errors of metabolism, it is invaluable as a record of congenital infections, especially cytomegalovirus (Chapter 2.10).

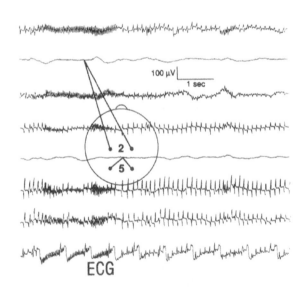

Figure 1.1.1 A section of cassette EEG/ECG recorded during a severe non-epileptic convulsive syncope in a neonate with hyperekplexia due to a dominant negative mutation in the GlyT2 gene *SLC6A5*. Note that the 'spikes' – which are giant repetitive compound muscle action potentials (CMAP) – whether very rapidly recurring at 30Hz ('tonic') or at around 8Hz ('clonic'), are confined to scalp areas overlying muscle and so are absent at the vertex (channels 2 and 5, arrowed). Similar repetitive CMAP 'spikes' are seen on the ECG channel. The EEG is virtually isoelectric because of the profound syncope, and for the same reason the ECG shows severe bradycardia with absent P waves and junctional escape rhythm. This appearance has only been reported in (neonatal) hyperekplexia.

## Clinical vignettes

### 1.1.1 'Sporadic' case

A boy had frequent episodes of grunting with intense stiffening and deep cyanosis from the neonatal period. He received a diagnosis of hyperekplexia (Fig. 1.1.1) and was kept in hospital for the first four months of his life. His parents had always denied any family history but many years later his mother revealed that she herself had been hospitalized for four months from the neonatal period. Family honour had prevented disclosure of this information previously. It turned out that both he and his mother had a pathogenic dominant mutation in the gene encoding the glycine transporter GlyT2.

### 1.1.2 You have got to see it[1]

A schoolboy presented with a history that he would suddenly stiffen, particularly when he moved suddenly. These episodes would last a minute or so and then he was alright. It almost seemed from the way he described it as a sort of cramp, but he wasn't able to describe it very well and his mother was rather reluctant to imitate his abnormal movements. In any event the boy was entirely normal; no abnormal movements could be reproduced. However, as the boy got out of his chair to leave he suddenly twisted his neck, stiffened his left arm and turned his body around in a grotesque posture which lasted 20 or 30 seconds and then stopped. The doctor immediately recognized paroxysmal kinesigenic dystonia, and asked the young man how often he had this problem and he said he had it two or three times a day. The doctor asked if it was a problem for him and he said it wasn't much of a problem but it was embarrassing sometimes. Then his mother interjected and said, "Of course we would like him treated because it must be quite painful for him." The doctor then asked her why she thought it was painful, if he himself hadn't said so. The conversation then went something like this:

Mother – "It is obvious that it must be painful to be in such a position."

Doctor – "But he didn't say so himself."

Mother – "But I know it must be."

Doctor – "How do you know that?"

Mother – "Because when I had it it was very painful."

The doctor stopped in his tracks: "When you had it?" he said to the mother.

Mother – "Yes – I had it from the age of 10 to about 23. It stopped when I had my children."

Doctor – "What did the doctor think it was?"

Mother – "I don't think I saw a doctor."

Doctor – "What did your parents think about it?"

---

1 This is a Stuart Green vignette, reproduced from Deonna and Stephenson (2008), with permission.

Mother – "Well, it didn't happen very often and I used to try and hide it with other movements. I never actually told my parents so nobody knew about it."

Doctor – "So you are telling me you had this abnormal movement for 10 to 15 years and now it has gone away but you never mentioned it to me until now?"

Mother – "Well, I never really thought about it until we were talking about the subject and I really saw what happened to my son."

He was put on carbamazepine and did very well.

COMMENT
For a variety of reasons family members don't always tell you the critical information which gives the diagnosis.

## Further reading

Berkovic SF, Harkin L, McMahon JM, et al. (2006) De-novo mutations of the sodium channel gene SCN1A in alleged vaccine encephalopathy: a retrospective study. *Lancet Neurol* **5**: 488–492.

Deonna T, Stephenson JBP. (2008) Stuart Green's vignettes 3 and 4. *Eur J Paediatr Neurol* **12**: 153–154.

Kempster PA. (2006) Looking for clues. *J Clin Neurosci* **13**: 178–180.

Macleod S, Ferrie C, Zuberi SM. (2005) Symptoms of narcolepsy in children misinterpreted as epilepsy. *Epileptic Disord* **7**: 13–17.

Robson P. (1984) Prewalking locomotor movements and their use in predicting standing and walking. *Child Care Health Dev* **10**: 317–330.

Scheffer IE, Berkovic SF. (1997) Generalized epilepsy with febrile seizures plus. A genetic disorder with heterogeneous clinical phenotypes. *Brain* **120**: 479–490.

Stephenson JBP. (1990) *Fits and Faints*. London: Mac Keith Press.

Van der Knaap MS, Vermeulen G, Barkhof F, et al. (2004) Patterns of white matter abnormalities at MR imaging: use of polymerase chain reaction testing of Guthrie cards to link pattern with congenital cytomegalovirus infection. *Radiology* **230**: 529–536.

# Chapter 1.2
## Examination Essentials

Much of the examination is by observation of the child from the moment that clinical contact is made. This is particularly so in the case of toddlers. One pays attention to dysmorphology, development, neurology and any general paediatric abnormalities. It is obvious that the features of the child must be interpreted in the context of the parents, and this is particularly important in the case of the head circumference. Charts allowing a plot of the child's and parental head circumference are helpful in this respect.

We will make mention of various directed examination techniques in the appropriate chapters in Part 3, but would say now that in the early preschool age group the provision of symbolic play materials gives an opportunity to observe important aspects of development and neurology.

If there is a facet of the neurological examination that we would most prize it is the examination of the eye movements. So much neurology is exposed when one explores saccades, ocular pursuit, optokinetic nystagmus, rotational nystagmus and the myriad subtleties of the motion of the eyes. The eyes are the mirror of the soul, the eye movements the mirror of the brain.

In the 'hard' neurology of the periphery the elicitation of reflexes is paramount. Not that one should use a hard red triangular tendon hammer almost as frightening as the scissor-man in Struwwelpeter. If one can provoke tendon reflexes in a profoundly hypotonic neonate with Prader–Willi syndrome then one may be confident that when one finds tendon reflexes to be absent in a child then that child has peripheral neuropathy or at any rate a lesion in the reflex arc.

The same attention to detail allows the distinction between the extensor plantar response and the striatal toe. The Babinski response may be old-fashioned but it says something about the pyramidal tract that no other sign does.

With respect to the finding of incidental 'abnormalities' the same caveats apply as to the significance of abnormal findings in a screening battery (Appendix 1). To take the skin examination as an example, hypopigmented macules are more common in those without tuberous sclerosis, café au lait spots in those without neurofibromatosis type 1, and inverted nipples in those without congenital defects of glycosylation (CDG1a). However, when a finding has a specificity of 100% – such as facial angiofibromata in tuberous sclerosis – then the diagnosis becomes certain.

We mentioned in Chapter 1.1 the use of home video/audio in the expansion of the clinical history. Likewise, these same observational tools (and also old family photos) may allow retrospective examination and the recognition of details not appreciated even by the family member holding the camera.

## Clinical vignettes

### 1.2.1 Covert microcephaly
A 2-year-old girl was brought to the clinic for an opinion as to whether she had Rett syndrome. Having reached the developmental stage of being able to give a toy back to her parents but not to the level of brushing the little doll's hair, she had lost purposeful use of her hands early in the second year of life. She would clap her hands together in front of her mouth, alternately pant and hold her breath, and grind her teeth. Unexpectedly, her head circumference was 49.5cm.

On examination of her parents, her father's head circumference was 63.0cm and her mother's 62.5cm.

COMMENT
Although this girl's head circumference was 0.5cm above the expected value for a girl of 2 years, in the light of the parents' head circumference measurements she had relative microcephaly entirely in keeping with Rett syndrome. Some years later an *MECP2* gene mutation was detected.

### 1.2.2 Eye to eye
A 21-month-old girl had been unsteady on her feet for 2 weeks. On first examination there was nothing definite apart from cerebellar ataxia, but she was shy and disliked close examination of her eyes. Prolonged observation of her eye movements via a glass partition and through binoculars from a distance revealed at first ocular flutter and then occasional opsoclonus.

COMMENT
Opsoclonus–myoclonus syndrome may need sustained but sensitive examination for detection. Neural crest tumours are not necessarily discovered.

## Further reading

Gamstorp I (1995) Child neurology – from my point of view. *J Child Neurol* **11**: 394–399.

Leigh RJ, Zee DS. (2006) *The Neurology of Eye Movements. 4th edn.* Oxford: Oxford University Press.

# Chapter 2.1
## Video with Audio

### Video

Video recording has been used for many years as an aid to diagnosis, particularly in video telemetry and in EEG departments, but this chapter is about video recording as a neurological investigation in its own right. Home video recording using a video camera or more recently a mobile phone is becoming an almost indispensable tool in discerning the nature of paroxysmal events (see especially Chapters 3.12–3.15).

There is little scientific or evidence-based information in the literature, but our experience is that such recordings are of immense value.

Most simply, the parent picks up a video camera or mobile phone and records an event, and on playback the physician is able to see and hear what has been recorded. If further events need to be captured the parents may be advised on recording techniques: for example, whether to focus on an infant's face or eyes or whatever is likely to answer the diagnostic question.

If episodes are nocturnal and not easily predictable, then arrangements may be made for prolonged bedtime video recording without the parents being present.

As with family history, it may be necessary to obtain home video recordings of relatives with similar paroxysmal events to complete the diagnosis.

As mentioned in Chapter 1.1, a family collection of home videos may allow a retrospective review of the child's development.

### Audio

The video emphasizes the visible aspects of the movie, but often the audio component is as important as what one sees, sometimes more so. A compulsive Valsalva manoeuvre may be difficult to recognize from video alone, but the sound of the hyperventilation and then the *lack* of sound in the 11 seconds silence during the Valsalva manoeuvre makes it clear why the syncope follows. Equally helpful is the sound of the intermittent hyperventilation heard in Rett syndrome and in Pitt–Hopkins syndrome. The quality of the sound of a gelastic–dacrystic (laugh–cry) seizure from a hypothalamic hamartoma is another good example: the subtle transition from laughter to crying gives the diagnosis.

Not only is the responsible clinician able to watch and listen to what has been recorded (as often as is needed) at the first encounter, but also he or she may return with further questions in mind as the diagnostic process evolves. Most importantly, the capture of a video allows it to be shared with more experienced colleagues at home or abroad (using, for instance, http://www.rapidshare.com), provided consent has been obtained. This is an additional reason for taking an instant video of a condition which manifests in the consulting room, such as myoclonus–dystonia (Chapter 3.21).

## Clinical vignettes

### 2.1.1 Is it epilepsy?
A developmentally normal 9-month-old girl was brought to the clinic with the question, was it epilepsy or a movement disorder? The parents had a home video of episodes which showed rhythmic adduction of the thighs associated with back arching and a vacant expression lasting some minutes. Episodes were captured while in a car seat. The girl cried if interrupted.

COMMENT
Home video alone enabled the diagnosis of infantile masturbation without need for further investigations (Chapter 3.14).

### 2.1.2 From home video to channelopathy diagnosis
An infant boy with no family history began having apparently unprovoked episodes since the first day of life. Secure diagnosis was made after observation of a home video recording at the age of 4 months.

The infant was observed to be crying in a gurgly manner and looking distressed for several minutes, with few limb movements. Colour change alternated between the right and left side of the face (the rest of him was enclosed in a babygrow). On the side of the face which was pale, the eye was open and the pupil large, while on the side of the face that was flushed there was ptosis and the pupil was small. Tears were more obvious on the side of the face with pallor and large pupil. Before one half of the face would become flushed, the eyelid on that side would droop and the pupil contract giving an appearance of Horner syndrome.

COMMENT
The appearances shown indicated alternating increase and decrease of sympathetic

outflow to the sides of the face. The sound and sight of the child's cry suggested that he was in pain, and the quality of his grunts indicated that he might have been defaecating, even though this had not actually occurred.

From this home video alone the diagnosis of the non-epileptic condition now known as paroxysmal extreme pain disorder could be established conclusively (Chapter 3.14) irrespective of other investigations. As expected, he improved markedly on carbamazepine.

### 2.1.3 It's a seizure isn't it?
A boy had an earlier history of epileptic infantile spasms. These spasms remitted, but he was left asymbolic (i.e. with no understanding of meaning). His main enjoyments were twirling plates, hyperventilating and holding his breath. He was referred because of new tonic seizures that were seen both at home and at his school for children with severe learning disability. Video recording was undertaken by one of the nursery nurses in the playroom of the paediatric neuroscience unit. Two episodes were captured, with video and audio. At first he hyperventilated loudly while twirling a plastic plate on the table in front of him, then made a strong Valsalva manoeuvre, most obvious in the 11 seconds silence before he groaned and collapsed in tonic extension. His mother then said, "It's a seizure isn't it?"

COMMENT
Yes, it was a seizure but an anoxic seizure not an epileptic seizure. Video with sound is an excellent way of demonstrating such Valsalva-mediated syncopes (Chapter 3.14).

### 2.1.4 'Epilepsy' with regression
This boy posed considerable diagnostic problems to his physicians abroad. He first presented with toe walking at the age of 2 years. At that stage he could reproduce a sentence spoken by his father. At around 2½–3 years of age his development seemed to plateau and regress and he began to have seizures. At first he would pant and then appear to stop breathing, and then later he would fall to the floor. He would be clumsy at these times. Often he would fall back or stagger and his speech was garbled for a few seconds. He became disruptive and hyperactive. The seizures developed so that they were characterized by one or two deep breaths, and then a staring look for 10 seconds and then a straight backward fall. Over time the seizures became more pronounced and came to include both tonic and vibratory components and what appeared to be a clonic component, aside from the loss of postural control which was a feature from early on.

INVESTIGATIONS (1)
*EEG* – A small number of EEGs were said to contain multifocal spikes, especially in sleep.

*Brain magnetic resonance imaging (MRI)* – Normal.

*Urinary dolichols* – 5.9µg/mg (control range 1.0 ± 0.7).

*Skin biopsy* – A single curvilinear cytoplasmic profile was seen on electronmicroscopy.

COURSE (1)
His parents were told that his epilepsy was secondary to late infantile neuronal ceroid lipofuscinosis (LINCL). The seizures did not respond consistently to any type of antiepileptic medication.

INVESTIGATIONS (2)
*EEG* – Normal recordings were obtained.

*Electroretinogram (ERG)* – Normal flash and flicker responses.

*Urinary dolichols* – Repeat estimation normal.

*Skin biopsy* – Repeat examination showed no abnormality.

COURSE (2)
He did not regress further, but seizures continued.

INVESTIGATIONS (3)
Home video with audio was recorded. This showed an apparently autistic boy with compulsive Valsalvas, but unlike the situation in clinical vignette 2.1.3 the tonic syncope of the Valsalva manoeuvre was followed by an epileptic seizure, that is to say these were anoxic–epileptic seizures (Chapter 3.15).

COMMENT
This boy had a mild form of autism spectrum disorder with considerable language and communication difficulties. LINCL was diagnosed on the basis of an inadequate battery of tests. His recurrent seizures were misinterpreted as epilepsy, an understandable difficulty for physicians who had not seen the onset of the episodes. Home video with audio that included the onset allowed confident clinical diagnosis.

### 2.1.5 Focal seizures but video-EEG did not help
The parents were concerned about their 6-month-old son's very frequent shivering episodes and brought a home video to the consultation. Episodes lasted 5–15 seconds, began with a slight deviation of the eyes, head and mouth to the right and stopped abruptly. Some were preceded by a jerk of the mouth, and in all of them shivering movements above the neck and shoulders predominated.

INVESTIGATION (1)
*Video-EEG* showed only 'muscle artefact'.

COURSE (1)
Episodes recurred intermittently, sometimes provoked by voluntary actions.

INVESTIGATIONS (2)
Home video recordings were shared with an international panel of paediatric neurologists who had an interest in movement disorders.

COURSE (2)
Normal development continued. An episode was noted after coming out of the bath at about the age of 2 years.

COMMENT
Shuddering attacks are rarely reported but are not uncommon. If the child is otherwise normal no additional investigations are indicated. In this the video-EEG did not help, but the video did.

### 2.1.6 Alarming spasms
A 9-month-boy had runs of spasms especially when sitting in his high chair. The paediatrician told his parents that his chance of being cognitively normal later was only 10%.

INVESTIGATIONS (1)
Video showed repeated spasms while he was in a high chair. More than 10 episodes occurred in succession, with flexion of the neck, upward deviation of the eyes and extension elevation and abduction of his upper extremities. Each spasm was long, over one second. The run of spasms was terminated when he was offered a toy.

COURSE (1)
Runs of spasms continued.

INVESTIGATIONS (2)
Ictal EEG showed no change during spasms. The interictal EEG was of course normal.

COURSE (2)
Episodes remitted after several weeks and development continued normally.

COMMENT
Benign non-epileptic infantile spasms is a better term than benign infantile myoclonus for this sort of harmless behaviour that is only hazardous when misdiagnosed as epileptic infantile spasms. To be certain of the diagnosis (and rule out epileptic spasms without interictal hypsarrhythmia – see Clinical Vignette 2.2.3) an EEG (preferably with EMG from both deltoids) has to be recorded *during* the spasms. However, video alone is usually enough to make this diagnosis with high probability.

### 2.1.7 It's easier to run without an EEG attached
This boy presented at 4 years of age with a history of clumsiness and walking awkwardly with frequent falls from when he started walking between the ages of 12 and 18 months. He was said to tire easily, and tended to swing his left leg out occasionally when walking. The symptoms fluctuated and were not always present. The paternal grandmother reported that her son, the child's father, had similar symptoms which eased in adolescence and early adulthood. The paternal grandfather died at 39 years from an alcohol related illness. Apart from mild clumsiness there were no abnormal neurological signs.

INVESTIGATIONS (1)
Video-EEG showed mild slowing of the background with rare occipital sharp waves. Episodes of falling or unsteadiness or shakiness did not occur over a 24 hour period.

COURSE (1)
The symptoms persisted over the following months with no new signs noted at clinic visit.

INVESTIGATIONS (2)
Home video captured the intermittent 'swaggering' gait due to foot dystonia which was elicited on running.

COURSE (2)
He was investigated for dystonia.

INVESTIGATIONS (3)
*Brain MRI* – Normal.

*Karyotype* – Normal.

*Dystonia 1 (DYT1) mutation analysis* – Negative.

*Blood* – Urea and electrolytes, creatine kinase, ammonia, lactate, transaminases, amino acids, all normal.

*Urine* – Amino acids and organic acids normal.

COURSE (3)
At 4½ years myoclonic jerks were noted, particularly during fine motor tasks such as cutting shapes, drinking from a beaker and writing. Often there were several minutes between individual jerks.

INVESTIGATIONS (4)
Mutation analysis of the epsilon-sarcoglycan gene (*SGCE*) confirmed a heterozygous 5bp deletion in exon 7, known to be pathogenic in myoclonus–dystonia. The same mutation was detected in the boy's father.

COMMENT
Home video alerted the physician to the presence of a movement disorder. In myoclonus–dystonia, gait disturbance may be the only symptom for several years before the appearance of the lightning-like jerks of myoclonus. The dystonia might be seen only during or after prolonged motor activity such as running long distances. Likewise the myoclonic jerks may be absent at onset or not detected during a clinic visit if the assessment does not include complex motor tasks. The typical alcohol responsiveness, a clue to diagnosis in adults, may have been a factor in the paternal grandfather's illness.

### 2.1.8 'Epilepsia partialis continua'
A 6-year-old previously healthy left-handed boy presented with a 2-week history of

jerking of his left hand. This consisted of a rhythmical flexion movement of the fingers at around 1Hz which was continuous while awake and asleep and decreased in amplitude while writing. There were no other abnormal signs; in particular, there was no weakness or sensory disturbance. A diagnosis of epilepsia partialis continua was made.

INVESTIGATIONS (1)
*Video* in hospital confirmed the occurrence in sleep.

*Video-EEG* did not show any electrographic change; the movement continued in all sleep stages

*Brain MRI* – Normal.

*Brain proton magnetic resonance spectroscopy (H-MRS)* – Normal.

*Plasma and urine amino acids* – Normal.

*Plasma lactate* – Normal.

*Urine organic acids* – Normal.

*CSF protein, glucose, lactate* – Normal.

COURSE (1)
He was started on oxcarbazepine without any change over the first week.

INVESTIGATIONS (2)
*MRI of the cervical cord* showed an intramedullary lesion at the level of C6–7. There was no contrast enhancement. The appearances were suggestive of a low-grade glioma.

COURSE (2)
Biopsy/surgical intervention was deferred because of the risk of impairment of hand function.

COMMENT
While continuous and paroxysmal myoclonus is well recognized in spinal cord lesions, the movement in this boy was more suggestive of epilepsia partialis continua from a lesion in the cerebral cortex rather than of spinal myoclonus. However, the lack of any change between waking and all stages of sleep as shown on video and video-EEG argued for a subcortical lesion.

## Further reading

Fertleman CR, Ferrie CD, Aicardi J, et al. (2007) Paroxysmal extreme pain disorder (previously familial rectal pain syndrome). *Neurology* 69: 586–595.

Kaufman DM. (1995) Videotape quality. *Mov Disord* 10: 803–804.

McLellan A, Phillips HA, Rittey C, et al. (2003) Phenotypic comparison of two Scottish families with mutations in different genes causing autosomal dominant nocturnal frontal lobe epilepsy. *Epilepsia* 44: 613–617.

Nechay A, Ross LM, Stephenson JB, O'Regan M. (2004) Gratification disorder ("infantile masturbation"): a review. *Arch Dis Child* **89**: 225–226.

Sheth RD, Bodensteiner JB. (1994) Effective utilization of home-video recording for the evaluation of paroxysmal events in pediatrics. *Clin Pediatr* **33**: 578–582.

Stephenson JBP. (2001) Anoxic seizures: self-terminating syncopes. *Epileptic Disord* **3**: 3–6.

Stephenson J, Breningstall G, Steer C, et al. (2004) Anoxic–epileptic seizures: home video recordings of epileptic seizures induced by syncopes. *Epileptic Disord* **6**: 15–19.

Taylor DC. (2003) Narrative based medicine. *Dev Med Child Neurol* **45**: 147.

Tibussek D, Karenfort M, Mayatepek E, Assmann B. (2008) Clinical reasoning: shuddering attacks in infancy. *Neurology* **70**: e38–41.

# Chapter 2.2
## Electroencephalography

Electroencephalography (EEG), aside from video, is the most commonly requested neurological investigation. It should never be 'routinely' ordered without having some sort of question in mind. Furthermore, the question must be one which the type of EEG requested may be able to answer.

### What is the EEG?
The electrical activity of the brain used to be recorded on paper in a number of channels (commonly 8 or 16) using one of several montages (a montage is a topographical arrangement of electrodes, making it easier to see the location on the scalp of the various electrical rhythms or discharges). In many countries today EEG is in digital form, often with simultaneous video registration.

Rhythms are conventionally described in terms of frequency, ranging from fast activity (beta) at 14–30Hz (equals cycles per second or c/s) through alpha at 8–13Hz and theta at 4–7Hz to slow or delta at 0.5–3Hz. Activity faster than beta activity is commonly not true EEG but rather a biological 'artefact' arising from a scalp muscle electromyogram (EMG). Very slow activity also results from biological artefacts related to respiration or sweating, often called sway.

Activity which is recurrent but not rhythmic may still be described in terms of its approximate frequency: for example irregular slow activity might be described as being predominantly 2–3Hz.

Rhythmic and non-rhythmic activity is also described in terms of amplitude. Amplitude is usually measured in microvolts (µV) and ranges from less than 2µV in electrocerebral silence ('flat EEG') to 400µV or more in high-voltage spike discharges.

Spikes are transients with a pointed appearance and a duration of less than 80 milliseconds (ms). They are often associated with a longer duration slow wave-form and the combination is described as a spike-and-wave complex. Very short duration transients of a spike-like appearance of less than 30ms duration are likely to be scalp compound muscle action potentials.

Sharp waves have a duration of 80–200ms but have a similar pointed shape. There is no standard term for longer duration steeply pointed waves but they may be referred to as sharp or sharply contoured components.

Polyspikes are multiple closely spaced spikes, and may be followed by a slow wave as in polyspike and wave. High-voltage beta activity may be difficult to distinguish from polyspike. Polyspike bursting (lateralized serial clustered closely spaced spikes) is a feature of the mitochondrial disorder due to *POLG1* deficiency, though with much higher specificity than sensitivity.

In children the EEG is often recorded with a bipolar derivation. In this the montage involves the connection of adjacent electrodes consecutively. If the slow (delta) waves in two such adjacent channels deflect towards each other in opposite directions that is commonly called 'phase reversal'. Similarly, in a bipolar montage, if spike discharges in adjacent channels point towards each other they are commonly referred to as negative spikes. By contrast, when spikes point away from each other they are called positive spikes.

## Provocations
Many factors influence the EEG, such as age, state of consciousness, temperature and metabolic balance. Certain stimuli are deliberately employed to provoke abnormalities which would otherwise be missed.

In *photic stimulation* (stroboscopic activation) pulsed light is flashed at varying rates into the child's open eyes to detect photosensitivity. It is important to have an ECG channel in place, since photic stimulation may also provoke cardiac asystole that will affect the EEG!

*Eye closure* is an important provocation which is sometimes omitted because the young child may not close his or her eyes on command. However, the eyes may always be closed passively. Spike-and-wave or sharp components not otherwise obvious may be induced by this manoeuvre.

*Fixation-off* is a technique for eliminating visual fixation without either closing the eyes or turning off the light. Occipital paroxysms of spike-and-wave are induced in certain epilepsies, in particular Panayiotopoulos syndrome and Gastaut-type occipital epilepsy (Chapter 3.12).

*Hyperventilation* (induced in young children by having them blow tissues or mobiles) is most useful for provoking the regular high-amplitude spike-and-wave of typical absence epileptic seizures. Hyperventilation is also helpful in reproducing non-epileptic 'absences' with diffuse slow (delta) activity in older children. As with photic stimulation, it is essential to have an ECG channel in place, since hyperventilation may induce cardiac arrhythmia (such as *torsades de pointes* in long-QT syndrome) that may itself cause EEG slowing.

*Sleep* may be induced naturally in the EEG department with kindness, time and patience, though occasionally sedation with chloral hydrate or melatonin may be necessary. Night-time natural sleep recording may be obtained with overnight video EEG. Sleep deprivation is employed to elicit spikes in other epilepsies, for example in the case of early morning tonic–clonic epileptic seizures in suspected juvenile myoclonic epilepsy (JME), and in suspected benign rolandic epilepsy.

### Special provocations
Modifications of photic stimulation are helpful in certain circumstances.

MONOCULAR OCCLUSION
Monocular occlusion is used when standard photic stimulation induces spikes or spike and wave, the so-called photoparoxysmal response in a child with television-induced epilepsy (this is more for management than diagnosis, in that if the photoparoxysmal response is prevented by monocular occlusion the same technique may be employed by the child to avoid television seizures).

PATTERN STIMULATION
Pattern stimulation using a large printed display or alternating black and white stripes may confirm and clarify a clinical diagnosis of pattern-sensitive epilepsy in a child whose eyes flicker in the presence of striped decorations.

SLOW STROBOSCOPIC ACTIVATION
Slow stroboscopic activation using a flash frequency of 0.5 cycles per second or less, induces large occipital spikes (which are giant visual evoked potentials) in one condition causing epilepsy and neurological deterioration (late infantile neuronal ceroid lipofuscinosis, LINCL, with the *CLN2* gene). Since LINCL is arguably the most common cause of epilepsy with regression, slow stroboscopic activation is of particular importance and should be requested specifically if the EEG department is not familiar with paediatric neurological disorders.

OCULAR COMPRESSION
Ocular compression has an indirect effect upon the EEG when it induces cardiac asystole due to an exaggerated vagal oculocardiac reflex. It is now only very rarely indicated (Chapter 3.14 and 3.15).

## Polygraphy: additional recordings
A single channel of ECG is always recorded at the same time as the EEG in case sudden changes in heart rate lead to changes in the EEG background activity which would not

otherwise be interpretable. ECG electrodes should be attached first as the placement of EEG electrodes is an occasional precipitant of syncopes (when the EEG has been requested for the wrong reason – see Indications for EEG, below) Likewise, a simple recording of respiration allows recognition of the usual forms of apnoea and respiratory rhythm disturbance. Additional recordings of eye movements, surface EMG and body movements may be helpful in certain clinical situations, particularly in the neonate in whom it is difficult to tell the stage within the sleep–wake cycle.

It is wise to record surface EMG from both deltoids in any child with very frequent seizures or when an ictal recording is anticipated. Ictal EMG is particularly useful in any type of fall or drop attack: with spasms or tonic seizures there is sudden increase in EMG whereas resting EMG tone disappears – the EMG line goes flat – in what are variously called atonic or astatic seizures or negative myoclonus.

## Digital ambulatory EEG
This allows continuous EEG (plus ECG and other physiological measurements) to be recorded for prolonged periods at home. The system uses a hard drive, and electrodes may be checked daily. This type of monitoring is suitable for children in whom events occur less often than daily.

## Video-EEG
Many units employ video during routine EEG recording. The technique is very useful for children with frequent events daily but also may capture events that occur by chance.

## Video telemetry
This inpatient technique provides continuous recording of simultaneous EEG with video. It is particularly used in children

- with frequent daily 'blanks' and normal interictal EEG with hyperventilation who may have a partial onset epilepsy

- with known epilepsy and behavioural or cognitive decline which may be due to continuous spike and wave discharges during slow-wave sleep (CSWS)

- when intractable epilepsy is being evaluated for surgery to determine localization of onset of seizures

- with bizarre stereotypies and/or non-epileptic attack disorder

- when clinical history and home video have not determined whether episodes are epileptic or non-epileptic.

## Cerebral function monitors (amplitude-integrated EEG or aEEG)
So-called cerebral function monitors are designed to be simple to use and record usually one or two channels of compressed EEG over hours and days. These monitors are used

25

in neonatal and intensive care units, and during anaesthesia. It is valuable to be able to record at least a single channel of proper EEG from the electrodes to confirm apparent abnormalities in the cerebral function monitor tracings, and if abnormalities seem likely then it is best to obtain some sort of 'standard' EEG.

### Indications for EEG

1. Clarification of the type of epilepsy once a clinical diagnosis of epilepsy has been made.

2. Management of epileptic encephalopathies (conditions in which there is a potentially reversible disorganization of the EEG).

3. Follow-up of non-lesional epilepsy, for example, focal epilepsies of childhood and other primary childhood epilepsies.

4. Any undiagnosed acute neurological illness or loss of skills (including mutism and suspect poisoning).

5. Unexplained developmental delay or intellectual impairment.

6. Suspect neurodegenerative disorder (subacute or chronic loss of skills).

Further details of these six EEG indications are now given.

*1. Clarification of the type of epilepsy once clinical diagnosis has been made*
Details are summarized in Table 2.2.1, which includes the EEG and clinical associations that make up the more generally recognized syndromes in infancy and childhood.

It is important to recognize that unless an epileptic seizure is recorded in a routine EEG, as is usual in absence epilepsy, the abnormalities found are not 100% specific for an epilepsy diagnosis.

*2. Management of epileptic encephalopathies*
• Hypsarrhythmia – chaotic high-voltage slow waves mixed with spike and sharp activity – often coexists with epileptic infantile spasms and developmental arrest.

• Hypsarrhythmia which has been abolished by corticosteroids may reveal focal spikes or slow activity suggesting underlying pathology.

• Frequent bilateral spike and wave complexes commonly without epileptic seizures are associated with acquired apparent 'deafness', loss of language or 'elective mutism' in Landau–Kleffner syndrome. In some cases the disappearance of this abnormality is accompanied by improved language comprehension but often no such benefit is seen.

• Long runs of slow (2 per second) spike and wave, often irregular, may be associated with fluctuating impairments of awareness and cognitive and motor skills, and with progressive decline in mental ability.

• CSWS requires monitoring by night-time sleep recordings.

Table 2.2.1 Electroclinical syndromes (see Table 3.12.1 for more details)

| EEG | Clinical | Syndrome |
| --- | --- | --- |
| Suppression–burst | Fragmentary myoclonus/early spasms | 'Ohtahara syndrome' but more important to recognize metabolic encephalopathies especially pyridoxal phosphate responsive and glycine encephalopathy (see Table 3.1.1 for details) |
| Generalized spike–wave, polyspike, focal spikes, photosensitivity – but often normal at first | Generalized or unilateral clonic seizures with fever (febrile status). Later multiple seizure types | Dravet syndrome (*SCN1A* mutations usually) |
| Hypsarrhythmia | Infantile spasms | West syndrome |
| 2Hz spike–wave; high-voltage 10Hz bursts in sleep | Learning disability. Atypical absences/tonic seizures in sleep | Lennox–Gastaut syndrome |
| Ictal 3Hz spike–wave | Typical absences, hyperventilation-induced | Childhood absence epilepsy |
| Spikes/polyspikes only with photic stimulation | Seizures *only* with flicker | Photosensitive epilepsy |
| 4–6Hz multiple spikes and polyspikes | Early morning jerking and generalized tonic–clonic seizures ± absences | Juvenile myoclonic epilepsy |
| Broad focal sharp waves centrotemporal | Nocturnal hemifacial salivatory seizures often with speech arrest ± tongue tingling | Benign childhood epilepsy with centrotemporal spikes (benign rolandic epilepsy) |
| Spikes/sharp waves (focal or generalized); often continuous spike and wave during slow sleep | Verbal auditory agnosia ± subtle seizures | Landau–Kleffner syndrome |

### 3. Follow-up of non-lesional ('primary' epilepsy)

In benign focal epilepsy of childhood with rolandic spikes there is evidence the seizures remit before rolandic spike complexes disappear. Thus, disappearance of the rolandic spike suggests that remission has occurred. However, this does not mean that one has to wait until the spikes have gone to discontinue therapy.

In childhood absences with 3 per second regular spike and wave, disappearance of spikes from the EEG *might* also suggest that the epilepsy has remitted.

In most other epilepsies there are inadequate data to make clear inferences with respect to prognosis from the EEG appearance. On the one hand patients with JME (with early morning tonic–clonic seizures with or without myoclonic jerks) may show a normal EEG after valproate therapy but will probably relapse in due course without treatment, while, on the other hand, some epilepsies remain in remission despite the persistence of spikes at the time of stopping therapy.

### 4. Acute undiagnosed neurological illness (including loss of skills)

In the term neonate, a suppression–burst pattern with very low voltage alternating with high-voltage irregular spikes may be seen in severe asphyxia, in glycine encephalopathy, and in pyridoxal phosphate-responsive seizures and many cases of pyridoxine-responsive epilepsies. Other causes are listed in Table 3.1.1.

Periodic lateralized epileptiform discharges may be seen in herpes encephalitis but also occur in asphyxia and in other static encephalopathies.

Spike–wave complexes, often asymmetrically distributed, are the usual accompaniment to verbal auditory agnosia in Landau–Kleffner syndrome (see Chapter 3.11). 'Mutism' is sometimes a feature.

General slowing of the background despite focal neurological signs is a nonspecific feature: it might be seen in meningitis, including tuberculous meningitis, but is of no precise diagnostic value.

Focal slow activity may be seen with *any* focal pathology including cerebral abscess and cerebral tumour, and often after prolonged partial status epilepticus in young children.

Focal flattening (reduction in amplitude of the background) is seen in subdural haemorrhage or effusion, but is also nonspecific.

Multiple spikes superimposed on rhythmic lateralized large slow waves suggest progressive neuronal degeneration of childhood, i.e. Alpers disease, and/or a mutation in mitochondrial *POLG1* (Fig. 2.2.1).

A very low-amplitude EEG indicates impaired cerebral perfusion often with raised intracranial pressure due to a variety of causes including hypoxia/ischaemia, barbiturates, hypothermia, etc.

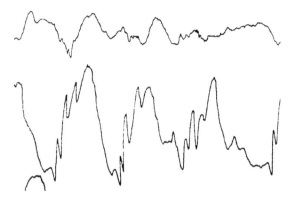

Figure 2.2.1 Classical appearance of multiple spikes superimposed on rhythmic slow waves (RHADS), as in this child with Alpers disease due to a *POLG1* mutation (NB diagnostic sensitivity low but specificity high).

Diffuse moderate-amplitude beta activity is often a drug effect and in this context may be a manifestation of drug intoxication, particularly by benzodiazepines.

### 5. Severe global developmental delay or intellectual impairment
High-voltage or very high-voltage posterior spike and wave accentuated by passive eye closure, the waves being high-voltage sharp components (broader or wider than sharp waves), is a feature of Angelman syndrome and may be present well before other signs and behavioural features of the syndrome are obvious. In the Angelman-like syndrome due to mutations in the *SCL9A6* gene, runs of 10Hz activity at an early age have been reported.

Trains of spike or sharp waves particularly in the central regions and at first only in sleep with poorly organized background activity may develop in Rett syndrome.

Slow background with little reactivity is a feature of *MECP2* duplication in boys.

Whether or not modern imaging has been done to disclose lissencephaly or other diffuse cortical dysplasias, EEG is likely to show diffuse high-voltage activity in the alpha frequency.

### 6. Suspect neurodegenerative disorders (subacute or chronic loss of skills)
Progressive reduction in EEG amplitude after infancy is typical of infantile neuronal ceroid lipofuscinosis (INCL).

Very high-voltage posterior complexes induced by slow strobscopic activation at 0.5Hz or less are typical of LINCL.

Diffuse beta activity of moderate amplitude, usually developing after the age of 18 months, is suggestive of infantile neuroaxonal dystrophy (INAD).

Multiple spikes superimposed on rhythmic lateralized large slow waves in Alpers disease have been mentioned in the previous section.

CSWS are seen in Landau–Kleffner syndrome and many other conditions, including neuroserpinopathy.

Stereotyped high-voltage polyphasic complexes repeated every several seconds and often associated with subtle transient reduction in tone and EMG are typical of post-measles subacute sclerosing panencephalitis (SSPE) – very rare indeed in the authors' countries but tragically common in others (Chapter 3.22).

### EEG in the paediatric intensive care unit
In the paediatric intensive care unit an additional indication for EEG is to demonstrate ongoing EEG activity in children who are totally paralysed, such as the infant with severe Guillain–Barré syndrome described in Clinical Vignette 2.8.3.

### Video telemetry and other prolonged EEG recordings to capture episodes
Unlike most 'routine' EEG, video telemetry or ambulatory recording systems aim to capture episodes to make a specific diagnosis. What is recorded depends on several factors including the age of the child. Various physiological and psychological non-epileptic events may be captured as often as epileptic seizures. The differential diagnosis of the well-known epileptic infantile spasms is a good example: epileptic spasms sometimes occur with an ictal discharge but without interictal hypsarrhythmia, but in non-epileptic infantile spasms the ictal EEG remains normal.

### Hazards of EEG
There are no absolute contraindications to EEG. However, serious potential dangers arise from misinterpretation of the findings when these are conveyed from the electroencephalographer to the clinician. Most frequently this arises when EEGs are requested for the wrong reasons, particularly in normally developed children with febrile seizures, in convulsive syncope (anoxic seizures), and in behaviour disorders (especially conduct disorders) without dementia or other neurological deviations. The difficulty arises because EEG spikes characteristic of epilepsy are found in a small proportion (1–2%) of children who do not have epilepsy. Therefore, if EEGs are carried out for the wrong indications, a small proportion will show spikes and it will be difficult to hide this fact from the parents. To make matters worse, normal phenomena may be misinterpreted as abnormalities. For example the shifting 'small sharp spikes of light sleep' may be reported as multifocal spikes, or the high-voltage sharp notched slow bursts of a young child's drowsy state (hypnagogic–hypersynchrony) are misinterpreted as generalized spike and wave.

EEG should be employed with great caution in children with cerebral palsy, because the findings are even more easily misinterpreted. A high proportion of children with cerebral palsy have spike discharges on routine EEG and so the finding cannot be used to assist the diagnosis of epilepsy or other paroxysmal events. Those with cerebral palsy may have non-epileptic events such as reflex syncopes like anyone else. However, if the child with cerebral palsy does have epilepsy, a lack of spikes on a routine EEG does not predict that remission has occurred.

Similar considerations apply to autism. There is therefore no justification for requesting an EEG in autism spectrum disorder when there are no other specific indications such as emergent epilepsy.

In the neonatal period misinterpretation of normal phenomena is a particular hazard. Background discontinuity, suppressions, asymmetries, asynchronies and sharp waves may all be normal phenomena, depending on gestational age and state. Sharp waves in particular do not have the same implications as at older ages.

From school age onwards a 'routine' EEG involves hyperventilation unless the EEG technician is warned against this. There is a potential hazard of cerebral ischaemic attacks if hyperventilation is performed in those with sickle cell disease and it is probably wise to avoid hyperventilation in such child patients. In moyamoya disease EEG signs of focal ischaemia may be induced by hyperventilation: it is not established that this is a true hazard, but it is enough to make one wary of continuing hyperventilation when there is a huge asymmetrical slow build-up.

**Requesting a 'routine' EEG**
We conclude with practical remarks on requesting an EEG, now that the indications and the relevant clinical problems are understood.

The interpretation of the EEG depends on both the problem to be solved and the state of the child, so EEG requests should contain a certain minimum of information:

- Age (and gestational age) in young infants
- Mention of fever, biochemical upset (in particular blood glucose level) or systemic illness at the time of the recording
- A detailed history of any seizures (including the date and time of the last seizure before the EEG recording)
- Up-to-date information on medications
- A statement on what the problem is: that is, the question or questions to be answered by the EEG. 'Query epilepsy', 'query a normal EEG' or 'recurrent febrile convulsions' are not appropriate reasons for requesting this investigation.

Some examples of the type of EEG which might be requested are listed in Table 2.2.2.

Table 2.2.2 Choice of EEG: some examples

| Type of EEG | Clinical situation | Findings | Interpretation |
|---|---|---|---|
| Routine (without provocations but with video if practicable) | Sick neonate with hiccups | Burst–suppression | Glycine encephalopathy |
| | Nocturnal hemifacial salivatory seizures | Rolandic spike–wave (S/W) clusters | Benign rolandic epilepsy (BRE) / benign epilepsy with centrotemporal spikes (BECTS) |
| | Acute ataxia | Diffuse beta activity | Benzodiazepine ingestion |
| | Acute regression/myoclonus/epilepsia partialis continua | Polyspikes on upstroke of rhythmic slow waves | Alpers (*POLG1* mutation likely) |
| | Autonomic status epilepticus | Spike complexes, varied sites | Panayiotopoulos syndrome |
| | Loss of skills | Periodic complexes | Subacute sclerosing panencephalitis |
| | | Diffuse beta activity | Infantile neuroaxonal dystrophy |
| | History of any type of paroxysmal event | Event captured on video with EEG/ECG/EMG | Diagnosis of epileptic or non-epileptic event established |
| Serial routine | BRE/BECTS | Spikes no longer | Epilepsy remitted |
| | 'Autistic' state | Decline of voltage | Infantile neuronal ceroid lipofuscinosis |
| Routine with hyperventilation | Blanks | 3/s symptomatic S/W | Absence epilepsy |
| | Stroke-like episodes (caution!) | Huge asymmetrical slow build-up | Moyamoya |

Table 2.2.2 continued

| Type of EEG | Clinical situation | Findings | Interpretation |
|---|---|---|---|
| Routine with photic stimulation | Infantile hemiclonic or atypical febrile seizures | Photoparoxysmal response | Dravet syndrome |
| | Television seizures | Photoparoxysmal response abolished by monocular occlusion | Simple television epilepsy |
| Pattern stimulation | Pattern sensitive | Spikes induced | Pattern-sensitive epilepsy |
| With slow strobe (0.5Hz) | Mixed epilepsy, ataxia, cognitive decline | Giant occipital spikes at 0.5Hz | Late infantile neuronal ceroid lipofuscinosis |
| Routine with repeated passive eye closure | Unexplained delay/ seizures with fever in first year of life | High-voltage 3–4/s sharp components maximal posteriorly mixed with smaller spikes or sharp waves | Angelman syndrome |
| Fixation-off (Frenzel glasses) | Ictus emeticus | Occipital S/W induced | Panayiotopoulos syndrome |
| | Migraine-like seizure | Occipital S/W induced | Gastaut-type occipital epilepsy |
| Sleep EEG | Clinically diagnosed epilepsy with infrequent seizures; normal routine EEG with standard provocations | Various | Depends on epilepsy type (e.g. increased S/W in BRE/BECTS) |
| | Cognitive decline | CSWS | Landau–Kleffner syndrome and other causes of CSWS |

(continued over)

Table 2.2.2 continued

| Type of EEG | Clinical situation | Findings | Interpretation |
| --- | --- | --- | --- |
| Sleep deprivation EEG | Early morning myoclonus and/or generalized tonic–clonic seizures | Fast spikes then rhythmic slow, polyspike and wave, 4–6/s S/W | Primary generalized epilepsy, especially juvenile myoclonic epilepsy |
| With ocular compression (by physician) | Unusual seizure including prolonged unresponsiveness after head bump or other stimulus | Identical episode reproduced after cardiac asystole | Reflex anoxic seizure/reflex asytolic syncope or anoxic–epileptic seizure (if rhythmic S/W follows EEG flattening) |
| Short video-EEG with suggestions: (1) suggest in clinic event will occur in EEG department; (2) suggest again in EEG dept; use usual provocation; have witness present | ? Non-epileptic attack disorder | Seizure induced without EEG change and recognized by witness as typical (from direct observation and review of video) | Non-epileptic attack disorder |
| EEG polygraphy | 'Breath-holding' seizures | Apnoea, QRS complex amplitude reduction, slow burst on EEG | Compulsive Valsalva manoeuvres |

### Three concluding comments

Despite all we have written, there will be some who are still tempted to request a routine EEG to answer the question, "Is it epilepsy?" This temptation should be strongly and completely resisted!

All in all, it is best if the doctor who has the clinical care of the child patient is the one who 'reads' the EEG.

Be good to your EEG technicians/technologists: they deserve to be cherished!

Table 2.2.2 continued

| Type of EEG | Clinical situation | Findings | Interpretation |
|---|---|---|---|
| Digital ambulatory recording | Daily 'blanks' not defined | Focal origin ictal spikes | Partial seizures |
| | Acquired mutism | CSWS | Landau–Kleffner syndrome ('acquired epileptic aphasia') |
| Video telemetry | Nodding attacks | Atonia with S/W | Astatic seizure (negative myoclonus) |
| | Frequent daily 'blanks'; normal routine EEG with hyperventilation | Focal discharge during behavioural alteration | Complex partial epileptic seizure |
| | | No EEG change during bizarre stereotypy | Non-epileptic attack disorder |
| aEEG (if full EEG not available) | Unexplained unconsciousness | Beta activity prominent | Benzodiazepine poisoning |
| | | High voltage | Status epilepticus (obtain full EEG to clarify) |

# Clinical vignettes

### 2.2.1 Simple fainting fit

An intelligent 7-year-old girl blacked out while standing eating in the kitchen. She was pale with her eyes rolling and her teeth clenched. There were no clonic movements, incontinence or tongue biting but she was drowsy afterwards.

INVESTIGATION

The EEG showed frequent clusters of left rolandic spike and slow complexes, the amplitude of the spikes exceeding 200µV.

COMMENT

The clinical diagnosis was vasovagal syncope and the EEG examination was not appropriate. The hazard here was that the clinician might alarm the parents by disclosing the 'results' of the EEG or even suggesting to them that this was the beginning of epilepsy.

### 2.2.2 Lethal fainting fits

An 8-year-old boy had a clinical history suggestive of syncope, including an episode of collapse with stiffening when he was being chased. An episode of stiffness in the night was also reported.

INVESTIGATIONS (1)
The EEG showed very frequent right central spike–wave complexes.

COURSE
He was diagnosed with epilepsy, put on sodium valproate and had no further episodes for three years. He then collapsed again and the emergency services found ventricular fibrillation. He could not be resuscitated.

INVESTIGATIONS (2)
After death the previous EEG trace with the rolandic discharges was reviewed. On the ECG, the QTc was grossly prolonged at 0.6s (600ms). Analysis of DNA samples taken at post-mortem examination showed that he had a mutation in an *LQT* gene, as did one of his parents.

COMMENT
An EEG should not have been requested because none of the indications for EEG were satisfied. A history suggestive of syncope precipitated by excitement and exertion, together with an episode at night, pointed to long-QT syndrome type 1. In the event, the inappropriately requested EEG gave rise to the false diagnosis of epilepsy and the long QTc on the ECG channel was overlooked, with fatal consequences. (If DNA had not been taken at post-mortem examination, the neonatal Guthrie card would have been a suitable source.)

### 2.2.3 Spasms with white spots

An 8-month-old girl was referred for an EEG because of a history of 'infantile spasms'.

INVESTIGATIONS (1)
The routine EEG was completely normal.

COURSE (1)
The paediatrician telephoned to ask, "What about the white spots?"

INVESTIGATIONS (2)
*Video telemetry* confirmed that although the interictal EEG was normal each of her serial spasms was associated with a high-voltage biphasic slow complex on which beta activity was superimposed.

*Brain imaging* showed subependymal calcifications and a small number of cortical tubers.

COURSE (2)

The spasms ceased before therapy could be commenced. The course of her tuberous sclerosis was comparatively mild.

COMMENT

The lack of hypsarrhythmia on the 'routine' EEG led to doubt about the original diagnosis of epileptic infantile spasms. The ictal EEG recording confirmed that the spasms were indeed epileptic spasms. Records during an event are necessary when one has to be 100% specific about the diagnosis of a paroxysmal disorder.

### 2.2.4 'Elective mutism'

This boy was referred to a child and family psychiatric unit towards the end of his fourth year when he had stopped talking after a number of stressful events ("life events") within the family: "… there is little doubt that [he] is electively mute and that his symptoms give him a lot of power within the family."

When he was reviewed at the age of 4 years his parents said that his speech had begun to deteriorate when he was 3½ years old. Previously he could hold long conversations with adults about past and future events, face to face and on the telephone, using normal vocabulary and grammar. Over the weekend he was noted to be talking normally at times and at other times 'mumbling' and ignoring people who spoke to him. During the following week he seemed to be 'cut-off' at times: the 'mumbling' stopped, but no other sounds were made. Hearing was checked and found to be normal. Vocalization returned, described by his parents as "sounds like words but they weren't words: he sounded and acted like a child wanting to talk but not knowing how." He began to use pointing and developed his own gestures to communicate. His behaviour began to deteriorate and he became difficult to manage. Psychiatric treatment of his behavioural difficulties was effective but his speech did not return. He had no seizures of any kind.

On examination his success with performance items from the Stanford–Binet and Merrill–Palmer tests of intellectual function were at his age level; he played with toys appropriately; he followed gestures and pantomime and looked at faces and was aware of speech, but he gave no proper response to verbal labels for objects, miniature toys, or pictures. Otherwise he seemed neurologically intact.

INVESTIGATIONS

*EEG* – There were frequent bursts of spike and wave throughout a routine recording. The frequency was 2–3 Hz, and the distribution generalized with posterior and variably left-sided accentuation.

COURSE

A 2-week therapy trial of betamethasone abolished his EEG spikes but did not improve his language comprehension. Six months later occasional absences were reported, subsequently characterized on EEG by 2–3Hz spike and wave with small regular twitchings of his mouth. The absences were abolished by sodium valproate, once again with no improvement in auditory verbal understanding. His needs were met by a special school for children with severe language disorders.

COMMENT

The Landau–Kleffner syndrome commonly presents as if it were a psychiatric condition. In this context the EEG with bilateral spiking has very strong diagnostic power. All-night sleep EEG would probably have shown prolonged CSWS.

'Mutism' is one of the few indications for EEG, with sleep if necessary, in apparently psychiatric disorders.

### 2.2.5 Not familial rectal pain

At the age of 6 years this boy with mild learning disability began to have frequent – more than 3–5 attacks per day – very stereotypical 'attacks'. There would be 1–3 minutes of tonic posturing of both arms with trembling, but he remained completely conscious. There was always flushing at the start of the 'attack' and at the end he would start to cry because of pain around his anus.

INVESTIGATIONS (1)

*EEG* – On every (interictal) EEG recording there were almost continuous bifrontal spikes.

COURSE

There was no response to valproate, levetiracetam or topiramate. On carbamazepine, he clearly got worse. Partial response was obtained with phenobarbitone.

INVESTIGATIONS (2)

*Ictal video-EEG* showed that the episodes were frontal tonic epileptic seizures (and not compulsive Valsalvas as might have been an alternative diagnosis!).

*Karyotype* – In 4/100 mitoses a ring chromosome 20 was seen.

COMMENT

The exceedingly rare condition that used to be called familial rectal pain, but is now paroxysmal extreme pain disorder, seems always to begin in early infancy, usually on day 1.

Bizarre symptomatology and curious EEG appearances should make one wonder about chromosomal disorders. Rhythmic bifrontal slow activity is the best known EEG 'signature' of ring chromosome 20 but it may instead be rhythmic spike and wave. To confirm this not uncommon syndrome it may be necessary to examine 200 mitoses.

### Further reading

Asano E, Pawlak C, Shah A, et al. (2005) The diagnostic value of initial video-EEG monitoring in children—review of 1000 cases. *Epilepsy Res* 66: 129–135.

Bauder F, Wohlrab G, Schmitt B. (2007) Neonatal seizures: eyes open or closed? *Epilepsia* 48: 394–396.

Boyd SG, Harden A, Egger J, et al. (1986) Progressive neuronal degeneration of childhood with liver disease ("Alpers' disease"): characteristic neurophysiological features. *Neuropediatrics* **17**: 75–80.

Coutelier M, Andries S, Ghariani S, et al. (2008) Neuroserpin mutation causes electrical status epilepticus of slow-wave sleep. *Neurology* **71**: 64–66.

Dan B, Boyd SG. (2003) Angelman syndrome reviewed from a neurophysiological perspective. The UBE3A–GABRB3 hypothesis. *Neuropediatrics* **34**: 169–176.

McLellan A, Phillips HA, Rittey C, et al. (2003) Phenotypic comparison of two Scottish families with mutations in different genes causing autosomal dominant nocturnal frontal lobe epilepsy. *Epilepsia* **44**: 613–617.

Millichap JG. (2006) Electroencephalography hyperventilation and stroke in children with sickle cell disease. *Clin EEG Neurosci* **37**: 190–192.

North KN, Ouvrier RA, Nugent M. (1990) Pseudoseizures caused by hyperventilation resembling absence epilepsy. *J Child Neurol* **5**: 288–294.

Panayiotopoulos CP, Michael M, Sanders S, et al. (2008) Benign childhood focal epilepsies: assessment of established and newly recognized syndromes. *Brain* **131**: 2264–2286.

Stephenson JBP. (2008) Cerebral palsy. In: Engel J, Pedley TA, eds. *Epilepsy: a Comprehensive Textbook.* Philadelphia: Lippincott Williams & Wilkins, pp. 2631–2636.

Watemberg N, Tziperman B, Dabby, R, et al. (2005) Adding video recording increases the diagnostic yield of routhing electroencephalograms in children with frequent paroxysmal events. *Epilepsia* **46**: 716–719.

# Chapter 2.3

# Electromyography and Nerve Conduction Studies

### Nerve conduction studies
Many sophisticated methods of studying nerve and muscle are available. Indications and interpretation of the most commonly used methods are outlined here.

*Motor nerve conduction studies*
The painless magnetic stimulator has proved useful in the investigation of central motor pathways, and limited information may be obtained about proximal nerve function from F-wave analysis, but most techniques study that part of the motor nerve which begins quite a way from its origin in the anterior horn cells.

The principle of study is that the nerve is stimulated and the evoked potential recorded in a distal muscle. If the size of the resultant muscle action potential is smaller than expected this indicates that fewer axons are conducting, either because of degeneration of the axons themselves (axonal neuropathy) or because there has been degeneration of the anterior horn cells. If there is anterior horn cell disorder and/or proximal axonal degeneration, then distal muscles will show the changes of denervation on EMG as described below.

As normally measured, the velocity depends on the myelination of the largest and fastest conducting nerve fibres. Abnormalities of myelin, either congenital hypomyelination or demyelination, lead to slow conduction velocity throughout the measurable length of the nerve. Thus, the time taken for a proximal stimulus to reach the muscle (the proximal latency) and the time for a distal stimulus to reach the muscle (the distal latency) will be increased. The conduction velocity is calculated by subtracting the distal latency from the proximal latency and dividing this into the accurately measured distance between the two points stimulated. The conduction velocity is thus markedly reduced in hypomyelinating and demyelinating neuropathy.

If, in addition to demyelination, there is axonal damage, then EMG signs of denervation in the muscle are likely as well. In pure axonal neuropathy the (fastest) conduction velocity tends to be normal.

If demyelination is segmental or a nerve is compressed then 'conduction block' may be induced. In conduction block, when the nerve is stimulated proximal to the block the area under the curve of the evoked muscle potential will be less than if stimulation is carried out distal to the block. If conduction block exists at various levels, as may occur particularly in acquired demyelination (e.g. in Guillain–Barré syndrome), then muscle weakness may be considerable.

It should be remembered that if there is acute injury to a nerve in any part of its course, the appearance of the expected electrophysiological signs of the damage may be delayed for weeks.

*Sensory conduction*
Sensory nerve conduction is normally studied by applying a supramaximal electrical stimulus to a digit via a ring electrode or using a standard nerve stimulator. The small action potential may be amplified by averaging the response to a series of stimuli. The 'average' latency between the stimulus and the action potential divided into the distance gives a measure of the conduction velocity. A reduction in the size (peak-to-peak amplitude) of the sensory action potential has several causes, including axonal neuropathy, conduction block for any reason, and demyelination (when there is also marked slowing of conduction velocity).

*Repetitive nerve stimulation*
Repetitive stimulation of a motor nerve as in conduction studies may be used to study the neuromuscular junction. The muscle action potential is recorded on the surface or by a subcutaneous needle electrode over a distal muscle such as the abductor digitorum brevis in the case of ulnar nerve stimulation, and the extensor digitorum brevis in the case of stimulation of the lateral popliteal nerve. Slow and fast rates from 2 to 50/s assist in the diagnosis of myasthenia (in which repetitive stimulation leads to a decremental response) and infantile botulism (in which there is usually an incremental response).

In Lambert–Eaton myasthenic syndrome – which is rarely seen in childhood as a paraneoplastic complication of occult neural crest tumours (ganglioneuroblastoma) or lymphoproliferative disease – a low-amplitude compound action potential shows a marked increment on repetitive (tetanic) nerve stimulation.

# Electromyography
The type of EMG needed for the study of neuromuscular disorders involves recording from an intramuscular needle. Observations are made on the insertional electrical activity which accompanies the introduction of the needle, the spontaneous activity which occurs when the muscle is at rest, and the exertional activity which occurs during contraction.

The most important abnormality of insertional activity is the dive-bomber discharge (so-called because of the sound of the EMG) found in myotonic disorders including myotonic dystrophy and most often seen in the mothers of floppy neonates.

Abnormal spontaneous activity is less useful diagnostically than one might suppose. The regularly recurring short-duration transients known as fibrillations are unfortunately not only found in denervation of the muscle, but may also be present in myopathies, particularly myositis.

Abnormalities of exertional activity are more useful. In neurogenic lesions the interference pattern produced by all the available motor units is incomplete and the individual motor unit potentials tend to be of long duration and often of higher amplitude. By contrast, in myopathic conditions a full interference pattern of reduced amplitude may be seen and the individual motor units tend to be of short duration.

*Exercise EMG*
Exercise EMG, whereby the amplitude of the compound muscle action potential from a muscle such as the hypothenar is measured repeatedly before and after exercise, is a simple way of investigating muscle channelopathies, in particular the periodic paralyses and paramyotonias, and may be a guide to the type of mutation involved.


## Practical aspects of nerve conduction and EMG
Many variations of technique and the site of the study are possible in different clinical circumstances. The actual practice of EMG recording is fraught with difficulties which extensive practice reduces. In nerve conduction studies details are important. The skin temperature should be 37–38 °C. Cooler extremities may lead to falsely low conduction velocity and, in particular, increased distal latency. Errors of distance measurement have a proportionally greater effect on the calculated conduction velocity the smaller the child. There is an argument for using subcutaneous needle electrodes both for stimulation and for recording when this aspect is important. Some find that the discomfort from nerve stimulation is less when subcutaneous needle electrodes are used. Some operators seem to be able to 'hypnotize' their child patients to remain happy during needle electromyography; others use sedatives such as midazolam. The most accessible nerves for motor conduction studies are the ulnar, median, lateral popliteal (common peroneal) and (posterior) tibial. The most accessible for sensory studies are the median, sural and plantar.


## Notes on some clinical aspects

*Neonatal/congenital myasthenia*
The diagnosis of congenital myasthenic syndromes (CMS) may be particularly difficult. The technique of *stimulation single-fibre EMG (stimSFEMG)* is a promising advance. It has been found that stimSFEMG (of the orbicularis oculi or the frontalis muscle) has high specificity (~80%) and sensitivity (~90%) for the diagnosis of CMS.

*Paediatric intensive care unit*
Evaluation of critical illness polyneuropathy and myopathy is an important area.

In the critical care setting EMG may aid the diagnosis of axonal Guillain–Barré syndrome that may mimic brain death (see Clinical Vignette 2.8.3). EMG is also helpful in the floppy baby on a ventilator pending the results of *SMN* gene testing (in spinal muscular atrophy, type 1) and in myasthenia and spinal muscular atrophy with respiratory distress.

*Neurophysiology vs biopsy vs imaging*
EMG has a very high detection rate for neurogenic and neuromuscular junction disorders but a low rate of detection of myopathic motor unit potentials in infancy. By contrast, muscle biopsy is less good at detecting early neurogenic changes and better at revealing myopathy.

Direct comparisons of EMG and nerve conduction with imaging of muscle (altrasound and MRI) and nerve (MRI) are not available, but the clinician will as ever try to integrate the composite findings.

*Regression*
EMG is particularly important in conditions with axonal neuropathy, nerve conductions aiding the detection of demyelinating neuropathies. Such studies are most revealing when there is a combination of central and peripheral dysfunction, such as in mitochondrial disorders, infantile neuroaxonal dystrophy (INAD) and certain leukodystrophies.

*Intermittent disorders*

MYOKYMIA
In the clarification of episodic ataxia type 1, surface EMG may be all that is required to document myokymia. EMG is not usually needed for the diagnosis of myotonias and paramyotonias.

HYPEREKPLEXIA WITH SEVERE NEONATAL APNOEA
Surface EMG is probably diagnostic in the profound neonatal apnoeas that may be a manifestation of hyperekplexia. Whether separately recorded from deltoids or as an epiphenomenon on EEG and ECG leads, surface EMG demonstrates high-voltage repetitive compound muscle action potentials at 8–30Hz (see Fig. 1.1.1, p. 8).

*Functional disorders*
Although surface or needle EMG and nerve stimulation may contribute to the differential diagnosis of suspected 'functional' or psychogenic disorders, one should beware the potential exacerbating effect of the investigation itself.

## Clinical vignettes

### 2.3.1 Vaccine damage
A 6-month-old girl was admitted with a 4-day history of fever, lethargy, vomiting and inability to bear weight. She had received her first dose of oral polio vaccine 4 weeks previously and an intramuscular injection of DTP vaccine into her left thigh at the same time. She was irritable, dyspnoeic and hypertensive (blood pressure 130/70mmHg). All limbs were flaccid, the left more so and the left lower limb most so, with absent tendon reflexes. She had lost neck control and made no effort to sit. Facial muscles bilaterally and the right diaphragm were paralysed. On the third day in hospital scoliosis, ocular flutter and opsoclonus were observed. The eye movements resolved within a few days but the scoliosis persisted for several months. Sensation appeared normal.

INVESTIGATIONS
*EEG* – Normal.

*Nerve conduction and EMG* – Motor conduction velocity in the right common peroneal nerve was 44.5m/s with distal latency of 3.1ms. Sensory conduction velocity in the right median nerve was 37m/s. EMG was normal. The phrenic nerve was stimulated on the right, and a normal latency for diaphragmatic action potential was seen. Tetanic stimulation produced a visible diaphragmatic contraction on the right. F waves were not detected.

*Repeat EMG* was undertaken 2 months later in the left quadriceps and left tibialis anterior muscles. Spontaneous activity (fibrillation and positive sharp waves) was profuse in both muscles, particularly the tibialis anterior. Very few motor units could be found. Several long-duration polyphasic units were seen in the quadriceps, and one at 1.5mV was of abnormally high amplitude for her age.

*CSF* contained 39 polymorphonuclear cells per microlitre with a protein concentration of 0.48g/L and glucose 2.7mmol/L, blood glucose not being measured.

*Repeat CSF examination* 1 week later showed 37 white cells (96% lymphocytes) per microlitre, protein 0.86g/L and glucose 2.6mmol/L.

*Immunological studies* showed normal B-cell and T-cell numbers and function. Immunoglobulin A (IgA) was persistently low at 7.3mg/dL with an absent IgA using double diffusion immunoelectrophoresis in the saliva.

*Virology* – Tests for Coxsackie B and other enteroviruses were negative. Neutralizing antibody litres were raised to polio 1, polio 2 and polio 3, and these viruses were excreted in the stools, polio 2 virus up to 6 weeks after admission. The latter was identified by oligonucleotide mapping as vaccine strain, and types 1 and 3 were identified by intratypic serodifferentiation as vaccine strain.

COMMENT
Delayed appearance of nerve stimulation/EMG abnormalities are characteristic of both acute polyneuropathy (Guillain–Barré syndrome) and poliomyelitis. In this typical

vaccine-associated case of poliomyelitis, late EMG evidence of denervation was found in the muscles of the limb into which the DTP vaccine had been injected.

### 2.3.2 Falling from the knees down

A 2½-year-old girl, who walked on her own at 20 months, seemed to have poor balance and often stumbled and fell 'from the knees'. She complained that her legs hurt if she walked any distance (100 metres). Her divorced father had been diagnosed as having Friedreich ataxia, but was not accessible for examination.

INVESTIGATIONS
*Nerve conduction* – Right median nerve conduction velocity was 5m/s with distal latency of 16.4ms.

*CSF protein* – 0.49g/L.

*Sural nerve biopsy* – Axons and myelination were reported as normal.

*Gastrocnemius muscle biopsy* was normal on light and electronmicroscopy.

*Leukocyte arylsulphatase* was normal.

COURSE
Her paternal grandmother was contacted and found to have a conduction velocity of 15m/s in the right ulnar nerve with a distal latency of 9ms, and a distal latency of 11ms in the right median with no response obtainable from stimulation at the elbow. Sensory potentials could not be obtained from her. She had minimal wasting.

By examining family members an extensive dominant inheritance of hereditary motor and sensory neuropathy – Charcot–Marie–Tooth type I – was determined. The girl, who was the index case, is employed with only minor physical difficulties 17 years later.

COMMENT
Ataxia with rombergism and tendon areflexia may be a presentation of Charcot–Marie–Tooth type I, but the diagnosis will be missed (as in the case of her father) if nerve conduction studies are not undertaken. Genetic studies (*PMP22*) will provide definitive diagnostic information in 70% of cases.

### 2.3.3 A hoarse, floppy infant with a treatable condition

This previously normal infant presented at 10 months with motor delay, feeding difficulty and a weak, hoarse cry. She was generally weak, especially in nuchal muscles, but alert and visually attentive with normal eye movements. Reflexes were normal. A paternal uncle had died in infancy having had a similar disorder. The father, now asymptomatic, had been treated with quinine during childhood for muscle cramps.

INVESTIGATIONS (1)
*Brain MRI* – Normal.

*Creatine kinase* – Normal.

*Muscle ultrasound* – Normal.

*Initial nerve conduction studies and EMG,* including *repetitive stimulation studies* were normal.

*Muscle biopsy* – Normal.

COURSE (1)
A trial of pyridostigmine had no effect and she remained hypotonic and weak.

INVESTIGATIONS (2)
At 20 months (while still on pyridostigmine) *nerve conduction studies* were repeated. An impressive double depolarization was seen with 'giant F-waves'.

COURSE (2)
Slow channel syndrome was suspected and, after withdrawal of pyridostigmine, quinidine was introduced. Within 2 days she sat unaided for the first time and walked a week later. Aged 10 years she has normal strength and stamina but becomes weaker if she misses a dose of quinidine.

COMMENT
Having excluded brainstem glioma, a neuromuscular disorder was suspected but could not be confirmed initially. The effect of pyridostigmine may have been to 'uncover' the electrophysiological expression of the ion channel dysfunction. DNA studies have not so far identified a pathogenic mutation, although, as expected for this disorder, inheritance appears to be dominant with variable expression. Even rare disorders should be pursued vigorously if potentially treatable (Chapter 3.23).

### 2.3.4 Infant desaturation
Severe episodes began at age 5 months but previously feeding was poor and later on his mother said that he had had "no clue about bottle".

During episodes he would become less active and drop his dummy (comforter) from his mouth, which would become circular. His face became grey, pale, sweaty and blue, with rapid shallow respirations and then sudden stiffening – dramatic tonic spasm – with apnoea.

Provocations included any disturbance, in retrospect anything that made him work harder.

In an episode his heart rate would be rapid at first then slow (bradycardia), with cardiac arrest on occasions. Maximum asystole was several minutes (!) during which he required major cardiopulmonary resuscitation. After the most prolonged asystole he was in a coma and brain MRI showed symmetrical increased signal in the basal ganglia (resolved on follow-up MRI).

Congenital myasthenia was considered.

INVESTIGATIONS (1)
*Repetitive nerve stimulation* – Normal.

*Carbamazepine trial* (given in case a variant of paroxysmal extreme pain disorder) led to some improvement.

COURSE (1)
Much later he developed ptosis, reversed by ice pack application.

INVESTIGATIONS (2)
*Edrophonium (Tensilon) test* (Chapter 2.16) – Positive.

*Molecular genetics* – Mutations were not found in *RAPSN* but were in *CHAT*.

COURSE (2)
He has done well on pyridostigmine.

COMMENT
Congenital myasthenic syndomes may elude detection unless actively sought. Published evidence suggests that stimSFEMG is more sensitive than repetitive nerve stimulation. Therapeutic trials other than those listed in Table 2.16.1 are to be discouraged.

### 2.3.5 Not cerebral palsy
This boy, the first child of first cousins, was the product of an uneventful pregnancy and had normal developmental milestones until the age of 1 year. There was developmental arrest around the age of 1 year and at 15 months he was referred to the local paediatrician. Mild hypertonia was noted and a diagnosis of evolving cerebral palsy was made and a programme of developmental therapy commenced. He was alert and interactive with good social responses and feeding but no symbolic play. Over the following 9 months there was no developmental progress.

At 2½ years he was referred for neurological opinion. There was marked axial hypotonia with evolving spasticity, absent tendon reflexes (except for ankle jerks), very low amplitude ocular oscillations, optic atrophy, strabismus, drooling of saliva and feeding difficulties. There was also evidence of cognitive decline.

INVESTIGATIONS
*EEG* showed excess fast activity in the beta range.

*EMG* showed features of denervation.

*Nerve conduction studies* showed findings in keeping with a sensorimotor axonal neuropathy.

*MRI* showed cerebellar atrophy with abnormal signal in the basal ganglia on T2 flair.

*H-MRS* did not show any abnormality.

*Blood amino acids, ammonia, lactate, creatine kinase, transaminases, urea, creatinine* – Normal.

*Urine* amino acids and organic acids – Normal.

*CSF* protein, glucose, lactate and amino acids – Normal.

*Genetic studies* – A homozygous pathogenic mutation was found in *PLA2G6* (on chromosome 22q12–q13).

COMMENT

In the absence of a clear cause and a period of follow-up a diagnosis of cerebral palsy should be resisted. In this case, the clinical picture – which included developmental arrest, ocular 'wobble', and central and peripheral deficits including absent tendon reflexes – was in keeping with INAD. Although the brain MRI did not show the hyperintensity of the cerebellar cortex expected in INAD, the EEG and EMG (and nerve conduction) studies together with the clinical presentation pointed strongly to this devastating autosomal recessive neurodegenerative disorder. If INAD had not been confirmed by finding a *PLA2G6* mutation, then spheroids would have been sought in biopsy of skin or conjunctiva. This is an excellent example of the Aicardi dictum on the clinical integration of data from all sources, as spelt out in the first paragraph of 'Philosophy of tests' in the Introduction to this handbook.

## Further reading

Cardamone M, Darras, Ryan MM. (2008) Inherited myopathies and muscular dystrophies. *Semin Neurol* **28**: 250–259.

Fournier E, Arzel M, Sternberg D, et al. (2004) Electromyography guides toward subgroups of mutations in muscle channelopathies. *Ann Neurol* **56**: 650–661.

Gaebler JW, Kleiman MB, French MLV. (1986) Neurological complications of oral polio vaccine recipients. *J Pediatr* **108**: 878–881.

Harper CM, Engel AG. (1998) Quinidine sulfate therapy for the slow-channel congenital myasthenic syndrome. *Ann Neurol* **43**: 480–484.

Pascotto A, Coppola G. (1992) Neonatal hyperekplexia: a case report. *Epilepsia* **33**: 817–820.

Pitt M. (2008) Neurophysiological strategies for the diagnosis of disorders of the neuromuscular junction in children. *Dev Med Child Neurol* **50**: 328–333.

Rabie M, Jossiphov J, Nevo Y. (2007) Electromyography (EMG) accuracy compared to muscle biopsy in childhood. *J Child Neurol* **22**: 803–808.

Royden Jones H, DeVivo DC, Darras BT. (2003) *Neuromuscular Disorders of Infancy, Childhood and Adolescence: a Clinician's Approach.* Philadelphia: Butterworth Heinemann.

Scarcella A, Coppola G. (1997) Neonatal sporadic hyperekplexia: a rare and often unrecognized entity. *Brain Dev* **19**: 226–228.

# Chapter 2.4
## Evoked Potentials

Evoked potentials are generated by sensory stimuli. They may be measured from a sense organ, such as the retina or the cochlea, or from the neural pathway, or from the brain itself.

### Electroretinogram

As an aid to diagnosis in paediatric neurology the electroretinogram (ERG) is commonly measured by averaging the response to repeated light flashes, either using a surface electrode at the nasion or, more sensitively, using a gold foil electrode inserted into the fornix of the lower eyelid. Increasingly, contact lens electrodes are preferred and are well tolerated even in young children. Measurements are made of the photopic and scotopic (dark adapted) response. Sometimes the term 'mesopic' is used when the eye is considerably but not totally dark adapted.

Disorders involving the nervous system in which the ERG response is low or extinguished are listed in Table 2.4.1. In this table conditions with a low or extinguished ERG response are divided into those in which there is congenital low vision and those in which low vision becomes manifest later, or is indeed never noticed. In the first group of conditions other disabilities may be so severe that the visual disturbance is not recognized unless the ERG is done. It is important to recognize that the ERG has substantial amplitude at birth and there should not be a difficulty in detecting these congenital retinopathies which are further discussed in Chapter 3.6. These are autosomal recessive in inheritance, except for mitochondrial cytopathies which may also have other inheritance patterns. In osteopetrosis (marble bones disease) the retinal defect may be limited to cone dysfunction at first, but the flash ERG becomes extinguished with time.

Unfortunately one of the common causes of a very low ERG associated with neurological disorder is retinopathy of prematurity, often associated with the neurodevelopmental consequences of periventricular leukomalacia. In this sequel of preterm birth the low ERG response is associated with blindness, but in several of the

Table 2.4.1 Low or extinguished ERG response in genetic neurological disorders

| Condition | | Clues |
|---|---|---|
| 1. Congenital low vision | Leber amaurosis complex | Blindness predominates |
| | Osteopetrosis | Low vision is more often acquired. Skull radiograph dense |
| | Joubert syndrome | Panting tachypnoea |
| | Walker–Warburg syndrome | Ocular abnormalities, cobblestone lissencephaly, high creatine kinase |
| | Peroxisomopathies (several disorders) | Zellweger-like, hepatosplenomegaly may not be present |

genetic conditions it has to be looked for, since there may be no obvious visual defect to provide a clue.

### Visual evoked potentials

Visual evoked potentials (VEPs) are recorded from surface electrodes over the visual cortex in response to either repetitive flash or pattern-reversal stimulation. In children it is often helpful to record the ERG and the VEP at the same time, and if possible the EEG also to clarify the site and the type of lesion. Pattern VEP allows more precise quantitation of the results, but although possible in young infants is usually confined to the older child who can fixate.

With diffuse retinal disorders involving the macula as well as the periphery, not only will the ERG response be absent but the VEP will be absent also, as in retrolental fibroplasia.

In disorders of the peripheral retina, although the ERG response may be absent the VEP may be normal, as in the early stage of retinitis pigmentosa. As the retinal damage becomes more severe, the VEP will become affected.

If the retinal ganglion cells degenerate, the ERG response is normal but the VEP may be absent. This situation is found in infantile GM2 gangliosidosis (Tay–Sachs disease).

Lesions of the anterior visual pathway, optic nerves and chiasm lead to abnormalities or complete loss of the VEP. An oversimplified interpretation of the different findings suggests that in disorders of the axons, for example with optic hypoplasia or compressive lesions, the VEP amplitude is reduced and its shape distorted, whereas in disorders of myelination such as optic neuritis, the latency is increased though the

Table 2.4.1 continued

| Condition | | Clues |
|---|---|---|
| 2. Later onset low vision or vision unremarkable | Osteopetrosis | Skull radiograph dense |
| | Bardet–Biedl syndrome | Polydactyly, obesity, hypogenitalism |
| | Laurence–Moon syndrome | Obesity, learning disability, ataxia |
| | Neuronal ceroid lipofuscinosis | |
| | – Infantile (INCL) | Rett-like loss of skills and hand 'knitting' |
| | – Late infantile (LINCL) | Seizures, ataxia and regression |
| | – Juvenile (JNCL) | Blindness, then slowing up, mumbling (both LINCL and JNCL *may* have bull's-eye maculopathy) |
| | Mitochondrial cytopathy | Multisite involvement (central nervous system, peripheral nervous system, etc.) |
| | DNA repair disorder | Cockayne phenotype |
| | Refsum disease | Deafness, neuropathy and ichthyosis |
| | Chronic global peroxisomal deficiency | Deafness, failure to thrive |
| | Bassen–Kornzweig syndrome (abetalipoproteinaemia) | Ataxia, previous steatorrhoea |
| | Hunter syndrome (mucopolysaccharidosis type 2) | Deafness, hepatosplenomegaly, short stature, face coarsening |
| | Mucolipidosis type 4 | Corneal clouding, neurodevelopmental regression |
| | Hallervorden–Spatz disease (pantothenate kinase 2 deficiency) | Rigidity, dystonia |

amplitude and waveform may be normal. Pathologies more posteriorly in the visual pathways are likely to show not only alterations in VEP but disturbances in the EEG, for example occipital spikes in association with periventricular leukomalacia.

Lesions of the visual cortex may be present without any appreciable change in the VEP as ordinarily detected, but with flattening of the occipital EEG.

Maturation of the VEP may be delayed so that the latency is increased for the first months of life.

Pathologies at more than one site commonly coexist and lead to more than one of these appearances being found in the same child. For example, preterm hypoxic–ischaemic damage may lead to optic nerve hypoplasia with abnormality or even loss of the VEP together with the periventricular leukomalacia associated with posterior high-voltage EEG spikes. Such a situation is one of the outcomes of the survivor when one of a pair of monozygotic twins has died in utero.

The combination of ERG, VEP and EEG changes and their time course is very helpful in the diagnosis of certain neurodegenerative disorders, in particular the various types of neuronal ceroid lipofuscinosis. In the infantile variety (INCL), the ERG response becomes progressively smaller until it is extinguished, and the VEP becomes smaller also. The EEG then also progressively diminishes until it becomes virtually isoelectric (flat). In the late infantile type (LINCL), the ERG response disappears early but the VEP is grossly enlarged. These giant VEPs can be seen on the ordinary EEG during photic stimulation at slow rates. In the juvenile form (JNCL), the ERG response also disappears early, with later reduction in amplitude of VEP and diffuse abnormality of the EEG.

### Brainstem auditory evoked potentials
Brainstem auditory evoked potentials (BAEPs) are employed both in detecting sensorineural deafness and in demonstrating abnormalities of conduction through the auditory pathway. For the test a series of monaural clicks is delivered to one or other ear. In the evaluation of hearing, the threshold in decibels at which the resulting wave forms are seen is estimated. For the analysis of the BAEP itself, the clicks are delivered to an intensity of about 70dB (or higher if considerable sensorineural deafness is discovered). The most important and easily discriminated waves are wave I from the auditory nerve and wave V from the midbrain (inferior colliculus). The most valuable measurements are first the interwave latency between wave I and wave V, and secondly the amplitude ratio of wave V to wave I (wave V divided by wave I). Increased latency will reflect a disorder of myelination, while a reduction in the wave V amplitude (and therefore a reduction in the wave V/wave I ratio) will result from problems of the axon.

### Somatosensory evoked potentials
The least pleasant of the evoked responses that may be undertaken in children is the somatosensory evoked potential (SSEP). A peripheral nerve is stimulated by trains of electrical impulses and the SSEP recorded from the surface or needle electrodes over the spinal cord or contralateral parietal cortex.

It is rather poorly tolerated in the young, but finds value during operations involving the spine and aorta, and in the intensive care unit in evaluating coma. Selective loss of lower limb responses may sometimes assist in the diagnosis of spinal tumour. Rarely the investigation may help in confirming the clinical diagnosis of non-organic sensory symptoms.

Subtle differences in SSEPs might assist in the differentiation between Unverricht–Lundborg and Lafora progressive myoclonic epilepsies (Chapter 3.22).

## Magnetic stimulation and central conduction time

This painless technique, whereby the motor cortex can be stimulated by brief alterations in the magnetic field in a painless manner and recordings made at various points on the pathway to a distal muscle, provides a safe and elegant technique for studying central motor pathways in childhood. Practical uses are limited and it is mainly a research tool. A promising potential application is evaluating children with severe dyskinesia who may benefit from deep brain stimulation if corticospinal tract function is well preserved.

## Clinical vignettes

### 2.4.1 Not Rett syndrome

An 18-month-old-girl had made reasonable progress in the first year of life and had got to the stage of saying three words and waving 'bye-bye', drinking from a cup without a lid and trying to walk, at any rate around furniture. She then stopped progressing and lost skills, had a tendency to scream and began to bring her hands together. Her head circumference declined from the 50th to the 2nd centile.

Her development did not plateau, but continued to regress. Intention tremor was evident when she put her thumb into her mouth and her plantar responses were extensor. She developed myoclonic jerks at the age of 2 years and thereafter her visual competence and head control declined, but her abilities fluctuated for a while.

INVESTIGATIONS

*EEG* – At 21 months the EEG was mildly slow with maximum amplitude of about 50μV. At 2 years slow activity was interrupted by low-voltage fast activity, and by 2½ years it was unequivocally of low voltage, associated with non-epileptic myoclonus.

*ERG* – At age 2 years was just within normal limits, with a corneal electrode amplitude of 30μV under mesopic conditions. By 2½ years there was marked reduction of amplitude to 8–9μV.

*CSF protein* – 0.05g/L.

*Conjunctival biopsy* – No abnormality of nerves or abnormal storage was detected.

*Rectal biopsy* (age 2½ years) – Histological sections showed foamy histiocytic cells particularly in the superficial parts of the lamina propria. Granular osmiophilic deposits

(GROD) were seen both in neurons and in the smooth muscle cells of the muscularis mucosae.

COMMENT
INCL may present as autistic regression with hand-washing stereotypies similar to those seen in Rett syndrome, but EEG and ERG evidence of cerebroretinal degeneration soon evolves. In this case example, diagnosis by the finding of GROD on biopsy was done before protein palmitoyl thioesterase (PPT) assays were available, but a belt-and-braces diagnosis would still involve the finding of both GROD and PPT deficiency in leukocytes.

### 2.4.2 'Ataxic cerebral palsy' with wobbly eyes
An 18-month-old boy had been noted to have multidirectional nystagmus from a few months of age. Visual, language comprehension and communication development were considered normal but he was only just able to sit unaided and had titubation and marked intention tremor. There had been no regression and he had normal hearing on behavioural testing.

INVESTIGATIONS
*EEG* was normal.

*ERG* was normal.

*VEP* was delayed and reduced in amplitude.

*BAEP* showed a normal wave I but no discernable later waves.

*Otoacoustic emissions* confirmed normal hearing.

*MRI* showed diffusely abnormal white matter signal but no loss of volume.

COMMENT
The diagnosis of Pelizaeus–Merzbacher disease – the paradigm example of hypomyelination – was confirmed by finding a pathological mutation in the *PLP* gene. The loss of later waves in the BAEP results from 'temporal dispersion' consequent on slow conduction through abnormally myelinated auditory pathways: hearing was not affected.

## Further reading

Aminoff MJ, ed. (2005) *Electrodiagnosis in Clinical Neurology, 5th edn.* New York: Churchill Livingston.

Fazzi E, Signorini SG, Scelsa B, et al. (2003) Leber's congenital amaurosis: an update. *Eur J Paediatr Neurol* 7: 13–22.

Laird PW, Mohney BG, Renaud DL. (2006) Bull's-eye maculopathy in an infant with Leigh disease. *Am J Ophthalmol* 142: 186–187.

Muntoni F, Brockington M, Godfrey C, et al. (2007) Muscular dystrophies due to defective glycosylation of dystroglycan. *Acta Myol* 26: 129–135.

# Chapter 2.5
## Structural Imaging

Modern structural imaging methods, in particular magnetic resonance imaging (MRI), computerized tomography (CT) and ultrasound, may allow appreciation of both anatomical detail and the effects of disease states. It should be recognized at the outset, however, that normal imaging does not equate with no neurological disorder.

**Magnetic resonance imaging**
MRI is the most useful technique for evaluating the structure of the central nervous system (CNS). It allows much better grey–white matter differentiation than CT with resolution of anatomy and pathology, and it does not have the (slight) hazard of ionizing radiation. In the newborn infant it competes with ultrasound as a safe method for study of the CNS.

There are many sequences available in MRI, each with its own advantages and disadvantages. Most information can be achieved when studies are individually tailored for each child. The clinical and laboratory information, the differential diagnosis and the ability of the child to cooperate all need to be taken into account in selection of appropriate sequences. The findings on the initial sequences can then also suggest modification of the remainder of the study. The optimal information can be achieved when the study is planned and supervised by a paediatric radiologist familiar with the clinical details and laboratory findings.

*Sequences*

T1-WEIGHTED SEQUENCES
T1-weighted sequences are used for delineation of anatomy, especially grey–white matter differentiation. T1-weighted imaging (susceptibility-weighted sequences) is useful also for detection of small amounts of blood, for example in non-accidental injury.

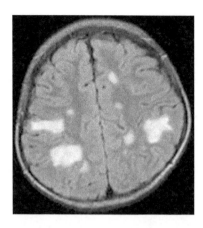

Figure 2.5.1 Brain MRI in 6-year-old girl with acute disseminated encephalomyelitis (ADEM) shows multiple discrete areas of high T2 signal in the cerebral white matter.

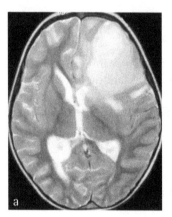 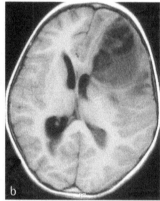 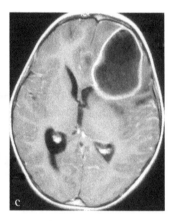

Figure 2.5.2 Brain MRI in 5-year-old boy shows large mass with mass effect and midline shift in the left frontal lobe. (a) T2-weighted sequence shows high T2 signal and (b) T1-weighted sequence shows low T1 signal. (c) Post-contrast sequence showing ring enhancement indicates that this is likely to be an abscess rather than a tumour.

T2-WEIGHTED SEQUENCES

On T2-weighted sequences water, including CSF, is bright. Oedema is also bright, making T2-weighted imaging sensitive to acute processes including infection, inflammation and tumours (Fig. 2.5.1).

CONTRAST ENHANCEMENT

Gadolinium compounds are used for intravenous contrast. A T1-weighted sequence is always used to obtain post-contrast images. Contrast enhancement indicates hypervascularity or breakdown of the blood–brain barrier (Fig. 2.5.2).

Recent evidence suggests that the cranial nerves enhance in both infantile Krabbe disease and in late infantile metachromatic leukodystrophy.

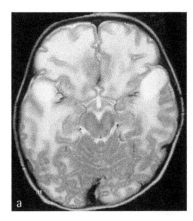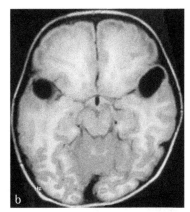

Figure 2.5.3 (a) Brain MRI in 2-year-old with microcephaly, deterioration of motor function and cerebellar ataxia. T2-weighted sequence shows abnormal high signal in white matter with brighter signal in both anterior temporal lobes. (b) Same child, T2 FLAIR sequence also shows abnormal high signal in white matter but in both anterior temporal lobes the signal has nulled (is dark) indicating that this has free fluid and is cystic. Cysts were also identified in both frontal lobes and a diagnosis of megalencephalic leukoencephalopathy with subcortical cysts was made.

### T2 FLAIR (FLUID ATTENUATED INVERSION RECOVERY)

This is a T2-weighted sequence which depicts free fluid, such as CSF in ventricles, as dark (fluid is said to be 'nulled'). FLAIR images are used to distinguish parenchymal lesions from adjacent CSF in ventricles. This sequence may also be used to show cystic versus solid intraparenchymal lesions – free fluid in cysts is nulled (becomes dark) while solid lesions remain bright (Fig. 2.5.3). Subdural collections may be more easily distinguished from subarachnoid fluid on this sequence. In addition to all this, bright white matter lesions are often more conspicuous on T2 FLAIR than regular T2-weighted sequences, making this the single most useful sequence in neuroimaging (Fig. 2.5.4).

### T1 INVERSION RECOVERY

T1 inversion recovery (sometimes confusingly called T1 FLAIR) produces more pronounced grey–white matter differentiation than regular T1-weighted images. This is very useful for focal cortical thickening or heterotopia (Fig. 2.5.5). T1 inversion recovery is a sensitive sequence for detection of ischaemia in the neonate (Fig. 2.5.6).

### FAT SUPPRESSION

This technique makes fat dark on all sequences and can be useful to determine the presence of fat in lesions such as a teratoma. It is used to darken the fat of the orbit to detect high T2 signal lesions within the fat, or in T1-weighted sequences with enhancement to demonstrate lesions in the orbit that would otherwise be indistinguishable from fat. Axial T1-weighted imaging with fat suppression can be helpful in identifying intramural haematoma in cases of cervicocephalic dissection.

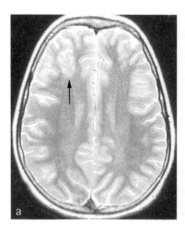 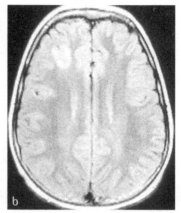

Figure 2.5.4 (a) Brain MRI in a 4-year-old boy. T2-weighted sequence shows an abnormal deep sulcus in the right frontal lobe (arrow). (b) Same child, T2 FLAIR sequence shows abnormal high signal in the lesion making it much more conspicuous.

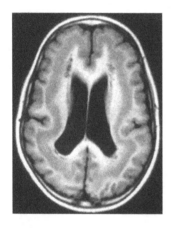

Figure 2.5.5 Brain MRI in an 8-year-old boy. T1 inversion recovery sequence increases the contrast between dark cortex and white matter which is very bright. In this child, the additional abnormal layer of cortical tissue deep to the true cortex, a band heterotopia, is very clearly visible as a result.

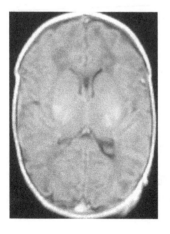

Figure 2.5.6 Brain MRI, T1 inversion recovery sequence in 5-day-old infant with grade II neonatal encephalopathy showing abnormal high T1 signal in the lateral aspect of both thalami and in the posterior aspect of both lentiform nuclei.

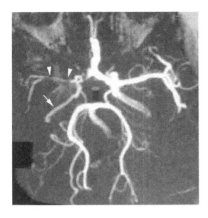

Figure 2.5.7 Magnetic resonance angiography in a 4-year-old with intracranial vasculopathy. The right internal carotid artery (arrow) is diffusely narrower than the left, as is the right middle cerebral artery. There are focal areas of signal drop-out in the right middle cerebral artery (arrowheads), suggestive of focal stenoses.

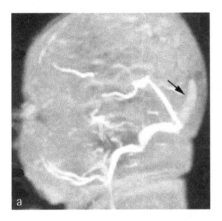
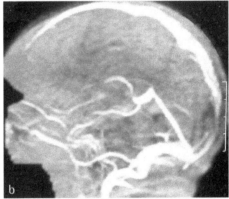

Figure 2.5.8 (a) Magnetic resonance venogram in neonate. No flow is seen in the sagittal sinus due to thrombosis. Some high signal posteriorly within the sinus is also due to thrombus rather than flow (arrow). (b) Magnetic resonance venogram in same child 3 months later after anticoagulation. Normal flow is now re-established in the superior sagittal sinus.

MAGNETIC RESONANCE ANGIOGRAPHY

MR angiography (MRA) of the cerebral arterial circulation may be done without intravenous injection and takes less than 3 minutes (Fig. 2.5.7). Lesions in the anterior circulation are better seen than in the posterior circulation. Contrast-enhanced MRA is a promising intraluminal vascular imaging modality but at present there is limited paediatric experience.

MAGNETIC RESONANCE VENOGRAPHY

MR venography (MRV) is also usually done without intravenous injection again in less than 3 minutes (Fig. 2.5.8). There may be some artefact due to signal loss from inplane flow in the vertical posterior part of the sagittal sinus. There are fewer artefacts when MRV is done with intravenous contrast.

DIFFUSION-WEIGHTED IMAGING (DWI)

This technique measures the diffusional motion of water. Where there is free diffusion such as water in the CSF in the ventricles, this is portrayed as dark, whereas brain parenchyma, where diffusion of water is more restricted, will be brighter. In acute ischaemia there is cytotoxic oedema, and failure of the ATP pump results in water accumulating in cells where its motion is restricted by membranes and organelles, etc. This restricted diffusion is shown as bright areas in diffusion imaging. Later cell breakdown frees water again, reflected as low signal on DWI. In the evolution of ischaemic brain injury affected areas will progress from initial brightness, through a phase of relatively normal signal intensity ('pseudonormalization'), to low signal intensity – this temporal sequence is helpful in timing lesions and identifying whether multiple lesions occurred simultaneously. DWI is also helpful in distinguishing acute ischaemia from other acute pathologies, e.g. infection or posterior reversible leukoencephalopathy syndrome. DWI is positive in acute ischaemia within minutes of the ischaemic insult, before changes are detectable by T1- or T2-weighted sequences (Fig. 2.5.9).

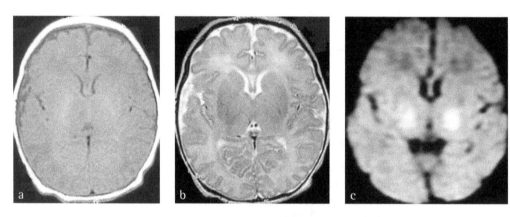

Figure 2.5.9 Brain MRI in 4-day-old infant with grade 2 neonatal encephalopathy. (a) T1-weighted and (b) T2-weighted sequences show normal signal in the thalami, but (c) diffusion-weighted imaging clearly shows abnormal signal in both thalami consistent with acute ischaemia.

An *ADC map* (ADC = apparent diffusion coefficient) is a form of diffusion imaging with brightness due to T2 bright areas (T2 shine through) eliminated. By unfortunate custom, free diffusion such as is seen in CSF is bright on ADC map and restricted diffusion is dark, which is the converse to the signal characteristics of a DWI image.

*Diffusion tensor imaging* uses information about diffusion in white matter tracts to produce complex 3D images of fibre tract anatomy and disruptions of this anatomy by disease. This may be very useful prior to surgery for tumours to detect the alignment of clinically important fibre tracts around and through the tumour.

WHOLE-BODY MRI
This is a technique that applies T2 fat saturation sequences to image the entire body. Coronal sequences allow coverage of relatively large areas of the body in short times. Sagittal sequences of the spine are usually added. The technique is best done with a special moving MRI table in adult work but in paediatrics can be done in a standard scanner.

Whole-body MRI is used in a whole-body search for a an occult neoplasm such as neuroblastoma that presents with neurological paraneoplastic phenomena (see Clinical Vignettes 2.6.1 and 2.12.3) or in the evaluation of a systemic disease such as leukaemia or metastatic tumour that may present to the paediatric neurologist.

MAGNETIC RESONANCE SPECTROSCOPY
See Chapter 2.6.

### Limitations of MRI
Movement during a sequence degrades all the images of that sequence in MRI, and a child must stay still for three or more minutes at a time to achieve the longer sequences in an MRI study. This may result in the need for sedation or general anaesthetic for young or developmentally delayed children.

Metal objects within the body may move within the magnetic fields, with possibly serious consequences. Metal objects that can't move such as dental braces may degrade the study with artefact (Fig. 2.5.10).

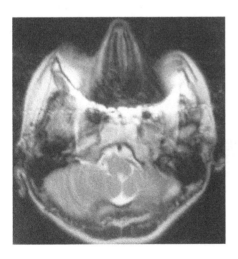

Figure 2.5.10 Dental braces artefact resulting in severe distortion of the anterior part of this brain image. Streaks extend posteriorly through the temporal lobe images and also superiorly (not seen on this slice) into the frontal lobe area.

Compared with CT especially, MRI is not good for the detection of calcification (Fig. 2.5.11), which may be important in neuroimaging, such as the pattern of calcification resulting from in utero infection of the brain or Aicardi–Goutières syndrome.

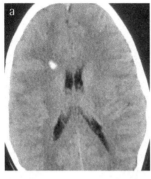
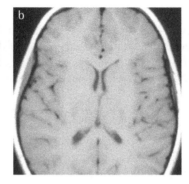
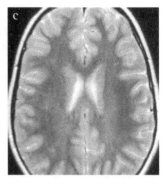

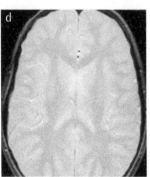

Figure 2.5.11 (a) A relatively large focus of calcification seen on CT is not visible on (b) T1-weighted or (c) T2-weighted or (d) gradient sequences on MRI.

*Normal myelination for age*

An important part of interpretation of any imaging, but in particular neuroimaging in children, is recognition of what the normal appearance is for any given age. The infant brain is quite different in appearance on MRI to the brain of an adult. The white matter of the infant brain is less myelinated than that of an adult, making it darker on T1-weighted and brighter on T2-weighted sequences than the mature brain. This makes detection of oedema more difficult in infants. Other lesions including cortical dysplasias may also become more conspicuous with maturation.

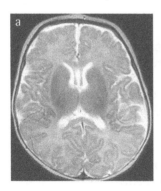
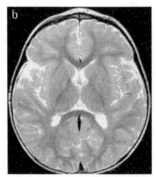

Figure 2.5.12 Brain MRI, normal T2-weighted image (a) at birth, and (b) at 22 months.

In the term-born infant, part of the posterior limb of the internal capsule, the corpus callosum and the posterior part of the midbrain as well as the cerebellar peduncles are myelinated (Fig. 2.5.12a). As the baby grows, myelination progresses in a predictable pattern from deep to superficial, from posterior to anterior, and from caudal to cephalad.

At 1 year of age the T1-weighted images are like those of an older child or adult.

At 2 years of age most of the white matter is dark on the T2-weighted sequence (Fig. 2.5.12b).

Some residual brightness on T2 in the posterior cerebral deep white matter is normal in older children.

*An approach to MRI interpretation in paediatric neurology*
The following approach to interpretation of MRI studies in paediatric neurology is suggested.

- First assess whether the study is adequate and not unduly degraded by motion or other artefacts.

- Next look at overall structure and whether any structure such as the corpus callosum or septum pellucidum is absent. Gross structural abnormalities such as schizencephaly may be obvious but focal cortical dysplasia or transmantle dysplasia may be very subtle. Wide sylvian fissures may be associated with glutaric aciduria type I. A small cerebellum may prompt the measurement of transferrin as a marker for congenital defects of glycosylation (CDG).

- Next look for areas of abnormal signal and determine their distribution. Is the abnormality predominantly in the white matter such as is seen in leukodystrophy or ADEM, in the white matter and basal ganglia such as might be seen in Krabbe disease, in the cortex or in the cerebellum?

- Look at the appearance of the abnormality on a variety of sequences.

  - Low T1, high T2 abnormalities are seen in acute lesions, inflammatory lesions and most tumours.

  - High T1, low T2 abnormalities are seen with calcification or iron deposition. MRI has a low sensitivity for detection of calcium deposits (CT or ultrasound may be better).

  - High T1 and high T2 areas within a tumour may indicate the presence of fat.

  - The appearance of blood products varies with the age of a bleed in a predictable fashion. Gradient-echo and susceptibility-weighted images may detect microhaemorrhages such as seen in vasculopathy.

  - Restricted diffusion within most or all of the area of abnormality may indicate acute ischaemia as the cause of the abnormality or in encephalitis or trauma may indicate the parts of the brain that have already undergone necrosis.

- Finally look again at the indication for the study and consider the MRI findings in the light of the clinical, laboratory and other information.

*MRI in neurological diagnosis*

The importance of pattern recognition – especially for white matter disorders – has been rightly stressed by van der Knaap (2005) but there remain few disorders in which the MRI appearances have a specificity of 1.0, that is to say they are pathognomonic of a particular condition. For instance, cysts in the temporal lobes may be seen in congenital cytomegalovirus infection, in Walker–Warburg syndrome, in megalencephalic leukoencephalopathy with subcortical cysts, and in Aicardi–Goutières syndrome.

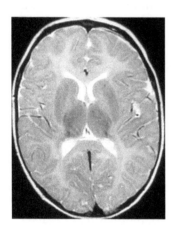

Figure 2.5.13 Brain MRI, T2-weighted sequence in child with Pelizaeus-Merzbacher disease at 22 months. The degree of myelination (darkening of white matter signal) is closer to that seen in the normal newborn infant than in the normally developing 22-month-old child shown in Fig. 2.5.12. Such severe lack of myelin in a 2-year-old suggests hypomyelination even without a follow-up MRI.

An approach to the diagnosis of white matter disorders has been elegantly described by Schiffmann and van der Knaap (2009). This involves the following:

- distinguishing hypomyelination (Fig. 2.5.13) from other white matter pathology; hypomyelination is defined as "an unchanged pattern of deficient myelination on two MRIs at least 6 months apart in a child older than 1 year"

- distinguishing confluent from isolated or multifocal lesions

- assessing the predominant distribution or localization of confluent abnormalities

- looking for other features such as megalencephaly, cystic white matter degeneration, anterior temporal cysts, increased perivascular spaces/cysts, grey matter abnormalities, calcification, microhaemorrhages and spinal involvement

- following the evolution of abnormalities over time.

Using this method the authors estimate that 60–70% of patients with white matter abnormalities will have a specific diagnosis.

We now discuss some selected MRI patterns.

CEREBELLAR ATROPHY

It is difficult to distinguish atrophy from hypoplasia except by serial imaging: in any case, hypoplasia and atrophy may coexist. Having said that, Table 2.5.1 summarizes the findings in cerebellar atrophy in the most common disorders – but bear in mind that there are many, many more!

HYPOMYELINATION

To diagnose hypomyelination, serial imaging is necessary to distinguish this from *delayed myelination* as seen in many cases of developmental delay, including that with *MCT8* mutations. The most important syndromes with hypomyelination that also have cerebellar atrophy are listed in column 2 of Table 2.5.1; molecular genetic confirmation is available in many.

When hypomyelination is associated with congenital cataracts, a defect may be found in the *FAM126A* gene, leading to a severe deficiency of hyccin. To make matters more difficult, cataracts may not appear until later, if at all.

MRI-BASED (AND CT-BASED) DIAGNOSES OF GENETIC DISORDERS

With the continuing advance of molecular genetics, the essential role of imaging in diagnosis declines. Two examples in which imaging has a primary role follow.

- *Leukoencephalopathy with brainstem and spinal cord involvement and elevated white matter lactate.* MRI of brain and spinal cord with H-MRS of white matter to identify the lactate peak were previously the sole basis of diagnosis, but now mutations in the gene *DARS2* coding for mitochondrial aspartyl-tRNA synthetase may be detected.

- *Cerebroretinal microangiopathy with calcifications and cysts (CRMCC).* In this condition both brain MRI and CT are necessary, together with skeletal survey. The brain imaging is completely specific and as yet no genetic investigations are helpful (see Clinical Vignette 2.5.5).

## Cranial ultrasound

Cranial ultrasound is useful in children in whom the anterior fontanelle is still open – i.e. approximately under 6 months of age. It allows visualization of most of the brain. No radiation is involved but the main advantage is that it can be easily done at the bedside. This is of particular advantage in the sick newborn or preterm infant in the neonatal intensive care unit.

The principal indications for cranial ultrasound are as follows:

- the evaluation of the preterm infant in the first week of life for intraventricular haemorrhage (Fig. 2.5.14) and after the first few weeks for periventricular leukomalacia (Fig. 2.5.15)
- the evaluation of the infant with a large head for hydrocephalus

**Table 2.5.1** Cerebellar atrophy (CA) and 'cerebellar atrophy plus'

| Pure CA | CA and hypomyelination | CA and progressive white matter abnormalities | | | CA and cerebellar cortex T2 hyperintensity | CA and basal ganglia (BG) involvement | | |
| --- | --- | --- | --- | --- | --- | --- | --- | --- |
| | | Periventricular | Diffuse | Subcortical | | BG calcification | BG atrophy | BG signal changes |
| Ubiquinone (CoQ10) deficiency | Pelizaeus–Merzbacher disease | Neuronal ceroid lipofuscinoses | VWM (eIF2B-related) | L-2-hydroxy-glutaric aciduria | Infantile neuroaxonal dystrophy | Kearns–Sayre syndrome | HABC | Mitochondrial |
| Ataxia-telangiectasia and ataxia-telangiectasia-like disorders | Pelizaeus–Merzbacher-like disease | Niemann–Pick disease, type C | | | Marinesco–Sjögren syndrome | Mitochondrial | Wilson disease | Wilson disease |
| Ataxia-oculomotor apraxia | Salla disease | Dentato-rubro-pallidoluysian atrophy | | | Mitochondrial | Cockayne syndrome | | 3-methyl-glutaconic aciduria |
| Late-onset GM2 | Leuko-encephalopathy with ataxia, hypodontia and hypomyelination | | | | | | | Infantile neuroaxonal dystrophy |
| CDG1a | Hypomyelination and atrophy of the basal ganglia and cerebellum (HABC) | | | | | | | L-2-hydroxy-glutaric aciduria |

- the initial or serial evaluation of the term infant with neonatal encephalopathy particularly for detection of thalamic echogenicity and middle cerebral artery infarcts. It is not a substitute for MRI in this setting, however, if the baby can be transported to the MRI unit (Fig. 2.5.16)

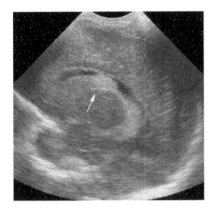

Figure 2.5.14 Cranial ultrasound, parasagittal plane, at day 3 in preterm infant born at 28 weeks' gestation, showing grade 2 intraventricular haemorrhage (arrow).

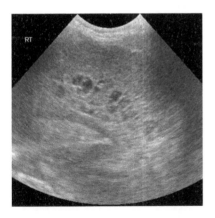

Figure 2.5.15 Cranial ultrasound, parasagittal plane lateral to the lateral ventricle, at day 28 in preterm infant born at 25 weeks' gestation. Multiple cysts are seen in the periventricular deep white matter consistent with periventricular leukomalacia.

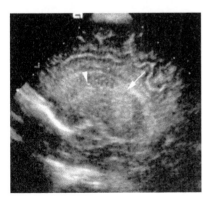

Figure 2.5.16 Cranial ultrasound, parasagittal plane, at day 2 in term infant with grade 2 neonatal encephalopathy showing abnormal high signal in the thalamus (arrow) and caudate (arrowhead).

- the detection of calcification, as in congenital infection and Aicardi–Goutières syndrome.

Cranial ultrasound is limited in these situations:

- detecting posterior fossa abnormalities; the vermis is normally echogenic and makes detection of echogenic abnormalities including haemorrhage difficult
- viewing the cerebral convexities; this makes it a poor test for the evaluation of trauma or possible non-accidental injury.

*Transcranial Doppler ultrasound* is a technique used even in older children in whom the fontanelle has closed. Ultrasound scanning through the relatively thin squamous temporal bone is used to evaluate the cerebral blood flow velocity in the vessels of the circle of Willis in a variety of disorders. It is widely used in the screening of children with sickle cell disease for vascular complications.

Recent studies have shown transcranial ultrasound to be helpful in visualizing the substantia nigra and raphe in the midbrain of adults with movement disorders. Increased or decreased echogenicity might be related to brain iron. It seems likely that this technique may soon be applied to older children with movement disorders.

**Brain CT**
Many of the indications for brain CT have been replaced by MRI. CT remains important for the evaluation of trauma, including non-accidental injury. It is also useful for the detection of calcification and for evaluation of the skull (Figs 2.5.17, 2.5.18). CT with or without contrast is a sensitive imaging modality for cerebral venous thrombosis. CT angiography holds promise as it is an intraluminal vascular imaging technique and has now supplanted the need for acute catheter cerebral angiography in the evaluation of children with acute intracranial haemorrhage.

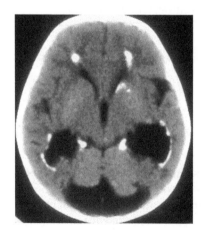

Figure 2.5.17 Brain CT in a 2-month-old infant who had congenital cytomegalovirus infection. Note the periventricular and parenchymal calcification as well as the cerebellar hypoplasia.

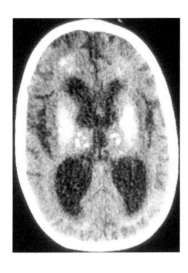

Figure 2.5.18 Brain CT in a 3-year-old boy with Aicardi–Goutières syndrome with dense calcification of the lentiform nuclei and less severe calcification of the thalami and of the white matter of the frontal lobes.

## Skull radiography

Skull radiographs are useful in the evaluation of

- trauma including non-accidental injury (Fig. 2.5.19)
- the 'funny shaped head' and craniosynostosis (Fig. 2.5.20)
- a very wide anterior fontanelle which may be part of bone dysplasia
- skull base abnormalities such as platybasia
- osteopetrosis
- CRMCC – previously known as 'Coats plus' – in which the tracery of the characteristic intracranial calcification may sometimes be nicely seen on lateral skull radiography.

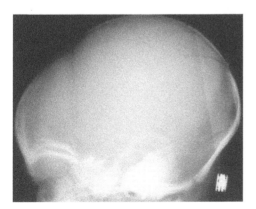

Figure 2.5.19 Parietal skull fracture on a radiograph of an infant following accidental injury – a fall from a height.

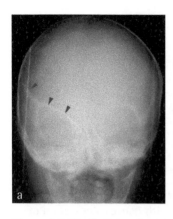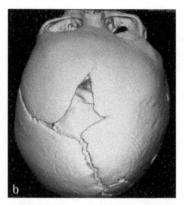

Figure 2.5.20 Unilateral coronal synostosis. (a) Postero–anterior skull radiograph shows elevation of the lesser wing of sphenoid (arrowheads) and distortion of the upper outer angle of the orbit – a Harlequin eye; (b) 3D CT of skull shows the fused right compared with the patent left coronal suture.

## Spinal imaging

### Spinal MRI
MRI is the best modality for imaging the spinal cord in children. Sagittal and axial T1- and T2-weighted images are most commonly used.

- A T2 fat-suppressed sequence or a STIR [short T1 or tau (inversion time) inversion recovery] sequence is particularly useful for oedema in the discs or vertebrae as in discitis.

- Coronal sequences are useful for children with scoliosis and for assessment of paravertebral plexiform neurofibroma in neurofibromatosis type I.

- Enhancement is used particularly with spinal tumours.

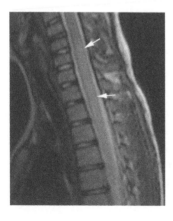

Figure 2.5.21 Spinal MRI in 6-year-old with ADEM showing abnormal high T2 signal in the cervicothoracic cord.

Abnormality of the spinal cord may be confined to the cord or may be associated with abnormality of the brain.

- The pattern of distribution of the abnormality may be diagnostic such as focal cord abnormalities associated with multiple foci of white matter abnormality in the brain in ADEM (Figs 2.5.1, 2.5.21).

- Periventricular abnormal T2 signal in addition to cord changes will prompt neuromyelitis optica (NMO) IgG studies (autoantibodies to aquaporin-4).

- Abnormal high T2 signal affecting the posterior columns may be seen in vitamin $B_{12}$ deficiency and in genetic cobalamin disorders.

- Spinal MRI should be added to brain imaging when ADEM, multiple sclerosis or non-accidental injury is suspected, or with Chiari I malformation.

- Imaging of the cord should also be added to initial assessment of midline cerebellar tumours in children since both medulloblastomas and ependymomas may have spinal metastases (so called 'drop mets') at diagnosis.

*Spinal CT*
CT is used more for imaging the vertebrae than the spinal cord. It can be used as part of the preoperative assessment of spinal developmental abnormalities and scoliosis. Its main role in paediatric neurology is the assessment of spinal trauma.

*Spinal ultrasound*
The spinal cord is at least partly visible by ultrasound in children of any age. However, by far the best views and the most information are achieved when ultrasound scanning is performed before the posterior elements of the vertebra ossify.

Ultrasound is most useful, therefore, in the neonate in the first few weeks of life. The technique uses no radiation, can be done at the bedside without sedation, and allows good visualization of the spinal cord and associated structures (Fig. 2.5.22). Some assessment can also be made of the mobility of the cord.

In the older child a limited view of the cord can be achieved by imaging between the ossified posterior elements.

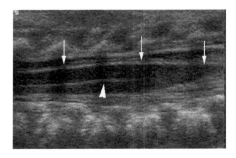

Figure 2.5.22 Normal ultrasound of spinal cord in 2-week-old infant. Dark conus (arrows) has a central echo (arrowhead), and nerve roots can be seen in the thecal sac distal to the conus.

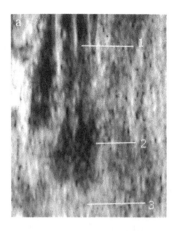 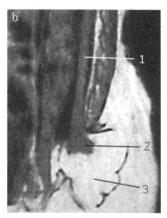

Figure 2.5.23 Infant with a lipomyelocele. (a) Spinal ultrasound at 3 weeks shows cord (1) ending in an expanded mass (2) within an echogenic fatty mass (3). (b) MRI at 6 weeks confirms the ultrasound findings and shows cord (1) ending in an expanded lower end (2) within a fatty mass (3) which is continuous with the subcutaneous lipoma.

The most common indication for spinal ultrasound is the detection of spinal dysraphism in the infant with a lumbosacral cutaneous abnormality (Fig. 2.5.23). Many studies have shown that spinal ultrasound has high sensitivity for detection of spinal dysraphism in the neonate. If ultrasound is normal, MRI is likely to be normal. MRI has been shown to give additional information among some of those in whom ultrasound detected some abnormality.

Many authors have shown that masses, raised lesions and haemangiomas have a significant association with spinal dysraphism. A simple dimple, however, has little if any risk and is not, therefore, an indication for investigation.

Dimples further from the anus are associated with greater risk of spinal dysraphism than those close to the anus. Sacrococcygeal sinuses rarely reach the spinal canal whereas thoracolumbar sinuses often do so.

## Other imaging in paediatric neurology

### Catheter cerebral angiography
Catheter cerebral angiography (CCA) is the criterion standard for imaging the cerebral circulation and has a continuing role despite advances in magnetic resonance and CT angiography, particularly in lesions confined to the posterior circulation. An example of its value in detecting arterial dissection in MRA-negative arterial ischaemic stroke is given in Clinical Vignette 2.5.3. In particular, CCA is useful in delineating the anatomy and haemodynamics of cerebrovascular malformations and for preoperative planning in patients with moyamoya disease. CCA may also be helpful in diagnosis of cerebral vasculitis, especially if this is confined to small vessels.

*Imaging of muscles*

Imaging of muscles may contribute to diagnosis as well as help identify a suitable site for muscle biopsy.

MRI allows direct visualization of muscles and muscle volume as well as detection of abnormal signals due to inflammation or to fat deposition.

Ultrasound is quicker and does not require any sedation even in very young children and babies. A high-frequency linear probe is used to obtain axial images of the mid-thigh and upper calf. Settings are fixed in the scanner corresponding to those needed to obtain a nearly black image of muscle in healthy volunteers.

Abnormal muscle has higher echogenicity with a finer granular pattern in myopathies as compared with a coarser brightness in neurogenic abnormalities (Fig. 2.5.24). Muscle ultrasound has been shown to have a high sensitivity and specificity for discrimination of normal versus abnormal muscle as well as for discrimination between myogenic and neurogenic causes of muscle abnormality.

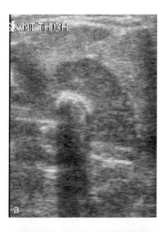
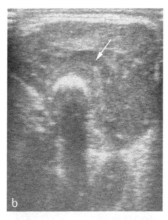
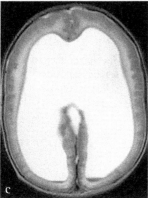
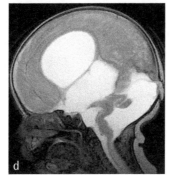

Figure 2.5.24 (a) Normal ultrasound of muscle of the anterior thigh in a term newborn infant. (b) Ultrasound of the anterior thigh of a newborn infant with Walker–Warburg syndrome. All the muscles are more granular in appearance, but the vastus intermedius in particular (arrow) is brighter than normal. (c) Brain MRI in same child shows hydrocephalus, agyria and cobblestone cortical dysplasia. (d) Sagittal MRI in same child also shows the occipital encephalocele as well as poor development and distortion of the brainstem and cerebellum.

*Brachial plexus imaging*

The brachial plexus can be imaged by ultrasound or MRI. In infants with brachial plexus injury due to birth trauma, imaging is focused on identification of the traumatic pseudomeningocele at the site of nerve root avulsion close to the cervical cord. Imaging can be confined to axial and oblique coronal views of the cord and spine using a heavily T2-weighted MR myelogram-type sequence (Fig. 2.5.25).

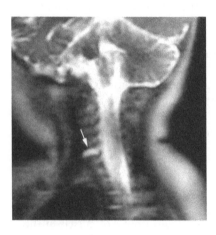

Figure 2.5.25 Brachial plexus injury with nerve root avulsion shown by pseudomeningocele formation (arrow) seen here on an oblique coronal heavily T2-weighted MR myelogram-type sequence.

## General imaging

In neurological investigation in children there are no organ-bound limits to where one searches for diagnostic clues to a neurological disorder. We list some examples in Table 2.5.2.

Table 2.5.2 General imaging in neurological disorders

| Region | Imaging method | Clinical situation | Finding | Inference |
|---|---|---|---|---|
| Heart | Echocardiography | Neonate with epileptic seizures | Rhabdomyomata | Tuberous sclerosis |
| | Echocardiography | Floppy baby | Cardiomyopathy | Mitochondrial or other metabolic disorder including Pompe disease |
| | Echocardiography | Unsteady primary school child | Thick septum | Friedreich ataxia |

Table 2.5.2 continued

| Region | Imaging method | Clinical situation | Finding | Inference |
|---|---|---|---|---|
| Heart | Echocardiography | Acquired chorea/ hemichorea | Valvular disease | Sydenham rheumatic chorea |
| | Echocardiography transoesophageal + bubble contrast | Arterial ischaemic stroke | Patent foramen ovale | Potential right to left shunt |
| Chest | Plain radiography | Floppy newborn infant | Raised right hemidiaphragm | Myotonic dystrophy |
| | Plain radiography | Floppy newborn infant | Thin horizontal ribs | Congenital myopathy or spinal muscular atrophy |
| | Plain radiography | Ataxia, opsoclonus; hypothalamic syndrome | Retrocardiac or paraspinal shadow | Neural crest tumour |
| | CT/MRI | Ataxia, opsoclonus; hypothalamic syndrome | Mass in sympathetic chain | Neural crest tumour |
| | MRI thymus | Myasthenia with +ve acetylcholine antibodies | Mass | Thymoma in myasthenia gravis |
| | Ultrasound diaphragm | Floppy baby with dyspnoea | Diminished movement | Spinal muscular atrophy with respiratory distress (SMARD1), etc. |
| Oesophagus | Barium swallow | Neck and upper trunk arching 'dystonia' | Gastro-oesophageal reflux/hiatus hernia | Sandifer syndrome |
| Liver | Ultrasound | Encephalopathy, delay, regression | Hepatomegaly ± abnormal echogenicity | Storage disorders, fatty acid oxidation defects, etc. |
| Kidney | Ultrasound | Suspect vision and tachypnoea | Cysts | Joubert syndrome |

Table 2.5.2 continued

| Region | Imaging method | Clinical situation | Finding | Inference |
|---|---|---|---|---|
| Kidney | Ultrasound | Gross hypotonia | Calcifications, cortex hyperechogenicity | Peroxisomopathy, severe GA2 (multiple coenzyme A dehydrogenase deficiency) |
| Ovary | Ultrasound | Encephalitis with oral dyskinesia, autonomic dysfunction, etc. | Teratoma | Anti-NMDA receptor antibody paraneoplastic encephalitis |
| Abdomen | CT/MRI | Ataxia, opsoclonus; hypothalamic syndrome | Paraspinal or perinephric mass | Neural crest tumour |
| Bones | Bone age | Delay | Retarded | Hypothyroidism, peroxisomopathy, etc. |
| | | | Advanced | *MCT8* mutations (hyperthyroidism, etc.) |
| | Skeletal survey | Subdural haemorrhage and encephalopathy | Metaphyseal corner fractures | Trauma |
| | Skeletal survey | Suspect storage | Dysostosis multiplex | Mucopolysaccharidoses, mucolipidoses |
| | Skeletal survey | Dysmorphism, delay, hypotonia | Epiphyseal stippling | Peroxisomopathy |
| | Skeletal survey | Ocular wobble, optic atrophy | ↑ Bone density | Osteopetrosis |
| | Skeletal survey | Coats retinopathy, cerebral calcification | Osteopenia, osteosclerosis, fractures | Cerebroretinal microangiopathy with calcification and cysts (CRMCC) |

## Clinical vignettes

### *2.5.1 Devastating congenital infection*
A baby girl born normally at 42 weeks' gestation weighed 3.4kg with head circumference 35cm and Apgar scores of 8 and 9 at 1 and 5 minutes respectively.

At 24 hours she had a dusky episode and was noted to have petechiae on the face and trunk. Platelet count was 23,000.

INVESTIGATIONS
*Cranial ultrasound* on day 2 showed periventricular foci of echogenicity (Fig. 2.5.26a).

*CT* on day 3 confirmed periventricular calcification. The cerebral white matter had abnormally low density (Fig. 2.5.26b).

*MRI* on day 7 showed severe diffuse white matter abnormality with poorly developed frontal gyral pattern suggesting an insult prior to 20 weeks gestation (Fig. 2.5.26c,d).

*Urine* was positive for cytomegalovirus, and cytomegalovirus DNA was detected in neonatal blood (>600 copies/mL).

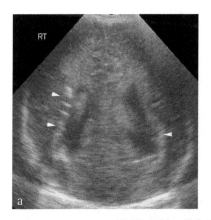

Figure 2.5.26 Congenital cytomegalovirus infection. (a) Cranial ultrasound, posterior coronal view showing periventricular echogenicity (arrowheads) due to calcification. (b) CT in same infant confirms periventricular calcification and also shows abnormal low density of frontal white matter. MRI on day 7 shows (c) severe diffuse white matter abnormality and (d) poorly developed frontal gyral pattern suggesting an insult prior to 20 weeks' gestation.

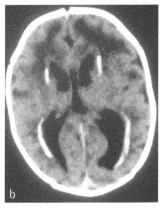
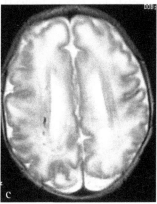
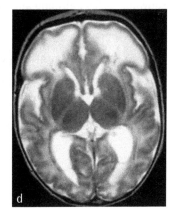

*Maternal blood sample* taken at 14 weeks in the pregnancy was retrospectively analysed: cytomegalovirus DNA was isolated, confirming early intrauterine infection.

COMMENT
In this book we show several examples of investigations in both true congenital infection and in congenital 'infection' where a genetic condition mimics a virus. In this case the virus was all too genuine.

### 2.5.2 Cherubic but not so happy

A 5-month-old boy presented following episodes of staring with unresponsiveness lasting up to 30 seconds. There was a background of recurrent infections and hypotonia. The baby had a cherubic appearance with coarse dry hair and lax skin. He was poorly responsive with tachypnoea, temperature instability and profound hypotonia.

INVESTIGATIONS
*Brain MRI with MR angiography* showed cortical atrophy with elongated tortuous cerebral arteries (Fig. 2.5.27).

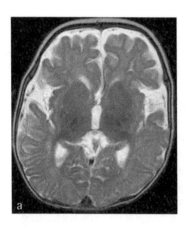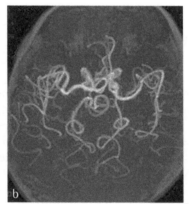

Figure 2.5.27 Menkes disease in 5-month-old. (a) Brain MRI and (b) MR angiography showing cortical atrophy and elongated and very tortuous cerebral arteries.

*Plasma copper* – 1.6mmol/L (13.1–19.7).

*Plasma ceruloplasmin* – 75mg/L (200–400).

*Microscopic hair analysis* showed pili torti and trichorrhexis nodosa.

*Mutation analysis* of *ATP7A* showed mutation c.1784_1785insG in exon 7.

COMMENT
As Menkes disease moves towards becoming a treatable disorder, diagnosis will have to be much earlier.

## 2.5.3 Pain in the face

A 7-year-old previously healthy boy with second cousin parents became unwell with vomiting some hours after playing unsupervised. Over the following three days he complained of pain on the left side of his head and face and was off form. Four days after onset of symptoms he became acutely confused, giggling inappropriately with slurred speech and unsteadiness "as if he was drunk". His responses were inappropriate. He had mild cerebellar ataxia and cerebellar dysarthria on examination in the accident and emergency department. The following morning there was significant improvement but by evening he deteriorated and had dysarthria with unsteadiness and inappropriate responses. On examination there was impaired one-leg stance and tandem gait. There was hesitancy and slowing of speech but content was appropriate and he was alert and orientated.

INVESTIGATIONS

*EEG* – Normal.

*Echocardiogram* – Normal.

*Brain MRI* showed a large area of infarction in the right cerebellar hemisphere with a smaller area of infarction on the left side. There was also some signal change in the midbrain and posterior corpus callosum.

*Intracranial MRA* – Normal.

*Thrombophilia testing* – Normal.

*Plasma lactate, creatine kinase, transaminases, ammonia and amino acids* – Normal.

*Urine amino acids and organic acids* – Normal.

*Catheter cerebral angiography* showed occlusion of a branch of the right posterior inferior cerebellar artery with narrowing of the right distal vertebral artery. The appearances were in keeping with a small vertebral dissection. There was no evidence of vasculitis or features to suggest a diffuse arteriopathy. The patient was anticoagulated and made a complete clinical and radiological recovery.

COMMENT

The history suggested a vascular event and it is possible that this was traumatic during unsupervised play. Facial pain is often a clinical clue in vertebral dissection. The case highlights the need for catheter cerebral angiography in otherwise unexplained arterial ischaemic events. An additional point: parental consanguinity does not always imply a genetic diagnosis!

## 2.5.4 Not too young for a puff of smoke

A 6-month-old girl presented to the local hospital having had an episode of staring with jerking of all four limbs for 1 minute. There were no abnormal neurological signs. Over the following months there were five similar episodes and one event in which there was jerking of the left arm with stiffening on and off over a period of 2 hours. There were no abnormal neurological signs.

INVESTIGATIONS (1)
*EEG – Normal.*

*Blood urea, creatinine, electrolytes, lactate, ammonia, creatine kinase and amino acids –* Normal.

*Urine amino acids and organic acids –* Normal.

COURSE (1)
Sodium valproate was commenced. New skills were acquired. She presented again at 8 months following a prolonged partial right-sided seizure in which her head and eyes were deviated to the right and the right arm was stiffened for almost 2 hours. There was a mild right-sided facial upper motor weakness. Focal, predominantly right-sided seizures continued over the following five days; these were unresponsive to multiple antiepileptic drugs.

INVESTIGATIONS (2)
*EEG* showed focal discharges in the left frontocentral region initially, followed by flattening of background rhythms on the left side.

*Brain MRI* showed abnormal signal in the cortex of the left hemisphere with abnormal diffusion on DWI. The features were consistent with acute ischaemia, a focal encephalitis, or an underlying mitochondrial disorder.

*Brain MRS –* Normal.

*Full blood count, coagulation and thrombophilia screen –* Normal.

*Autoantibody screen and immunoglobulins –* Normal.

*Urine –* Urea and electrolytes, creatinine, $B_{12}$, folate, thyroid function tests, ammonia, lactate carnitine, acylcarnitine, very long chain fatty acids, transferrin – Normal.

*CSF –* Glucose, lactate and protein all normal.

*Urine amino acids and organic acids –* Normal.

*Fatty acid oxidation studies on liver, muscle and fibroblasts –* Normal.

*Transaminases* were elevated (max. AST 192) and amino acids showed elevation of glutamate, glycine, alanine and proline.

*POLG1 mutation analysis –* Negative.

COURSE (2)
A metabolic disorder, possibly mitochondrial, was considered. The seizures ceased with a combination of phenobarbitone and phenytoin, and the child was commenced on coenzyme Q, biotin and carnitine supplementation. There were no further seizures but the child had significant cognitive and behavioural delay.

INVESTIGATIONS (3)
*Intracranial MRA* showed multiple abnormal anastomotic vessels consistent with moyamoya.

COURSE (3)
Bilateral extracranial/intracranial bypass procedures were performed over the following 6 months and at 2 years there is a right hemiplegia with moderate learning disability.

COMMENT
The abnormal liver function tests at the time of the acute encephalopathy were wrongly interpreted as implying a mitochondrial, possibly *POLG1*, mutation. Although the EEG and MRI during the period of epilepsia partialis continua were lateralized the shifting seizures from side to side pointed to a more diffuse process. Vasculopathies are probably as common as metabolic disorders in this clinical situation.

### 2.5.5 Coats plus
There was intrauterine growth retardation but this girl's early development was normal. She developed bilateral Coats disease at 3 years of age and underwent enucleation of the left eye. Vision was retained in the right eye. She also showed sparse hypopigmented hair, dysplastic nails, and transparent skin. A younger sister was then born and turned out to have the same condition. Both sisters acquired a movement disorder that was more severe in the younger of the two.

INVESTIGATIONS (1)
*Brain CT* (Fig. 2.5.28a) showed in both sisters extensive 'primeval' calcifications in irregularly contoured lumps. Mainly it was in the basal ganglia and thalami, in the cerebral hemispheres posteriorly and in the cerebellum.

*Brain MRI* (Fig. 2.5.28b) of both sisters showed a leukoencephalopathy in addition to the calcium deposition.

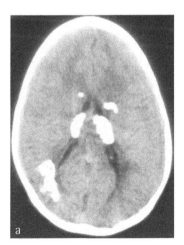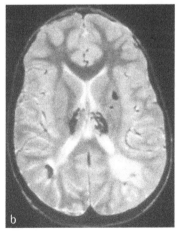

Figure 2.5.28 (a) Brain CT showing extensive 'primeval' calcifications in irregularly contoured lumps, mainly in the basal ganglia and thalami, in the cerebral hemispheres posteriorly and in the cerebellum. (b) Brain MRI showing a leukoencephalopathy with patchy signal change in areas abutting the low signal of the calcium deposition.

COURSE (1)
The younger sister fractured two limb bones while playing in a bouncy castle (trampoline-like structure).

INVESTIGATIONS (2)
*Skeletal survey* in both revealed diffusely osteopenic bones and sclerotic and lytic changes of the femoral metaphyses.

COURSE (2)
The elder sister had normal intellect and studied law at college, whereas her younger sibling had cognitive and behavioural problems and much more prominent asymmetrical dystonia.

The girls later developed signs of hepatic cirrhosis and portal hypertension which proved fatal in both.

COMMENT
This is one of the few conditions in which the brain imaging findings are completely specific. In some patients cerebral cysts are also seen, so the disorder is now called cerebroretinal microangiopathy with calcifications and cysts. The genetic basis and pathogenesis remain unknown at the time of writing.

### 2.5.6 Slowing down with a late diagnosis
This boy was already developmentally delayed at 10 months. He walked at 3 years, then being a bit shaky and speaking only a few words. By 5 years it was obvious that he had moderate learning disability. Occasional tonic–clonic epileptic seizures began at 14 years. By age 20 he was felt to be slowing down and had some rigidity and tremor. His head was large.

INVESTIGATIONS (1)
*Brain MRI* (Fig. 2.5.29) showed a disorder of white matter with high T2 signal maximal in the subcortical white matter, especially in the U-fibres. Cerebral hemispheric white matter was less affected more centrally and not at all in periventricular regions. An increased signal was also seen in the dentate nuclei.

*Lysosomal enzymes and very long chain fatty acids* – Normal.

COURSE (1)
The significance of the imaging findings was not recognized at the time by the adult neurological services.

Aged 24 years he was found on the ground poorly responsive and rigid. He was thought to have had a head injury, possibly related to a seizure. He remained akinetic for weeks, before gradual improvement to his previous state. In retrospect, his mother then said that he always slowed down with infections or head trauma.

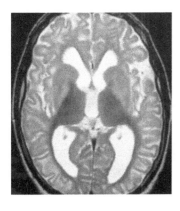

Figure 2.5.29 MRI at age 20 years showing abnormal high T2 signal in subcortical white matter with sparing of the deep white matter. There is also hyperintensity in the basal ganglia, especially in the globi pallidi.

INVESTIGATIONS (2)
*Brain MRI* was repeated and showed similar appearances to the earlier study.

COURSE (2)
The MRI was shown to a paediatric neurologist.

INVESTIGATIONS (3)
*Urine organic acids* – L-2 hydroxyglutaric acid was grossly increased at 1354μmol/mmol creatinine (reference range 0–5).

*Genetic studies* – Mutations in the *L2HGDH/DURANIN* gene were later detected.

COMMENT
The T2-weighted brain MRI appearance in L-2-hydroxyglutaric aciduria is completely specific but in the past adult neurologists were less aware of such genetic metabolic diseases that begin in childhood. There appears to be clinical heterogeneity in this disorder which has presented as epilepsy and even as migraine.

## Further reading

Aviv RI, Benseler SM, Silverman ED, et al. (2006) MR imaging and angiography of primary CNS vasculitis of childhood. *AJNR Am J Neuroradiol* 27: 192–199.

Barth PG, Aronica E, de Vries L, et al. (2007) Pontocerebellar hypoplasia type 2: a neuropathological update. *Acta Neuropathol* 114: 373–386.

Berg D, Godau J, Walter U. (2008) Transcranial sonography in movement disorders. *Lancet Neurol* 7: 1044–1055.

Biancheri R, Rossi A, Alpigiani G, et al. (2007) Cerebellar atrophy without cerebellar cortex hyperintensity in infantile neuroaxonal dystrophy (INAD) due to PLA2G6 mutation. *Eur J Paediatr Neurol* 11: 175–177.

Biancheri R, Zara F, Bruno C, et al. (2007) Phenotypic characterization of hypomyelination and congenital cataract. *Ann Neurol* 62: 121–127.

Brenner DJ, Hall EJ. (2007) Computed tomography—an increasing source of radiation exposure. *N Engl J Med* 357: 2277–2284.

Briggs TA, Abdel-Salam GM, Balicki M, et al. (2008) Cerebroretinal microangiopathy with calcifications and cysts (CRMCC). *Am J Med Genet A* **146A**: 182–190.

Brockmann K, Becker P, Schreiber G, et al. (2007) Sensitivity and specificity of qualitative muscle ultrasound in assessment of suspected neuromuscular disease in childhood. *Neuromuscul Disord* **17**: 517–523.

Budde BS, Namavar Y, Barth PG, et al. (2008) tRNA splicing endonuclease mutations cause pontocerebellar hypoplasia. *Nat Genet* **40**: 1113–1118.

Crow YJ, McMenamin J, Haenggeli CA, et al. (2004) Coats' plus: a progressive familial syndrome of bilateral Coats' disease, characteristic cerebral calcification, leukoencephalopathy, slow pre- and post-natal linear growth and defects of bone marrow and integument. *Neuropediatrics* **35**: 10–19.

D'Arrigo S, Vigano L, Buzzone MG, et al. (2005) Diagnostic approach to cerebellar disease in children. *J Child Neurol* **20**: 859–866.

Dick EA, de Bruyn R. (2003) Ultrasound of the spinal cord in children – its role. *Eur Radiol* **13**: 552–562.

Fernando S, Obaldo RE, Walsh IR, et al. (2008) Neuroimaging of nonaccidental head trauma: pitfalls and controversies. *Pediatr Radiol* **38**: 827–838.

Gregory A, Polster BJ, Hayflick SJ. (2009) Clinical and genetic delineation of neurodegeneration with brain iron accumulation. *J Med Genet* **46**: 73–80.

Hayakawa F, Okumura A, Kato T, et al. (2007) Interpretation scheme for non-expert pediatricians evaluating magnetic resonance images of children with cerebral palsy. *Pediatr Neurol* **37**: 331–337.

Koltzenburg M, Bendsuzus M. (2004) Imaging of peripheral nerve lesions. *Curr Opin Neurol* **17**: 621–626.

Koltzenburg M, Yousry T. (2007) Magnetic resonance imaging of skeletal muscle. *Curr Opin Neurol* **20**: 595–599.

Maia AC Jr, da Rocha AJ, da Silva CJ, Rosemberg S. (2007) Multiple cranial nerve enhancement: a new MR imaging finding in metachromatic leukodystrophy. *AJNR Am J Neuroradiol* **28**: 999.

Najm J, Horn D, Wimplinger I, et al. (2008) Mutations of CASK cause an X-linked brain malformation phenotype with microcephaly and hypoplasia of the brainstem and cerebellum. *Nat Genet* **40**: 1065–1067.

Phelan JA, Lowe LH, Glasier CM. (2008) Pediatric neurodegenerative white matter processes: leukodystrophies and beyond. *Pediatr Radiol 38*: 729–749.

Poretti A, Wolf NI, Boltshauser E. (2008) Differential diagnosis of cerebellar atrophy in childhood. *Eur J Paediatr Neurol* **12**: 155–167.

Rohrschneider WK, Forsting M, Darge K, Troger J. (1996) Diagnostic value of spinal US: comparative study with MR imaging in pediatric patients. *Radiology* **200**: 383–388.

Scheper GC, Van der Klok T, Van Andel RJ, et al. (2007) Mitochondrial aspartyl-tRNA synthetase deficiency causes leukoencephalopathy with brain stem and spinal cord involvement and lactate elevation. *Nat Genet* **39**: 534–539.

Schiffmann R, van der Knaap MS. (2009) Invited article: an MRI-based approach to the diagnosis of white matter disorders. *Neurology* **72**: 750–759 (with supplementary material at: http://www.neurology.org/cgi/content/full/72/8/750/DC1).

Steinlin M, Klein A, Haas-Lude K, et al. (2007) Pontocerebellar hypoplasia type 2: variability in clinical and imaging findings. *Eur J Paediatr Neurol* **11**: 146–152.

van der Knaap MS, Valk J. (2005) *Magnetic Resonance of Myelination and Myelin Disorders, 3rd edn.* New York, Berlin, Heidelberg: Springer.

van der Knaap MS, Pronk JC, Scheper GC. (2006) Vanishing white matter disease. *Lancet Neurol* **5**: 413–423.

Wolf NI, Harting I, Boltshauser E, et al. (2005) Leukoencephalopathy with ataxia, hypodontia, and hypomyelination. *Neurology* **64**: 1461–1464.

Zara F, Biancheri R, Bruno C, et al. (2006) Deficiency of hyccin, a newly identified membrane protein, causes hypomyelination and congenital cataract. *Nat Genet* **38**: 1111–1113.

# Chapter 2.6

## Functional Imaging

A number of imaging techniques can combine spatial resolution and functional information during specific brain activities. These include positron emission tomography (PET), single photon emission computed tomography (SPECT) and other nuclear imaging, functional MRI (fMRI) and magnetic resonance spectroscopy (MRS). Other functional neuroimaging techniques such as multichannel electroencephalography (EEG), magnetoencephalography (MEG), and near-infrared spectroscopic imaging (NIRSI) will not be discussed further here.

### Single photon emission computed tomography

SPECT is a nuclear medicine tomographic imaging technique using a gamma ray emitting radionuclide given to the patient, usually intravenously. SPECT is performed using a multiheaded gamma camera which rotates around the patient and acquires images from multiple angles. A computer then applies a tomographic reconstruction algorithm to yield a 3D dataset which is manipulated to form thin slice images in any chosen plane of the body, similar to those obtained from other tomographic techniques such as MRI or CT. In functional brain imaging $^{99m}$Tc-HMPAO (hexamethylpropylene amine oxime) is the radionuclide used. This is taken up by brain tissue proportional to brain blood flow, thus allowing images of local distribution of brain metabolism and energy use. In paediatric neurology SPECT is most widely used for detection of the focal origin of epileptic seizures. These typically have reduced metabolic activity between seizures compared with the rest of the brain and increased metabolic activity during seizures (Fig. 2.6.1).

### MIBG (meta-iodobenzylguanidine) scanning

MIBG scanning uses an agent that is tagged with technetium 99m, given intravenously and preferentially taken up by neuroendocrine cells. It is used in particular for the

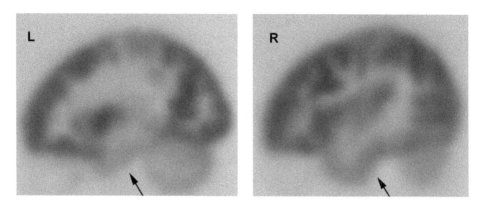

Figure 2.6.1 SPECT in child with temporal lobe epilepsy. Reduced activity is seen in left temporal lobe (L, arrow) compared with normal right temporal lobe (R, arrow).

detection of neuroblastomas. Neural crest tumours can present with a variety of paraneoplastic phenomena that manifest as neurological problems including opsoclonus–myoclonus, cerebellar ataxia and hypothalamic syndromes (see Clinical Vignette 2.6.1).

## Positron emission tomography

PET is also based on the administration of a radioactive tracer to the patient and the determination of its distribution by detecting the emitted gamma rays. However, both the radionuclide and the scanner are quite different to those used in other forms of isotope imaging. PET uses radioisotopes that undergo positron emission decay (also known as positive beta decay). After travelling up to a few millimeters positrons encounter and annihilate with electrons, producing a pair of gamma photons moving in opposite directions. The technique depends on simultaneous or coincident detection of the paired photons. In neurology the nuclide most widely used is fluorine-18 fluorodeoxyglucose (FDG), called FDG-PET. This tracer is a glucose analogue and FDG-PET is therefore a means of imaging the regional uptake of glucose in the brain. This in turn results in images of relative brain metabolic activity. As in SPECT, PET in paediatric neurology is most widely used for detection of seizure foci. These typically have reduced metabolic activity and reduced glucose and FDG uptake between seizures and increased glucose uptake during seizures.

SPECT uses a gamma camera and technetium-based radionuclides which are available in most hospitals, as opposed to PET which requires more expensive technology including a nearby cyclotron for production of positron emitting imaging agents.

Magnetic resonance spectroscopy

MRS can measure the concentration of certain metabolites in a selected location of the brain. Unfortunately, the number of metabolites that can be studied is limited.

Proton magnetic resonance spectroscopy (H-MRS) is most often used. This technique may give diagnostic information such as a glycine peak in glycine encephalopathy (Fig. 2.6.2), absence of the creatine peak in cerebral creatine deficiency syndromes (Fig. 2.6.3), or characteristically elevated NAA peak in Canavan disease (Fig. 2.6.4). Insofar as some creatine deficiency syndromes are treatable (Chapter 3.23), H-MRS should not be omitted in the appropriate clinical context.

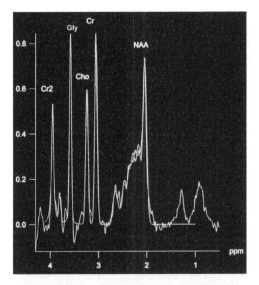

Figure 2.6.2 Term neonate with seizures. MRS on day 2 shows an abnormal peak 3.56ppm consistent with a glycine peak (Gly). Serum glycine levels were also high. A diagnosis of glycine encephalopathy was made. (Cr and Cr2 = creatine, Cho = choline, NAA = N-acetyl aspartate.)

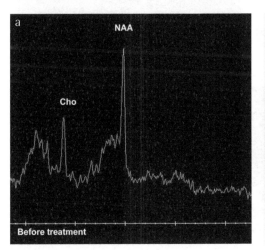

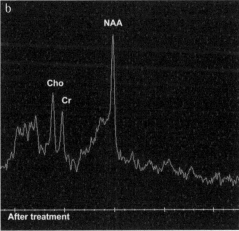

Figure 2.6.3 MRS in 13-year-old girl with developmental delay, done because of GAMT deficiency in an older sister. (a) No creatine peak is evident at 3.04ppm. (b) Repeat scan 4 months later after treatment with creatine monohydrate shows appearance of the creatine peak. (Cho = choline, NAA = N-acetyl aspartate, Cr = creatine.)

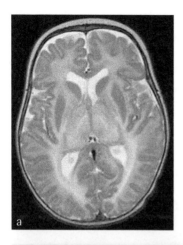

Figure 2.6.4 6-month-old boy with loss of motor skills and feeding difficulties. (a) T2-weighted MRI shows abnormal white matter and thalami. (b) MRS shows characteristically high N-acetyl aspartate peak. (c) MRS of a normal 6 month old for comparison. Note the relationship of the peak heights compared with (b). (Cho = choline, Cr = creatine, NAA = N-acetyl aspartate.)

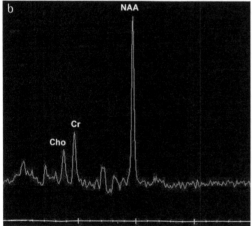

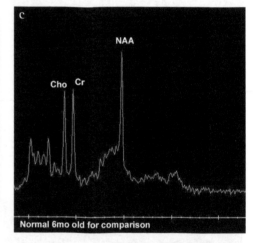

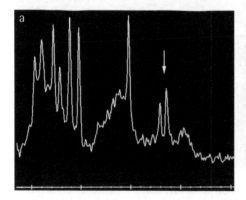

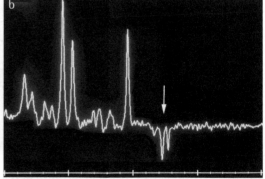

Figure 2.6.5 6-month-old with cytochrome oxidase deficiency. (a) MRS at short TE (TE=35) shows a double peak at 1.33ppm. (b) At longer TE (TE=144) the double peak at 1.33ppm inverts, characteristic of lactate (arrowed).

H-MRS may also give useful though less specific information such as the detection of lactate in the brain. In the clinical setting of hypoxic–ischaemic encephalopathy, the detection of lactate is a predictor of poor outcome. Outside the setting of acute ischaemia, the detection of lactate in the brain of a child may be an indicator of a mitochondrial disorder (Fig. 2.6.5) or Aicardi–Goutières syndrome. Lactate elevation is a specific component of the diagnosis of mitochondrial aspartyl-tRNA synthetase deficiency.

Phosphorus magnetic resonance spectroscopy ($^{31}$P-MRS) has been employed to demonstrate increased pH in episodic ataxia type 2, but at present is little used as a clinical neurological investigation.

### Magnetic resonance perfusion imaging

Magnetic resonance perfusion imaging provides information about cerebral haemodynamics; there are data suggesting it may be useful in evaluating cerebral perfusion in children with sickle cell disease and moyamoya.

### Functional MRI

The most widely used form of fMRI is the blood-oxygen-level dependent or BOLD fMRI. This is based on detecting changes in local MRI signal due to changes in the relative concentration of oxyhaemoglobin and deoxyhaemoglobin. When the cortex of the brain is activated there is a local increase in blood flow with an increase in the local concentration of oxyhaemoglobin and a decrease in deoxyhaemoglobin. This results in an increase in local signal activity. When the resting state image is subtracted from the image during activity the precise location of cortical activity can be identified. Functional MRI is used to elucidate the mechanisms of diverse disorders but in contrast to MRS its value in answering the question "What is the diagnosis?" is limited.

### Clinical vignettes

*2.6.1 Pure cerebellar ataxia with a noninfective cause*
A 3-year-old girl presented to her local hospital with a 3-day history of falling over. There was a history of a viral illness two weeks earlier and contact with varicella. There was marked truncal ataxia with reduced reflexes and past pointing.

INVESTIGATIONS (1)
Brain CT and MRI were normal. A diagnosis of postinfectious cerebellar ataxia was considered.

COURSE (1)
There was no change over the following 2 months and the child was referred for neurological opinion. Examination showed marked ataxia with dysmetria, titubation and slowing of speech. There were no ophthalmological or behavioural signs.

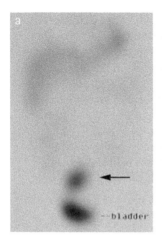
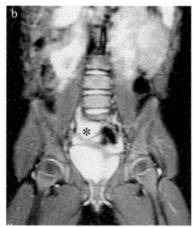

Figure 2.6.6 3-year-old girl with ataxia. (a) MIBG scan shows abnormal uptake above the bladder in the midline posteriorly. (b) Image from a whole-body MRI study initially reported as normal. Review of this in the light of the MIBG scan showed a mass above the bladder (asterisk) that had been mistaken for bowel loops.

INVESTIGATIONS (2)
*EEG* – Normal.

*Whole-body MRI* – Normal (Fig. 2.6.6b).

*Urine* – Urea and electrolytes, lactate, ammonia, carnitine, alpha 1 fetoprotein, immunoglobulin, vitamins $B_{12}$ and E, amino acids, organic acids and catecholamines were all normal.

*Plasma amino acids* – Normal.

COURSE (2)
There was no change over three weeks while investigations were being carried out.

INVESTIGATIONS (3)
MIBG scan showed abnormal uptake above the bladder in the midline posteriorly (Fig. 2.6.6a). Review of the whole-body MRI in the light of this finding showed a mass above the bladder that had been mistaken for bowel loops. The findings were in keeping with a paravertebral neuroblastoma. This was confirmed on histology.

COMMENT
Patients with paraneoplastic ataxia related to neural crest tumours may not have the full picture of opsoclonus, myoclonus, ataxia and behavioural changes. The paravertebral mass was misinterpreted as bowel on the whole-body MRI.

*2.6.2 Not a drug effect*
A girl had normal development until 1 year of age. She sat at 10 months, walked at 15

months, babbled and showed signs of nonverbal communication and symbolic play but lost these skills between 18 months and 2 years. At 2 years epileptic seizures emerged in the form of myoclonus and staring episodes.

INVESTIGATIONS (1)

*EEG* showed generalized spike and slow wave (3Hz) activity.

*Brain CT* – Normal.

*Karyotype* – Normal.

*Plasma* – ammonia, lactate, carnitine, acylcarnitine and amino acids all normal.

*Urine* – amino acids and organic acids normal.

*Serum creatinine* = 9–16mmol/L (normal 20–50mmol/L).

COURSE

The epilepsy was resistant to multiple drugs but was controlled eventually at 5 years by sodium valproate and vigabatrin. At 15 years there was severe learning disability with autistic features and impulsive behaviour. Expressive speech was limited to fewer than 10 words. At time of transfer to adult services a general slowing of mobility was noted followed by twisting movements of the mouth and face with bouts of anxiety and agitation. A drug effect was considered as the patient was on risperidone, sodium valproate and vigabatrin. The movements increased in severity and became ballistic and dystonic, affecting the face, neck and limbs leading to a flexed posture.

INVESTIGATIONS (2)

*MRI* at 17 years showed increased signal in the globus pallidus bilaterally.

*H-MRS* showed absence of a creatine peak. Biochemical testing showed elevated serum and urinary guanidinoacetate and urinary urate:creatinine ratio with low serum creatine and urinary creatinine. Guanidinoacetate methyltransferase (GAMT) activity in cultured fibroblasts was impaired, confirming GAMT deficiency. *GAMT* gene mutation analysis showed compound heterozygosity for two mutations considered pathogenic. After treatment including creatine supplements there was a reduction in seizure frequency and severity of movement disorder and creatine peak appeared on follow-up MRS. A 13-year-old sibling with a similar less severe course was subsequently found to have the same biochemical and genetic defect (Fig. 2.6.3).

COMMENT

Acquired movement disorder in children with a background of severe learning disability and early-onset epilepsy should prompt H-MRS to exclude this rare but potentially treatable disorder.

## Further reading

Bizzi A, Castelli G, Bugiani M, et al. (2008) Classification of childhood white matter disorders using proton MR spectroscopic imaging. *AJNR Am J Neuroradiol* 29: 1270–1275.

Boddaert N, Romano S, Funalot B, et al. (2008) 1H MRS spectroscopy evidence of cerebellar high lactate in mitochondrial respiratory chain deficiency. *Mol Genet Metab* **93**: 85–88.

Munson S, Schroth E, Ernst M. (2006) Role of functional neuroimaging in pediatric brain injury. *Pediatrics* **117**: 1372–1381.

Robertson NJ, Stafler P, Battini R, et al. (2004) Brain lactic alkalosis in Aicardi–Goutières syndrome. *Neuropediatrics* **35**: 20–26.

Sappey-Marinier D, Vighetto A, Peyron R, et al. (1999) Phosphorus and proton magnetic resonance spectroscopy in episodic ataxia type 2. *Ann Neurol* **46**: 256–259.

Scheper GC, Van der Klok T, Van Andel RJ, et al. (2007) Mitochondrial aspartyl-tRNA synthetase deficiency causes leukoencephalopathy with brain stem and spinal cord involvement and lactate elevation. *Nat Genet* **39**: 534–539.

# Chapter 2.7
## Cerebrospinal Fluid

The cerebrospinal fluid (CSF) is formed by the choroid plexuses within the ventricles, passes into the subarachnoid space around the spinal cord and finally over the surface of the brain, to be absorbed in the arachnoid villi in the sagittal sinus. The composition of the CSF changes during circulation from its creation to its final absorption. For example, the CSF protein is lowest in the lateral ventricles, intermediate in the lumbar subarachnoid space, and highest in the subarachnoid spaces over the surface of the cerebral hemispheres (where it is occasionally sampled in mistake for subdural fluid). Except when there is obstruction to the flow of CSF from the ventricular system or potential downward herniation of the brain, CSF is obtained by the lumbar route.

The technique of lumbar puncture should be too well known to require further description here, except to emphasize that needles must contain stylets to avoid the possibility of inducing implantation dermoids and leading to paraparesis some years later.

### Appearance
A cloudy appearance normally indicates infection. More important is the distinction between traumatic haemorrhage and subarachnoid bleeding. In subarachnoid haemorrhage the CSF, however red, runs like CSF and does not have the viscosity of blood. Xanthochromia of the supernatant may reflect bleeding several hours previously but a similar colour is seen when the protein content is very high from any cause. A 'shimmer' on flicking the tube suggests increased cells and/or protein >1.5g/L.

### Pressure
The opening pressure should always be measured using a manometer attached to the needle.

Pressure measurements obtained by the usual manometric method will be in centimetres of water ($cmH_2O$), but those obtained with the aid of a transducer will be in milimetres of mercury (mmHg). The conversion factor is approximately 1.3, by which the pressure in mmHg must be multiplied to give the value in $cmH_2O$.

The normal CSF pressure in a neonate is in the range 0–5.7mmHg, mean 2.8mmHg (0–7.6$cmH_2O$, mean 3.8$cmH_2O$). The upper limit of the CSF pressure in older children is said to be similar to the adult value of 14mmHg (19$cmH_2O$). The upper limit in the infant must be lower but information is limited.

## Cells
In the neonatal period and later, a white blood cell (WBC) count up to 5/$mm^3$ is normal. The distribution is skewed to smaller numbers, such that the median neonatal WBC count is 1/$mm^3$. It is wise to regard even 1 neutrophil/$mm^3$ as abnormal. The recognition of CSF malignant cells requires specialist expertise, but eosinophils are detectable with standard staining.

In the evaluation of CSF cell count when there has been a traumatic lumbar puncture haemorrhage, one retrospective study found that the CSF WBC count was only 20% of that expected by the number of red cells. However, inferences based on such calculations must be made with caution.

## Protein
The protein in the CSF consists mostly of albumin, synthesized entirely extrathecally, and immunoglobulins – IgG, etc. – synthesized both extrathecally and intrathecally.

Many laboratories even in children's hospitals give the upper limit of normal as the adult value of 0.45g/L (45mg/dL) total protein. In fact, the total protein begins at a high level in the neonatal period and falls to a plateau between 6 months and 10 years, followed by a slight increase up to the age of 16 years. More details are given in Appendix 2, but for most of infancy and childhood the upper limit of normal is about 0.32g/L (32mg/dL).

Increase in CSF protein (albumin) occurs when there is disruption of the blood–brain barrier (and notably in polyneuropathy).

Traumatic blood contamination may be expected to increase the CSF protein by around 0.01g/L for each 1000 red cells/μL but, as with similar calculations on cell counts, caution is indicated.

## Albumin
Because albumin comes entirely from outside the CSF, its concentration reflects the blood–CSF barrier. The CSF:serum albumin quotient ($Q_{alb}$) = CSF albumin (mg/L)/serum albumin (g/L). A $Q_{alb}$ >9 indicates blood–CSF barrier impairment.

## Immunoglobulin – quantitative indices

Although immunoglobulins may be increased because of disruption of the blood–brain barrier an important cause is intrathecal synthesis of immunoglobulin. Various formulae or indices are used to give a quantitative measure of intrathecal synthesis of IgG, the most important of the immunoglobulins.

The CSF IgG : albumin ratio = CSF IgG (mg/L)/CSF albumin (mg/L). The upper limit of normal for children under 18 months is 0.17, and for children over 18 months 0.22. Values above these figures suggest intrathecal IgG synthesis.

The CSF:serum IgG quotient ($Q_{IgG}$) = CSF IgG (mg/L)/serum IgG (g/L).

The CSF:serum IgG index[1] = $Q_{IgG}/Q_{alb}$ = $\dfrac{\text{CSF IgG mg/L} \times \text{serum albumin g/L}}{\text{CSF albumin mg/L} \times \text{serum IgG g/L}}$ .

The 'normal' upper limit for the CSF:serum IgG index is 1.02 under the age of 18 months and 0.78 over that age, a higher value indicating increased intrathecal IgG synthesis. This is an index of focal IgG production, adjusted both for leakage of IgG due to blood–brain barrier dysfunction and for serum albumin and IgG concentration. With these upper limits, false positives occur in ~2% of cases.

In the above calculations the degree of intrathecal IgG synthesis may be falsely elevated when measurements are made after a traumatic lumbar puncture.

## Immunoglobulin – qualitative: oligoclonal bands

The presence of two or more bands of immunoglobulin on isoelectric focusing (IEF) of CSF is referred to as 'oligoclonal bands' (OCBs). This CSF oligoclonal banding is only indicative of local CNS IgG production when the banding pattern in the CSF is distinct from the pattern seen in the serum. For this reason a serum sample must be sent with a CSF sample, as is done of course for the CSF:serum IgG index.

While OCBs are well known to assist in the diagnosis of multiple sclerosis it is important to recognize that they are found in many other situations with infections (subacute sclerosing panencephalitis, rubella panencephalitis, neurosyphilis, neuroborreliosis) or autoimmunity (anti-NMDA receptor encephalitis).

## Immunoglobulin – quantitative and qualitative

Although it has been suggested that in adults – where multiple sclerosis is a predominant condition – it is only necessary to request IEF for OCB, in children it is wise to request *both* quantitative (CSF:serum IgG index) and qualitative (isoelectric focusing for OCB) measures to determine whether there is local CSF IgG synthesis.

---

1 Also known as CSF IgG index or simply as IgG index.

### Asialotransferrin

The proportion of asialotransferrin (desialotransferrin, tau protein, τ protein) to total transferrin may be measured simply, quickly and cheaply by 2D gel electrophoresis. Normally asialotransferrin forms more than 8% of CSF transferrin, but in eIF2B-related disorders (vanishing white matter disease and several other phenotypes) it is below 8%. Although this test has not yet been validated in infancy, from toddlerhood onwards it has a high degree of sensitivity and specificity to predict mutations in the genes responsible for one of the five subunits of eIF2B. It may be a first-line investigation once a leukoencephalopathy has been detected on MRI/MRS.

### Myelin basic protein

This component of myelin may be found in increased quantities at the time of acute demyelination (as in acute disseminating encephalomyelitis), but data on sensitivity and specificity are limited.

### Cytokines

Although cytokines may be estimated fairly readily by means of commercially available kits, such estimations are not particularly helpful in clinical diagnosis.

### Interferon-alpha

The most important cytokine that is involved in certain virus infections and autoimmune disorders is interferon-alpha (IFN-α). The normal IFN-α value is less than 2 IU/mL. A serum sample is helpful but not always necessary for interpretation of CSF IFN-α. CSF IFN-α is raised acutely in herpes encephalitis and in cerebral systemic lupus erythematosus. It is consistently elevated for the first 12 months of life in Aicardi–Goutières syndrome.

### Glucose

The normal CSF glucose is two-thirds of the blood glucose level, which must always be estimated simultaneously, the blood sample taken *immediately before the lumbar puncture*.

Various degrees of low CSF glucose may be found in all inflammatory meningeal disorders whether infective or autoimmune, and in malignant meningitis. Low CSF glucose may also be seen after subarachnoid haemorrhage.

An important cause of low CSF glucose is GLUT1 deficiency. This is an important treatable cause of early-onset epileptic seizures, hypotonia, movement disorders, learning difficulties and microcephaly. A 4–6 hour fast is recommended with a blood glucose measurement immediately before the lumbar puncture for the CSF glucose estimation. In GLUT1 deficiency the CSF/blood glucose ratio has a mean of 0.35 with a range 0.19–0.49, and the lactate is always normal or low.

**Special biochemistry** (see also Table 2.14.4 in Chapter 2.14)

*Lactate*
Paired samples of fasting serum and CSF are taken for lactate. The upper limit of normal is usually given as 2.4mmol/L for serum and 2.2mmol/L for CSF lactate. CSF lactate is often but by no means always increased in mitochondrial disorders, and in certain organic acidaemias. It is normal or reduced in GLUT1 deficiency.

In certain circumstances the lactate/pyruvate (L/P) ratio is estimated. It is normally <20. The L/P ratio is increased in mitochondrial disorders but not in pyruvate dehydrogenase or pyruvate carboxylase deficiency.

## Amino acids
In some disorders the CSF:plasma ratio is diagnostic while in others the level of a particular amino acid may be abnormal. For example, in glycine encephalopathy the CSF:plasma glycine ratio is elevated to 0.1 or more (normal <0.025).

In pyridoxal phosphate-responsive seizures (pyridox(am)ine phosphate oxidase deficiency) causing neonatal seizures, threonine may be elevated in CSF and glycine in plasma.

In serine biosynthesis disorders (in particular 3-phosphoglycerate dehydrogenase and phosphoserine amino transferase deficiency), CSF serine and glycine are reduced while fasting plasma serine *may* be reduced less obviously.

In creatine synthesis disorders (especially guanidinoacetate-methyl transferase deficiency), CSF creatine is reduced, but brain MRS to see the absent creatine peak is the best investigation.

## Biogenic amines
Measurement of these metabolites may be of value in patients with

- hyperphenylalaninaemia and suspected disorders of biopterin metabolism
- movement disorders such as dopa-responsive-dystonia
- suspected pyridox(am)ine-5´-phosphate oxidase (PNPO) deficiency causing neonatal seizures responding to pyridoxal phosphate (see Chapters 2.14, 2.16, 3.1, 3.23).

NB *Pyridoxal-5´-phosphate* itself may be conveniently measured in the CSF in the same specimen used for detection of biogenic amines.

## Pterins
Pterins should *always* be measured in the same specimen of CSF as biogenic monoamines, but their estimation is also important in suspected inflammatory disorders, whether infective or autoimmune.

*Neopterin* in particular is increased in virtually all inflammatory and immune-mediated disorders (including Aicardi–Goutières syndrome). Neopterin, which has a short half-life, is a significantly more sensitive marker of CNS inflammation than CSF pleocytosis.

### Succinylpurine
Succinylpurines are increased in adenylosuccinate lyase deficiency in which there is early-life epileptic encephalopathy.

### Microbiology
All doctors are familiar with general techniques of microscopy and culture and serology in the diagnosis of infectious diseases which involve the CSF (see also Chapter 2.9).

IFN-α has been mentioned under cytokines. IFN-α is increased in congenital rubella, in CNS human immunodeficiency virus (HIV) infection, in the acute phase of herpes simplex encephalitis (in the infectious but not in the parainfectious relapse of that condition) and in Aicardi–Goutières syndrome in the first year of life. IFN-α is also increased in acute neurological systemic lupus erythematosus.

### Blood sampling with all diagnostic lumbar punctures
While it has been indicated in the various sections above it cannot be overemphasized that blood must be taken at the same time as lumbar puncture (preferably immediately before) to allow proper interpretation of CSF findings.

### Indications for CSF examination
Lumbar puncture is indicated in all cases of suspect meningitis or encephalitis, except when skin petechiae make meningococcal infection virtually certain, or if brain swelling, mass lesion, or obstructive hydrocephalus is thought likely (see below, Contraindications).

The remaining indications may be summarized as follows (with findings in parentheses).

- Acute polyneuropathy or Guillain–Barré syndrome (increased total protein without increased cells).
- Suspect poliomyelitis (increased cells – lymphocytes and/or polymorphs).
- Subacute polyneuropathy (increased total protein and increased immunoglobulin synthesis).
- Acute disseminated encephalomyelitis (increased total protein, increased immunoglobulin synthesis, mild or moderate increase in lymphocytes).
- Multiple sclerosis (OCBs).
- Benign intracranial hypertension, after MRI (increased pressure).

- *Suspect regressive disorder:*
  - Subacute sclerosing panencephalitis and rubella panencephalitis (OCBs; paired blood and viral titres)
  - Krabbe disease and metachromatic leukodystrophy (increased protein)
  - Mitochondrial (increased lactate, protein)
  - Aicardi–Goutières syndrome (increased lymphocytes or neopterin and IFN-α).
- *Early-onset epileptic seizures:*
  - Glycine encephalopathy (increased glycine and increased CSF/serum glycine ratio)
  - GLUT1 deficiency (decreased glucose, decreased CSF/blood glucose ratio, normal lactate)
  - Pyridox(am)ine oxidase deficiency (elevated threonine in blood and CSF, decreased CSF pyridoxal-5′-phosphate).
- *Movement disorders* – both hypo- and hyperkinetic forms have specific abnormalities, in particular:
  - Dopa-responsive dystonia
  - Tyrosine hydroxylase deficiency
  - Aromatic acid decarboxylase deficiency (see Chapters 3.7, 3.21).

## Contraindications to lumbar punctures

The most important contraindication to lumbar puncture is the suspicion of an intracranial mass lesion, brain swelling, obstructive hydrocephalus, spinal cord mass or spinal cord swelling. Clinical judgement is necessary here because no single sign or constellation of signs is consistently present in any of these situations. In the acute situation, where the history is measured in hours or days and the symptoms suggest bacterial meningitis, a critical matter is to select those few children in whom immediate diagnostic lumbar puncture is not indicated. Failure to localize a painful stimulus applied to the head (using Glasgow Coma Scale methodology) is an absolute contraindication to lumbar puncture. Tonic *non*-epileptic seizures or deterioration in the Glasgow Coma Scale score are strong warning signs of impending brain herniation and indicate that lumbar puncture may be dangerous (or be falsely blamed for a catastrophic outcome). Treatment may be implemented, imaging performed and the need for a lumbar puncture reconsidered after several hours.

In the subacute situation, in which the history is of the order of 2–4 weeks, with features such as headache, vomiting, weight loss, behaviour change or intermittent fever, the differential diagnosis includes posterior fossa tumour, missed tuberculous meningitis or brain abscess. Evidence suggesting a risk of cerebral herniation includes a larger than expected head size, a cracked-pot percussion note over the coronal sutures (McEwan's sign), papilloedema, loss of retinal venous pulsation, and an abnormal head posture, either tilted or held stiffly in an anxious-looking manner.

## Clinical vignettes

### 2.7.1 Roast beef seizures

A 3-year-old girl had seizures in the morning, mainly brief absences. She also had developmental delay with ataxia and dysequilibrium. Her mother volunteered that eating roast beef the night before might bring her seizures on.

INVESTIGATIONS

*EEG* – Interictal spike discharges over left centrotemporal region, phase reversing at C3, with biparietal paroxysmal sharp and slow acticivity.

*Blood glucose* at time of lumbar puncture = 4.2mmol/L.

*CSF glucose* = 1.9mmol/L.

*CSF/blood glucose ratio* = 0.45.

*CSF lactate* = 0.9mmol/L.

*Genetic study* – GLUT1 (*SLC2A1*) mutation was detected.

COURSE

She improved on a ketogenic diet, though relapsed when it was briefly withdrawn. Seizures that were 20–30/day before the diet became very rare. Mobility, which had been grossly impaired, slowly improved to walking with a frame and some support to her hip girdle, and with speech being mostly comprehensible to her parents by age 5 years (by then she could count to 10).

COMMENT

As we emphasized in Chapter 1.1, the clinical history is a major signpost to diagnosis and to the appropriate investigations along the route. Anything to do with feeds or diet or meals or food may be a clue to GLUT1 (*SLC2A1*) deficiency, although as in the present example the exact mechanism may not always be obvious. Lumbar puncture may be an invasive procedure but when it reveals a treatable disorder it must be worth the effort.

### 2.7.2 'Cerebral palsy' twice in the same family

Brothers in a family presented considerable diagnostic problems.

*First brother:* This boy, first child of healthy first-cousin parents, presented at the age of 1 year with developmental delay. He was not sitting independently but was acquiring new skills. There was lower-limb hypertonia with brisk tendon reflexes and extensor plantar responses.

INVESTIGATIONS (1)

*Brain CT* at 1 year showed calcification in the globus pallidus and white matter of the frontal lobes.

*CSF examination* at 1 year showed lymphocytosis with 16 WBC/mm³.

COURSE
At age 5 years he had a nonprogressive spastic diplegia with normal head growth and intelligence.

INVESTIGATIONS (2)
*Brain MRI* at 9 years showed high T2 signal in the centrum semiovale.

*CSF analysis* showed 8 WBC/mm$^3$.

*Serum and CSF interferon-alpha (IFN-α)* were normal (<2 IU/mL).

**Second brother:** A brother, born 7 years later, presented aged 1 year with severe developmental delay. At age 2 years he had dyskinetic–spastic cerebral palsy with poor postnatal head growth and learning disability.

INVESTIGATIONS
*Brain CT* at 1 year showed areas of microcalcification bilaterally in the region of the basal ganglia and widening of the sylvian fissures.

*Brain MRI* at 21 months showed ventricular dilatation with high signal in the frontal and periventricular white matter on T2-weighted imaging.

*CSF analysis* at 21 months revealed a lymphocytosis with a white cell count of 13/mm$^3$.

*Serum IFN-α* – Normal (<2 IU/mL).

*CSF IFN-α* was elevated at 25 IU/mL (normal <2 IU/mL).

The above findings were in keeping with Aicardi–Goutières syndrome. Subsequently a mutation in the *RNASEH2B* gene confirmed the diagnosis in this family.

COMMENT
The phenotype of Aicardi–Goutières syndrome is varied and it is now known that many patients may not have a progressive course. This family has a milder variant more often seen with an *RNASEH2B* mutation. The diagnosis may be missed if CSF examination of white cells and IFN-α is delayed beyond the first year.

A good resource is http://www.ncbi.nlm.nih.gov/bookshelf/br.fcgi?book=gene&part=ags.

### 2.7.3 Epilepsia partialis continua
A previously healthy 10-month-old girl presented with focal clonic seizures affecting the left side of her body and becoming bilateral over days. There was no response to benzodiazepines, phosphenytoin, phenobarbitone or paraldehyde. Elective intubation and thiopentone infusion resulted in cessation of seizures.

INVESTIGATIONS (1)
*Transaminases* – mildly elevated (AST 94).

*EEG* – discontinuous with frequent right sided spike discharges.

*CSF protein* was elevated at 742mg/L (normal for age <350mg/L).

*Brain MRI* – Normal.

COURSE
After extubation there were clinical signs of a double hemiplegia and brainstem dysfunction. The child died several weeks later. An autopsy was not performed.

INVESTIGATIONS (2)
The girl was found to have a mutation in the *POLG1* gene [compound heterozygote 4p.A467T/p.G848S resulting from base changes in exon 7 and exon 16 (c.2824g > A) of the *POLG1* gene].

COMMENT
Elevated CSF protein was the clinical clue to a diagnosis of Alpers disease in this girl in whom brain imaging was normal at presentation. Rapid confirmation of the diagnosis enabled appropriate family management.

### 2.7.4 Toe-walking explained
A 21-month-old girl, the first child of unrelated parents, was referred with a 6-week history of poor feeding, and loss of ability to roll, crawl, sit or stand or hold on to objects. She was severely emaciated. The social circumstances were very difficult. The child was last seen by the health services at the age of 1 year when she was crawling and walking on her toes holding onto one finger. She walked independently at 14 months and at 18 months was feeding herself with a spoon, speaking single words and had symbolic play. Six weeks before admission she developed a respiratory tract infection and was given an antibiotic and over the following 50 days she did not speak, roll, crawl, sit or stand. She stopped reaching out for objects and was less interactive, moaning a lot of the time. She stopped taking solids and reverted to feeding by bottle.

The toe-walking with otherwise normal development was confirmed on home video taken by parents 6 weeks earlier.

On examination she was not dysmorphic, with head circumference on the 50th centile. There was marked emaciation. She was crying and arching backwards. The upper limbs were extended and the hands fisted, and the lower limbs extended, inverted and somewhat rigid. The tendon reflexes were brisk, there was no ankle clonus and plantar responses were extensor. The optic discs were pale. There were normal eye movements, gag reflex and cough.

INVESTIGATIONS
*Brain MRI* showed abnormal high signal throughout the cerebral deep white matter. The cortical sulci were deep and there was dilatation of the lateral third and fourth ventricles suggestive of atrophy. There was low T2 and high T1 signal in the thalami. Contrast was not given.

*CSF protein* was elevated at 663mg/L.

*Motor nerve conduction velocity* (medial and tibial) was low, 50% of normal value for age.

*Lysosomal arylsulphatase A* was 0.8μmol/g/hr (reference 50–250), in keeping with the composite clinical diagnosis of metachromatic leukodystrophy.

COMMENT

Toe-walking may very rarely be the initial manisfestation of a progressive disorder. The unfavourable social circumstances were considered relevant at initial presentation, but home video confirmed the parental history including the very rapid decline occasionally seen with late infantile metachromatic leukodystrophy. Urine sulphatides and metachromatic granules would have given additional support, as would cranial nerve enhancement on brain MRI. The clinician must encourage laboratories to support the full range of neurological investigations, as we outline in this Handbook. In this situation the elevated CSF protein was an additional plank of evidence in a condition where one aims for complete diagnostic certaintly.

## Further reading

Biou D, Benoist JF, Huong CNX. (2000) Cerebrospinal fluid protein concentrations in children: age-related values in patients without disorders of the central nervous system. *Clin Chem* **46**: 399–403.

Carraccio C, Blotny K, Fisher MC. (1995) Cerebrospinal fluid analysis in systemically ill children without central nervous system disease. *Pediatrics* **96**: 48–51.

Crow YJ, Livingston JH. (2008) Aicardi–Goutières syndrome: an important Mendelian mimic of congenital infection. *Dev Med Child Neurol* **50**: 410–416.

Dale RC, Brilot F, Fagan E, Earl J. (2009) Cerebrospinal fluid neopterin in paediatric neurology: a marker of active central nervous system inflammation. *Dev Med Child Neurol* **51**: 317–323.

Deisenhammer, F, Bartos A, Egg R, et al. (2006) Guidelines on routine cerebrospinal fluid analysis. Report from an EFNS task force. *Eur J Neurol* **14**: e14.

Hoffmann GF, Surtees RAH, Wevers RA. (1998) Cerebrospinal fluid investigations for neurometabolic disorders. *Neuropediatrics* **29**: 59–71.

Hutchesson A, Preece MA, Gray G, Green A. (1997) Measurement of lactate in cerebrospinal fluid in investigation of inherited metabolic disease. *Clin Chem* **43**: 158–161.

Hyland K. (2003) The lumbar puncture for diagnosis of pediatric neurotransmitter diseases. *Ann Neurol* **54** Suppl 6: S13–17.

Jones CM, Smith M, Henderson MJ. (2006) Reference data for cerebrospinal fluid and the utility of amino acid measurement for the diagnosis of inborn errors of metabolism. *Ann Clin Biochem* **43**: 63–66.

Link H, Tibbling G. (1977) Principles of albumin and IgG analyses in neurological disorders. III. Evaluation of IgG synthesis within the central nervous system in multiple sclerosis. *Scand J Clin Lab Invest* **37**: 397–401.

Martín-Ancel A, García-Alix A, Salas A, et al. (2006) Cerebrospinal fluid leucocyte counts in healthy neonates. *Arch Dis Child Fetal Neonatal Ed* **91**: 357–358.

Portnoy JM, Olson LC. (1985) Normal cerebrospinal fluid values in children: another look. *Pediatrics* **75**: 484–487.

Rubenstein JS, Yogev R. (1985) What represents pleocytosis in blood-contaminated ("traumatic tap") cerebrospinal fluid in children? *J Pediatr* **107**: 249–251.

Rust RS Jr, Dodson WE, Trotter JL. (1988) Cerebrospinal fluid IgG in childhood: the establishment of reference values. *Ann Neurol* **23**: 406–410.

Scholl-Burgi S, Haberlandt E, Heinz-Erian P, et al. (2008) Amino acid cerebrospinal fluid/plasma ratios in children: influence of age, gender, and antiepileptic medication. *Pediatrics* 121: e920–926.

Vanderver A, Hathout Y, Maletkovic J, et al. (2008) Sensitivity and specificity of decreased CSF asialotransferrin for eIF2B-related disorder. *Neurology* 70: 2226–2232.

# Chapter 2.8
## Cardiac Tests and Autonomic Function

In this chapter a summary of the contribution of cardiological investigations to neurological diagnosis is followed by an outline of some tests of autonomic nervous function.

### Electrocardiography (ECG)

The heart rhythm as shown on ECG may be altered in paroxysmal disorders. The common difficulty relates to the distinction between syncopes and epileptic seizures (Chapters 3.12–3.15).

### Primary rhythm disturbances

REFLEX ASYSTOLE
Reflex cardiac asystole is not uncommon (see Chapter 3.14). If a good history is obtained, ocular compression to induce vagocardiac inhibition will *not* be necessary.

LONG-QT (LQT) SYNDROME
A QTc interval of 0.44s or over suggests LQT syndrome. It is simple to determine whether the QTc is prolonged on the ECG channel of an EEG, provided one does not over-read the QT interval by including a normal U-wave in the measurement. Automated computer analysis of routine ECGs may miss LQT, and if the LQT is suspected (see Chapter 3.14) the child should be referred urgently to a paediatric cardiologist. Aside from genetic causes of LQT syndrome, the QT interval may be prolonged in various metabolic derangements such as the hypocalcaemia of hypoparathyroidism.

In case of sudden death in supposed 'epilepsy', mutations in LQT genes may be tested for in the neonatal Guthrie card.

*Secondary rhythm disturbances*

EPILEPTIC ASYSTOLE

Epileptic seizures may lead to cardiac rhythm alterations of which asystole is the most dramatic. When this occurs the clinical manifestations of the epileptic seizure itself may be minor, whereas the effects of the prolonged cardiac asystole (loss of consciousness, stiffening and spasms) may dominate.

PANAYIOTOPOULOS SYNDROME

In this benign epilepsy of early childhood the pale and still appearance of the child during an epileptic seizure has been called 'ictal syncope'. In fact ictal cardiorespiratory dysfunction – with cardiac standstill – giving rise to true syncope is rare.

*Complex patterns*

VALSALVA

Compulsive Valsalva manoeuvres may be extremely frequent in some children with autism spectrum disorders and not only in those with severe learning disability. If an episode is recorded there will be a diminution of the amplitude of the QRS complex to 50% of its baseline level with tachycardia, followed within about 10 seconds by generalized EEG slowing with increased EEG amplitude, while the ECG shows a combination of restoration of the normal QRS complex amplitude and bradycardia. Home video of events may assist this diagnosis (see Clinical Vignettes 2.1.3, 2.1.4).

UPPER AIRWAYS OBSTRUCTION

If an infant is being serially suffocated by his or her parent (usually the mother), the parent is likely to ensure that any video component of the recording system is not in action during the event. However, the recording will have a complex appearance that includes sudden change in the ECG baseline coincident with generalized EMG on the ECG and EEG channels, and the development of bradycardia and EEG slowing over a period of up to 2 minutes. At about the time that the EEG becomes isoelectric with absent EMG, the ECG will accelerate and then the ECG and EEG will return to normal over several seconds.

*ECG findings in hereditary disorders*

- *Muscular dystrophy*

  Deep left ventricular Q waves in Duchenne muscular dystrophy

  Heart block or arrhythmia in Emery–Dreifuss muscular dystrophy (older patients)

- *Myotonic dystrophy*

  Conduction defects, often asymptomatic

- *Spinal muscular atrophy*

  Tremulous baseline from chest muscle fasciculation (superimposed EMG)

- *Friedreich ataxia*

  Inverted left ventricular T waves

- *Glycogenosis type 2*

  Short P-R interval, depressed S-T segments, inverted T waves

- *Mitochondrial cytopathy*

  Heart block, often complete; Wolff–Parkinson–White syndrome.

Most of these disorders have specific molecular genetic tests for confirmation of diagnosis but ECG findings may lend support to the diagnosis pending the genetic results.

### Echocardiography

RHABDOMYOMATA

Echocardiography is the method of choice for detecting rhabdomyomata in infancy. Such rhabdomyomata may be detected in a high proportion of infants with *tuberous sclerosis* at a time when other evidence of this disorder is lacking. Since these rhabdomyomata regress with time, early echocardiography is indicated in unexplained infantile epilepsy with suspect cerebral pathology (such as infantile spasms, simple or complex partial seizures).

SEPTAL HYPERTROPHY

A characteristic thickening of the interventricular septum is seen in *Friedreich ataxia* and may confirm that clinical diagnosis while the results of molecular genetic tests are awaited. Asymmetrical septal hypertrophy is also seen in neurofibromatosis, tuberous sclerosis, type 2 glycogenosis (Pompe disease) GM1 gangliosidosis and I cell disease, though these disorders are diagnosed by other methods.

VALVULAR DISEASE

The diagnosis of *Sydenham chorea* is often straightforward, but echocardiography may give additional evidence of acute rheumatic heart disease.

ACUTE SEVERE ILLNESS

In the intensive care unit, echocardiography may clarify the cause of a presentation, for example:

- in the unconscious child the discovery of cardiac tumours will point to a paroxysmal ventricular fibrillation

- in acute encephalopathy, the finding of cardiomyopathy with encephalitis suggest Coxsackie B infection

- in a child with arterial ischaemic stroke, valvular disease or vegetations may be relevant to the aetiology; the significance of patent foramen ovale is controversial.

## Autonomic function tests

Disorders of the autonomic nervous system in childhood are probably not rare but testing is difficult and rarely undertaken, outside of simple observations of pupil reactivity and arterial blood pressure.

Head-up tilt is used more as a method of reproducing syncopes (see below) than for exploring the autonomic system. Heart-rate variability has the potential for quantifying parasympathetic and sympathetic 'tone' but its interpretation is fraught with difficulties.

### Clinical situations

ACUTE PRESENTATION

Acute autonomic disturbance may be seen in *Guillain–Barré syndrome* or *traumatic spinal cord lesions*. The disturbance may be severe with rapid changes in heart rate and blood pressure and sometimes asystole.

In *Panayiotopoulos syndrome* autonomic epileptic seizures are the rule.

Prominent autonomic abnormalities are a feature of *anti-NMDA receptor encephalitis* with hypoventilation and cardiac dysrhythmias including asystole.

CHRONIC DISORDERS

Widespread autonomic dysfunction is a feature of the *Riley–Day syndrome* and is increasingly seen in *HIV infection*. It is likely to be a feature of mitochondrial disorders.

Autonomic impairments are also seen in the rare (in children) *Lambert–Eaton myasthenic syndrome* such as may be a clue to occult neural crest tumour.

LOCALIZED DISTURBANCES

Localized autonomic disturbances include Horner syndrome and Holmes–Adie pupil.

CONVULSIVE SYNCOPE

The term convulsive syncope is often used in a way that is ambiguous and may confuse. Most syncopes from infancy onwards are convulsive in the sense that non-epileptic jerks, spasms and extensions are manifestations of an anoxic seizure (Chapter 3.14). When syncopes induce epileptic seizures – anoxic–epileptic seizures – then the convulsion, now an epileptic one, may be much longer (Chapter 3.15).

Head-up tilt testing – tilting a patient 60° head up with ECG and continuous blood pressure trace, and preferably video and EEG – is a way of reproducing a neurally mediated syncope in a child of 7 years or older, but like ocular compression it should rarely be needed if the history is well taken. If head-up tilt is undertaken, it is important for a parent to be there to confirm that what is induced is identical to the natural episodes.

Swallow syncope and vomiting syncope are mediated by a *vagovagal reflex* that may be reproduced simply either by eating with EEG/ECG attached or more unpleasantly by a draught of ipecacuanha.

PAROXYSMAL EXTREME PAIN DISORDER

Paroxysmal sympathetic dysfunction is an increasingly recognized feature of the rare condition paroxysmal extreme pain disorder, previously known as familial rectal pain syndrome. In this sodium channelopathy (with mutations in *SCN9A*) of neonatal onset defaecation-triggered painful episodes are accompanied by flushing often with a Harlequin phenomenon. When the Harlequin phenomenon involves the face one sees sympathetic withdrawal with a transient Horner syndrome on the flushed hemiface and sympathetic overactivity with large pupil on the contralateral pallid hemiface. Prolonged cardiac asystole may complicate these attacks.

NEONATAL HYPEREKPLEXIA

In neonatal hyperekplexia, truly life-threatening syncopes associated with muscle hypertonia may be accompanied by junctional bradycardia and even asystole.

BATH-INDUCED PAROXYSMAL DISORDERS IN INFANCY

A common feature in all episodes induced by infant bathing is autonomic dysfunction. Home video is the simplest investigation.


# Clinical vignettes

## 2.8.1 Werdnig–Hoffmann-like syndrome with pneumonia

A 6-month-old boy had previously presented with constipation at the age of 4 weeks. The mother said that he had never kicked the covers off, couldn't hold his head straight and had had weak crying and whimpering for the previous 10 days. On examination he was an unwell baby with generalized floppiness and weakness: head control was absent. He was sweaty and his alae nasae were working. There were no mumurs but his heart seemed enlarged. The neurological findings were minor facial weakness, absent tendon reflexes and spontaneous clonus at the right ankle. Plantar responses were absent. A flare response to cutaneous stimulation was not elicited. His anus was lax.

INVESTIGATIONS

EEG was normal or showed a mildly slow background.

*Chest radiography* showed displacement of the heart to the left with cardiothoracic ratio of 56%.

*Echocardiography* showed extremely thickened septum and posterior left ventricular wall.

*CSF protein* was 0.21g/L.

*Muscle biopsy* showed glycogen storage.

*Leukocyte and fibroblast alpha-glucosidase (acid maltase)* was grossly deficient.

Neurophysiology and brain imaging were not performed.

COMMENT

An invasive course was taken to the diagnosis of Pompe disease in this floppy baby. The most direct route would be from echocardiographic and neurophysiological (denervation) data to the specific enzyme deficiency. In the event, antenatal enzyme testing was undertaken and the mother's second child was normal. Today, genetic analysis (alpha-glucosidase gene *GAA*) would be undertaken, and therapy would be potentially available.

### 2.8.2 Tilting for non-epilepsy

Two unrelated 11-year-old girls had virtually the same history. They both began to have episodes of unconsciousness with stiffening and some jerking from about the age of 2 years, in response to various unpleasant or painful stimuli. They had each been diagnosed with epilepsy and treated with antiepileptic medications without benefit.

INVESTIGATIONS

Both girls underwent head-up tilt-testing with EEG and ECG attached. The investigation was video-recorded and a parent was present. In each case after about 10 minutes there was brief bradycardia and then cardiac asystole for around 30 seconds. Both girls had the expected motor activity of a non-epileptic anoxic seizure, with predominant jerking or spasms in one and more prolonged tonic 'decerebration' in the other.

COMMENT

Sometimes it is difficult to reverse a long-term incorrect diagnosis of epilepsy in a child who has neurally mediated syncope. It is important to note that a 'positive' headup-tilt test – in the sense that syncope is induced – does not mean that the episodes complained of in everyday life are syncopal. It is essential, as in these girls, that the semiology is precisely reproduced and recognized by the parents as being identical to natural attacks.

### 2.8.3 Not brain-dead

A 1½-year-old boy was admitted with gasping respiration after a 10-day history of febrile illness with irritability and disinclination to move. He soon became completely paralysed in head, face, neck, trunk and limb muscles. There was complete external ophthalmoplegia and fixed dilated pupils. He was ventilated after i.v. midazolam but not anaesthetized.

INVESTIGATIONS

*EEG* showed prominent continuous diffuse fast (beta) activity which attenuated (reduced in amplitude) on nail-bed pressure.

*Ocular compression* during EEG/ECG led to cardiac asystole for 24s.

*Nerve conduction* – All peripheral nerves were very difficult to stimulate.

*CSF protein* = 0.25g/L.

*Brain MRI* – Normal.

*Microbiology* – *Campylobacter jejuni* was isolated from gastrointestinal secretions.

Course
He slowly recovered after prolonged illness, his only deficit being reduced movement at one ankle.

Comment
The motor axonal form of Guillain–Barré syndrome may come close to mimicking 'brain death'. EEG is helpful in revealing normal rhythms or as here the effect of benzodiazepines and alterations of EEG on sensory stimulus. Ocular compression is contraindicated in this situation where autonomic reflexes may be paradoxically exaggerated.

## Further reading

Aicardi J, Gastaut H, Misès J. (1988) Syncopal attacks compulsively self-induced by Valsalva's maneuver associated with typical absence seizures. A case report. *Arch Neurol* 45: 923–925.

Axelrod FB, Chelimsky GG, Weese-Mayer DE. (2006) Pediatric autonomic disorders. *Pediatrics* 118: 309–321.

Covanis A. (2006) Panayiotopoulos syndrome: a benign childhood autonomic epilepsy frequently imitating encephalitis, syncope, migraine, sleep disorder, or gastroenteritis. *Pediatrics* 118: 1237–1243.

Gastaut H, Broughton R, de Leo G. (1982) Syncopal attacks compulsively self-induced by the Valsalva manoeuvre in children with mental retardation. *Electroencephalogr Clin Neurophysiol Suppl* 35: 323–329.

Gastaut H, Zifkin B, Rufo M. (1987) Compulsive respiratory stereotypies in children with autistic features: polygraphic recording and treatment with fenfluramine. *J Autism Dev Disord* 17: 391–406.

Gospe SM Jr, Gabor AJ. (1990) Electroencephalography laboratory diagnosis of prolonged QT interval. *Ann Neurol* 28: 387–390.

Lempert T. (1996) Recognizing syncope: pitfalls and surprises. *J R Soc Med* 89: 372–375.

Morita H, Wu J, Zipes DP. (2008) The QT syndromes: long and short. *Lancet* 372: 750–763.

Nechay A, Stephenson JBP. (2009) Bath-induced paroxysmal disorders in infancy. *Eur J Paediatr Neurol* 13: 203–208.

Rosen CL, Frost JD Jr, Bricker T, et al. (1983) Two siblings with recurrent cardiorespiratory arrest: Munchausen syndrome by proxy or child abuse? *Pediatrics* 71: 715–20.

Salman MS, Clarke JTR, Midroni G, et al. (2001) Peripheral and autonomic nervous system involvement in chronic GM2-gangliosidosis. *J Inherit Metab Dis* 24: 65–71.

Stephenson JBP. (1990) *Fits and Faints.* London: Mac Keith Press.

Stephenson JB. (2008) Ocular compression a century on: time for a thumbs-off approach? *Epileptic Disord* 10: 151–155.

Taggart NW, Haglund CM, Tester DJ, Ackerman MJ. (2007) Diagnostic miscues in congenital long-QT syndrome. *Circulation* 115: 2613–2620.

# Chapter 2.9
## Microscopic Examinations: Cells and Biopsies

The microscopic and electronmicroscopic examination of many cells and tissues may assist in the diagnosis of childhood neurological disorders. While more specific investigations, whether microbiological, biochemical or genetic, may be necessary for the final diagnosis, these tests are helpful to the clinician. We list these tests here, beginning with the least intrusive.

### Hair
The twisted hair (pili torti) of Menkes disease and arginosuccinic aciduria may easily be demonstrated using a dissecting microscope. Trichorrhexis nodosa (intermittent swollen breaks) may be found in trichothiodystrophy, some cases of biotinidase deficiency, Menkes disease, and arginosuccinic aciduria.

### Blood (see also Chapter 2.11)

#### Red cells

ACANTHOCYTES
Neurological conditions associated with acanthocytes include what used to be called Hallervorden–Spatz disease with mutations in *PANK* (coding for pantothenate kinase) and in the allelic disorder HARP (hypoprebetalipoproteinaemia, acanthocytosis, retinitis pigmentosa and pallidal degeneration), in familial chorea–acanthocytosis and in hypo- or abetalipoproteinaemia.

ECHINOCYTES
Echinocytes (burr cells), which have shorter and more regular projections than

acanthocytes, have been found in the peripheral blood in a family with paroxysmal exertional dyskinesia (see Chapter 3.21) due to a mutation in *SLC2A1* encoding GLUT1. In the acute situation they are seen in haemolytic–uraemic syndrome.

MACROCYTOSIS
Evidence of macrocytosis will suggest vitamin $B_{12}$ deficiency and some disorders of cobalamin metabolism.

*White cells*

VACUOLATED LYMPHOCYTES
Examination of the *thin* part of a well-stained blood film by a haematologist will be sufficient to detect vacuolation in lymphocytes, which may be very numerous and small in the mucolipidoses (but *not* in the mucopolysaccharidoses) or larger and fewer in juvenile neuronal ceroid lipofuscinosis (JNCL) of classical type with *CLN3* mutations.

Vacuolated lymphocytes may also be found in a number of other disorders in which a specific lysosomal enzyme deficiency should be found. These include Pompe disease, GM1 gangliosidosis of the infantile type, Niemann–Pick disease type A, Gaucher disease, mannosidosis, fucosidosis, Wolman disease, aspartylglycosaminuria, sialidosis, sialic acid storage disease, and Salla disease.

BUFFY COAT ELECTRONMICROSCOPY
If neuronal ceroid lipofuscinosis (NCL) is suspected the buffy coat should be separated, fixed with glutaraldehyde, and examined by electronmicroscopy for membrane-bound granular osmiophilic deposits (GROD) that indicate protein palmitoyl thioesterase deficiency, as seen particularly (but not exclusively) in infantile NCL (INCL). In this situation yellow autofluorescence under ultraviolet light is sought. Curvilinear bodies may be seen in many lymphocytes in late infantile NCL (LINCL), and fingerprint bodies in the vacuoles of those with JNCL.

In many cases of NCL, compact electron-dense deposits with fingerprint profiles are found in the absence of vacuolated lymphocytes. These variant or atypical cases of NCL are important because they will not come to light on genetic testing (until every gene for NCL is known and searchable).

## Urine sediment

Golden-yellow metachromatic material within renal epithelial cells is found in all forms of metachromatic leukodystrophy. The second urine specimen of the day is the most useful but several specimens may be analysed so that renal epithelial cells are found and stained with toluidine blue.

Renal epithelial cells also show greenish birefringence in polarized light in metachromatic leukodystrophy, and yellow autofluorescence with ultraviolet light in INCL.

## Conjuctiva

The ophthalmologist will help with the procedure of conjunctival biopsy, which is actually neither difficult nor traumatic. Fixation for electronmicroscopy is essential. While it is helpful in a diagnosis of mucolipidosis IV (where multilaminate bodies may be seen in epithelial and endothelial cells), it is now seldom used where sophisticated biochemical and genetic methods are available. Spheroids may be sought in supect infantile neuroaxonal dystrophy (INAD) if gene testing is negative (see next section).

## Skin

Skin biopsy can be done at any site of the body with a disposable punch using a sterile technique and under local anaesthesia. The skin may also be sampled when underlying tissues are biopsied. The specimen may be processed for fibroblast culture at the same time. As with conjunctival biopsy its diagnostic value in countries or centres with more sophisticated biochemical and genetic methodologies is limited.

In clinically suspected INAD, skin biopsy to look for axonal spheroids is indicated if the genetic test for *PLA2G6* is negative.

In Lafora body disease skin biopsy may show characteristic inclusions but this test is not always positive. This makes for difficulties as the genetic analysis is not totally reliable either.

## Muscle

Although molecular genetic tests enable diagnosis of the more common neuromuscular disorders (70% of Duchenne muscular dystrophy, 95% of type 1 spinal muscular atrophy), muscle biopsy is needed for diagnosis and thereby genetic counselling in most other muscular dystrophies. Samples large enough for light and electron microscopy and histochemistry can be obtained using a needle (Bergström) or conchotome. If the possibility of a metabolic disorder such as a mitochondrial cytopathy exists an open biopsy may be preferred. Very rarely an open biopsy is required in suspected dermatomyositis where a needle biopsy has not yielded a satisfactory sample for histological examination.

It is important to select for biopsy a muscle which is involved clinically, is unlikely to be fibrotic and has not been used for EMG. To this end, muscle ultrasound or MRI may assist. Neuropathological processing of muscle using haematoxylin and eosin stain allows an overview of muscle structure such as distinguishing normal from dystrophic tissue. Muscle histochemistry for fibre type differentiation has largely been replaced by immunohistochemical evaluation for myosin heavy chain fast and slow isoforms which easily distinguishes muscle fibre types and is much less dependent on technical expertise.

Periodic acid Schiff staining is used for the detection of glycogen.

Sudan red is used for detection of excess lipid as in lipid myopathies.

Gomori trichrome stain is used to detect abnormal mitochondria beneath the muscle membrane which stain red and are known as 'ragged red fibres'.

Specific immunolabelling commonly used includes the following:

- dystrophin (rod; amino and carboxy terminals) – suspected Duchenne or Becker muscular dystrophy

- emerin – X-linked with elbow and neck contractures ± cardiac arrhythmia

- merosin (laminin) – suspected congenital muscular dystrophy

- alpha-dystroglycan – suspected congenital muscular dystrophy with dysmorphism

- sarcoglycans – limb–girdle muscular dystrophies

- collagen 6 – limb–girdle dystrophy with contractures.

Specific enzyme staining for cytochrome oxidase is performed in suspected Leigh disease or other mitochondrial disorders.

In vivo enzyme analysis for respiratory chain enzymes in muscle frozen immediately is performed at selected laboratories in patients with suspected mitochondrial disease.

### Nerve

The sural nerve is accessible and no important deficit follows its biopsy. A piece may be taken at the same time as a muscle biopsy. In rare situations, such as suspected giant axonal neuropathy (early-onset severe peripheral neuropathy with frizzy hair), nerve biopsy may be indicated if the mutation in the gigaxonin gene (*GAN*) is not found.

Small nerves in the skin may also be examined in a skin biopsy.

An argument has been made for combined skin, nerve and muscle biopsy in situations where either there is evidence for a peripheral process or there is a presumed central disorder with abnormalities of nerve conduction and/or EMG. The expansion of genetic testing possibilities makes this approach less and less necessary.

### Bone marrow

Bone marrow aspirate (or biopsy) may reveal characteristic cells that help in neurological diagnosis. Smears are stained by conventional Romanowski methods. A classic example is Gaucher disease but nowadays this test is rarely required.

- Niemann–Pick type C: foamy cells and sea-blue histiocytes are typical, though occasionally they may not be found.

- Haemophagocytic lymphohistiocytosis: typical marrow findings may point to this diagnosis in, for example, unexplained demyelinating peripheral neuropathy or encephalitis or atypical asymmetrical 'acute disseminated encephalomyelitis'.

## Liver

Although the liver may be safely biopsied by needle, provided coagulation is normal, this investigation is now rarely necessary where modern biochemical and genetic expertise is available. Liver biopsy may be combined with muscle biopsy in the evaluation of mitochondrial respiratory chain disease, to increase the diagnostic yield.

Measure of liver copper content may assist in the early diagnosis of Wilson disease (in which Kayser–Fleischer rings are almost always present).

## Rectum

In past decades the indications for diagnostic rectal biopsy have markedly reduced. When this technique is used it is essential to obtain sufficient biopsy thickness to include neurons of the myenteric plexus, that is to say a full thickness rectal biopsy is necessary.

At the time of writing, neuronal intranuclear inclusion disease has only been diagnosed in life through rectal biopsy: eosinophilic inclusions are seen in neurons. This disorder may present with ataxia, parkinsonism, dopa-sensitive dystonia, oculogyric crises and 'psychiatric' behaviour disorders.

Rectal biopsy to establish the diagnosis of NCL is now rarely required when biochemical and genetic evaluations are possible, but it is worth making sure that some material (such as a white cell pellet) for electron microscopy is available to supplement biochemical studies.

## Brain

Brain biopsy is also now seldom indicated but the following indications remain:

- *Primary angiitis of the central nervous system*

  This inflammatory vasculitis affects CNS vessels in the absence of an overt systemic inflammatory process. Catheter cerebral arteriography may be helpful but has a low sensitivity, and the diagnosis may only be made by *meningeal* or brain biopsy of affected tissue.

- *Haemophagocytic lymphohistiocytosis*

  If the diagnosis of haemophagocytic lymphohistiocytosis is not obvious from the general clinical picture (which would prompt mutation analysis in the perforin or related gene), a brain biopsy will show a necrotizing lymphocytic vasculitis.

- *Cerebellar leukoencephalopathy with presumed histiocytosis*

  In this recently described condition with prominent cerebellar white matter involvement, it is arguable that biopsy is not necessary to prove underlying histiocytosis.

- *Neuroserpinopathy*

  In regression with CSWS, biopsy may show Collins bodies, but if possible neuroserpin mutations should be sought in peripheral blood DNA.

- *Variant Creutzfeld–Jacob disease (CJD)*

  Suspected variant CJD is a rare candidate for brain biopsy, with special precautions against transmission. Tonsillar biopsy may, however, be sufficient.

- *Possible Rasmussen syndrome*

  In epilepsia partialis continua biopsy is sometimes needed when the clinical course is atypical before a decision on neurosurgical treatment.

- *Suspected subacute sclerosing panencephalitis (SSPE) with negative CSF*

  Demonstration of intranuclear measles inclusions and reverse transcriptase polymerase chain reaction for measles virus has been used to diagnose fulminant SSPE where CSF studies were 'negative' (Chung et al. 2004), but in the published case it was not specified whether oligoclonal bands were sought.

- *Unexplained brain imaging*

  Finally, it may be necessary to do a brain biopsy when there is a progressive disorder with unexplained imaging findings or when the diagnosis seems otherwise not possible. The pathology revealed might include glioblastoma multiforme, Schilder-type demyelination, Lafora disease, Whipple disease confined to the CNS, or other rare entities.

## Concluding comments on biopsies and tissue examinations

With advances in biochemical analysis and particularly in genetic testing, the role of microscopical examinations and biopsies has declined. Nonetheless, for diagnoses that have important implications there is an argument for 'diagnostic greed', that is to say having more than one piece of independent supporting evidence.

The value of post-mortem examination as an investigational tool needs to be emphasized. When the diagnosis cannot be made in life this is an option that deserves sensitive discussion well before the final illness.

## Clinical vignettes

### 2.9.1. Collapsed neonate

A 13-day-old infant was transferred because of acute collapse requiring intubation and resuscitation. On admission the baby was noted to be hypothermic and poorly responsive. There was gradual improvement with antibiotics and fluids, and an infectious cause was not confirmed.

INVESTIGATIONS
*Microscopic examination of hair shaft* showed evidence of pili torti and trichorrhexis nodosa.

*Plasma copper and ceruloplasmin* were low and a mutation was then found in the *ATP7A* (*MNK*) gene on Xq13.3, confirming the diagnosis of Menkes disease.

COMMENT
Although the hair may be normal in the neonatal period, in this case it provided an early clue to the diagnosis of this devastating disease.

In families with a previously affected child, neonatal plasma neurotransmitter evaluation (dopamine, norepinephrine and other neurochemicals dependent on the copper enzyme dopamine beta-hydroxylase) might allow an even earlier approach to the diagnosis and possible therapy. A raised urinary ratio of homovanillic to vanillylmandelic acid above 4.0 may be a simple clue.

### 2.9.2. Behavioural change in an 11-year-old boy
An 11-year-old boy presented with a 6-month history of subtle behaviour change with school refusal. There was associated headache on and off but no vomiting. There were no abnormal neurological signs.

INVESTIGATIONS (1)
*EEG and brain CT* were normal.

COURSE (1)
The boy became more withdrawn and irritable. A neurodegenerative disorder was suspected.

INVESTIGATIONS (2)
*Brain MRI* showed abnormal signal in the deep white matter posteriorly suggestive of adrenoleukodystrophy.

*Plasma very long chain fatty acids (VLCFAs)* – Normal.

*CSF cytology, protein, glucose* – Normal; no oligoclonal bands.

COURSE (2)
Over several weeks there was deterioration with difficulty feeding, emergence of pyramidal signs and poor responsiveness.

INVESTIGATIONS (3)
A brain biopsy was performed which showed features in keeping with glioblastoma multiforme.

COMMENT
This diagnosis is quite rare in children. The differential diagnosis on the initial MRI included adrenoleukodystrophy and SSPE, both of which were excluded on appropriate

testing (see Chapter 3.22). Tumours of this kind may be misdiagnosed as ADEM when there is steroid-responsiveness.

### 2.9.3 'Ohtahara syndrome'

A boy, the first of dizygotic twins, was born at 37 weeks' gestation by elective caesarean section for breach presentation. In retrospect his mother thought there may have been intrauterine jerks. There was a minor fall at 20 weeks in the pregnancy without any loss of consciousness. Birthweight was 2.92kg, length 47cm, head circumference 33.5cm. There was no significant family history, and two older siblings were healthy.

On day 3 the boy was admitted to the special care baby unit because of breathing difficulties. He settled and was discharged home but referred at 4 weeks of age because of evolving hypertonia with poor responsiveness and variable feeding.

On examination head circumference was on the 50th centile. There was marked general hypertonia with brisk reflexes, adducted thumbs, extensor posturing, excessive startle, myoclonic jerks and episodes of desaturation. There was no visual fixation or social interaction, and nasogastric feeding was required.

COURSE (1)

Over the next 7 months seizures continued and consisted of myoclonic, partial and tonic episodes. There was no response to clonazepam, clobazam, pyridoxal phosphate, pyridoxine, folinic acid, vigabatrin or valproate. There was no neurodevelopment and nasogastric feeding, suction and oxygen were required at home. At 7 months head circumference was between the 9th and 25th centiles.

INVESTIGATIONS (1)

*EEG* showed a suppression–burst pattern.

*Brain MRI and H-MRS* – Normal.

*Chromosomes* – Normal karyotype.

*Molecular genetic analyses* for mutations in *MECP2*, *CDKL5*, *SCN1A*, *ARX*, *PNPO* and *STXBP1* were all negative.

*Plasma* – Urea, creatinine, electrolytes, glucose, acid-base status, lactate, creatine kinase, transaminases, urate, amino acids, VLCFA, transferrins, acylcarnitine, carnitine, T3, T4, thyroid stimulating hormone, alpha aminoadipic semialdehyde ($\alpha$–AASA), ceruloplasmin and copper were all normal.

*Urine* – Organic acids, amino acids, $\alpha$–AASA, guanidinoacetate, creatinine were all normal.

*CSF* – Lactate, glucose, glycine (and CSF/plasma glycine and glucose ratios) were normal; protein was elevated at 936mg/L; threonine was mildly elevated at 83μmol/L (normal level <45).

*Fibroblast fatty acid beta-oxidation* – Normal.

COURSE (2)
The child died at 8 months of age.

INVESTIGATIONS (2)
Neuropathological examination of the brain showed a subtle cortical dysplasia in the form of blurring of the grey–white matter interface in the parietal regions with displacement of the grey matter into the subcortical white matter. Subpial heterotopic nodules were also noted, especially in both hippocampal regions.

COMMENT
It is best not to regard labels such as 'Ohtahara syndrome' as a final diagnosis. In this case example what was wrong could only be determined by post-mortem examination by a neuropathologist with special interest and competence in the neuropathology of infants. Post-mortem examination is still a most important neurological investigation.

### 2.9.4 Not Friedreich ataxia after all
An 8-year-old boy was referred by the school medical officer to the consultant paediatrician because of clumsiness and abnormal gait which had not been noticed at his school entrance examination. His parents agreed that his balance had deteriorated, but they also felt that he might be less clever than he had been. The educational psychologist and the paediatrician thought that the motor disability had contributed to the apparent lowering of his IQ. He was found to have a slow dysarthria, mild ataxia with possibly a sensory component, possible rombergism, absent tendon reflexes, extensor plantar reflexes, and pes cavus. Eye movements were entirely normal. ECG and spine radiograph were normal.

INVESTIGATIONS
*Echocardiography* did not show thickening of the interventricular septum.

*EEG* showed no definite abnormality.

*Nerve conduction velocity* was 28m/s in the right posterior tibial, with 10ms distal latency.

*Brain CT* showed areas of low attenuation in relation to the anterior horns and bodies of the lateral ventricles.

*CSF protein* was 0.53g/L.

*Urine* – Smears of centrifuged deposit of the second morning specimen stained with toluidine blue showed several aggregates of brown metachromatic granules, some of which appeared to be within the cytoplasm of epithelial cells of the upper urinary tract. These granules were not present in the lower urinary tract squamous cells or in polymorphs.

*Lysosomal enzymes* – Leukocyte arylsulphatase A was virtually absent, arylsulphatase B and beta-galactosidase being normal.

COMMENT
The clinical presentation of this boy with juvenile metachromatic leukodystrophy

resembled that of Friedreich ataxia, only the completely normal eye movements (various oculomotor control impairments characterize Friedreich ataxia) and the subtle intellectual deterioration arguing against the latter condition. The normal echocardiogram and the neurophysiological investigations also distinguished the two conditions.

### 2.9.5 Stiff baby, but not hyperekplexia
This girl was stiff at birth, but had no excessive startle, no head retraction reflex and no positive nose-tap response. The stiffness, which included limb flexion, did not abate, but was less prominent during sleep.

INVESTIGATIONS
Extensive investigations during life were unrevealing but when she died aged 4 months neuropathology was impressive, with no myelination of the pyramidal tracts.

COMMENT
Congenital absence of the pyramidal tracts has been rarely observed previously but disorders of this kind will not be detected without – as in this case – expert paediatric neuropathology.

## Further reading

Anderson G, Smith VV, Malone M, Sebire NJ. (2005) Blood film examination for vacuolated lymphocytes in the diagnosis of metabolic disorders; retrospective experience of more than 2,500 cases from a single centre. *J Clin Pathol* **58**: 1305–1310.

Anderson GW, Smith VV, Brooke I, et al. (2006) Diagnosis of neuronal ceroid lipofuscinosis (Batten disease) by electron microscopy in peripheral blood specimens. *Ultrastruct Pathol* **30**: 373–378.

Benseler SM, Silverman E, Aviv RI, et al. (2006) Primary central nervous system vasculitis in children. *Arthritis Rheum* **54**: 1291–1297.

Chung BH, Ip PP, Wong VC, et al. (2004) Acute fulminant subacute sclerosing panencephalitis with absent measles and PCR studies in cerebrospinal fluid. *Pediatr Neurol* **31**: 222–224.

Coutelier M, Andries S, Ghariani S, et al. (2008) Neuroserpin mutation causes electrical status epilepticus of slow-wave sleep. *Neurology* **71**: 64–66.

de León GA, Grover WD, Huff DS, et al. (1977) Globoid cells, glial nodules, and peculiar fibrillary changes in the cerebro-hepato-renal syndrome of Zellweger. *Ann Neurol* **2**: 473–484.

Duprez TP, Grandin CB, Bonnier C, et al. (1996) Whipple disease confined to the central nervous system in childhood. *AJNR Am J Neuroradiol* **17**: 1589–1591.

Feldmann J, Ménasché G, Callebaut I, et al. (2005) Severe and progressive encephalitis as a presenting manifestation of a novel missense perforin mutation and impaired cytolytic activity. *Blood* **105**: 2658–2663.

Harris NL, McNeely WF, Shepard JO, et al. (2002) Case Records of the Massachusetts General Hospital. Case 27-2002. *N Engl J Med* **347**: 672–680.

Kaler SG, Holmes CS, Goldstein DS, et al. (2008) Neonatal diagnosis and treatment of Menkes disease. *N Engl J Med* **358**: 605–614.

Krsek P, Maton B, Korman B, et al. (2008) Different features of histopathological subtypes of pediatric focal cortical dysplasia. *Ann Neurol* **63**: 758–769.

Kulikova-Schupak R, Knupp KG, Pascual JM, et al. (2004) Rectal biopsy in the diagnosis of neuronal intranuclear hyaline inclusion disease. *J Child Neurol* **19**: 59–62.

Lauria G, Lombardi R, Camozzi F, et al. (2009) Skin biopsy for the diagnosis of peripheral neuropathy. *Histopathology* **54**: 273–285.

Lohi H, Turnbull J, Zhao XC, et al. (2007) Genetic diagnosis in Lafora disease: genotype–phenotype correlations and diagnostic pitfalls. *Neurology* **68**: 996–1001.

Miller S, Shevell M, Silver K, et al. (1998) The diagnostic yield of the nerve–muscle skin biopsy in paediatric neurology practice. *Pediatr Rehabil* **2**: 95–100.

Roujeau T, Machado G, Garnett MR, et al. (2007) Stereotactic biopsy of diffuse pontine lesions in children. *J Neurosurg* **107** (1 Suppl): 1–4.

van der Knaap MS, Arts WF, Garbern JY, et al. (2008) Cerebellar leukoencephalopathy most likely histiocytosis-related. *Neurology* **71**: 1361–1367.

Venkateswaran S, Hawkins C, Wassmer E. (2008) Diagnostic yield of brain biopsies in children presenting to neurology. *J Child Neurol* **23**: 253–258.

Walker RH, Jung HH, Dobson-Stone C, et al. (2007) Neurologic phenotypes associated with acanthocytosis. *Neurology* **68**: 92–98.

Weber YG, Storch A, Wuttke TV, et al. (2008) GLUT1 mutations are a cause of paroxysmal exertion-induced dyskinesias and induce hemolytic anemia by a cation leak. *J Clin Invest* **118**: 2157–2168.

Yilmaz Y, Kocaman C, Karabagli H, et al. (2008) Is the brain biopsy obligatory or not for the diagnosis of Schilder's disease? Review of the literature. *Childs Nerv Syst* **24**: 3–6.

# Chapter 2.10
## Microbiology

Paediatricians together with microbiologists will be well able to deal with the diagnosis of most infections involving the nervous system. This chapter deals with some neurological aspects.

### Congenital infection and congenital infection-like disorder

*Presentation at birth*
When a baby is born with the phenotype of congenital infection – ill, rash, hepatosplenomegaly, thrombocytopenia – together with evidence of encephalopathy with or without epileptic seizures and intracranial calcification (on CT or more safely on ultrasound) then the investigations are TORCH [toxoplasmosis, rubella, cytomegalovirus (CMV), herpes simplex virus] screen serology on mother and baby, together with urine culture for CMV, and CSF examination in most instances. The HIV status of the mother is likely to be already known.

Congenital lymphocytic choriomeningitis with neonatal presentation, sometimes as jittery babies, also includes microcephaly and periventricular calcification but all have chorioretinitis. On follow-up there may be isolated cerebellar ataxia. Diagnosis is by anti-LCMV (lymphocytic choriomeningitis virus) antibody titres. Analysis of Guthrie card DNA has not been reported as we write.

VIROLOGY – NEGATIVE 'CONGENITAL INFECTION'
If all these microbiological studies prove negative, then in the past the condition would have been called pseudo-TORCH or congenital infection-like syndrome. With certain exceptions that is no longer regarded as a helpful diagnosis and one should now instead investigate the autosomal recessive congenital infection-like disorder Aicardi–Goutières syndrome. The diagnosis of Aicardi–Goutières syndrome may be made if the CSF

interferon-alpha (IFN-α) is raised in the absence of viral infection, but in this clinical scenario direct genetic testing for *TREX1* mutation is possible.

Another possibility is a haematological condition, such as neonatal alloimmune thrombocytopenia (NAITP).

*Later presentation*
If the infant presents at the age of a few months with developmental delay or regression and is found to have impaired head growth and intracranial calcification on imaging, the question of possible congenital infection will again arise. If there is deafness, congenital CMV will be strongly suspected and may be confirmed by the finding of CMV DNA on the Guthrie card that has been stored from the neonatal period.

If congenital CMV infection is excluded then once again the diagnosis of Aicardi–Goutières syndrome should be seriously considered, and whether or not there is CSF lymphocytosis, CSF IFN-α and pterins should be estimated. Again, direct genotyping may be possible.

## Acute herpes virus infections

*Herpes simplex*
The clinical diagnosis of herpes simplex encephalitis is normally confirmed by polymerase chain reaction of the CSF. IFN-α increases in the CSF at the time of acute herpes simplex virus infection and if there is a virological relapse then the IFN-α increases again. When there is a postinfectious relapse, characteristically with ballismus, then the IFN-α does not increase.

*Human herpes virus 6 (HHV6) and 7 (HHV7)*
HHV6 is increasingly recognized as a cause of encephalitis or encephalopathy with status epilepticus and later epilepsy, particularly mesial temporal lobe epilepsy. HHV7 is also likely to be a significant cerebral pathogen in children.

## Chronic viral infections

*Post-measles subacute sclerosing panencephalitis (SSPE)*
Throughout much of the world post-measles SSPE is not rare. Measles IgM in blood and increased CSF measles titres with intrathecal immunoglobulin production, together with periodic complexes on EEG, usually make the diagnosis clear.

*Chronic viral infection in hypogammaglobulinaemia*
Presumed chronic viral infections may occur in agammaglobulinaemia or hypogammaglobulinaemia, in so far as brain tissue has been shown to contain tubuloreticular inclusions, indicating production of IFN-α and, by inference, virus invasion.

*Borreliosis*
Although the neurological complications of Lyme disease, especially facial palsy, are well known it is important to mention this treatable and easily overlooked disorder.

## Sydenham chorea and possible related conditions
The ASO (anti-streptolysin O) titre and the anti-DNAase B titres are commonly increased in Sydenham rheumatic chorea but the connection is less secure in the case of PANDAS (paediatric autoimmune neuropsychiatric disorder associated with streptococcal infection), and even less so in the case of encephalitis lethargica.

## Other major infections
The diagnosis of tuberculosis meningitis, *Mycoplasma pneumoniae* infection, syphilis, trypanosomiasis and malaria should be well known to most physicians.

*Some comments on other infective agents*
Briefly we list some other infective agents that are that are not always thought of, with their associated disorder(s) and the usual diagnostic methods:

- *Varicella-zoster* – arterial ischaemic stroke and acute cerebellar ataxia – paired acute and convalescent viral titres blood and CSF

- *Campylobacter jejuni* – Guillain–Barré syndrome – campylobacter titres and/or culture

- *West Nile and enteroviral infections* – encephalitis [acute disseminated encephalomyelitis (ADEM)-like] and flaccid paralysis – nucleic acid amplification

- *Cat scratch fever* – status epilepticus – *Bartonella* serology

- *Whipple disease* – ADEM-like – polymerase chain reaction for *Tropheryma whipplei* in jejunal biopsy.

## Clinical vignettes

### 2.10.1 'Leukodystrophy' in an 11-month-old
This girl was the second child of healthy unrelated parents, weight 2.5kg at term. There were no perinatal problems and she was discharged home with her mother. At 6 months she was noted to have hypotonia with mild developmental delay. Persisting hypotonia at 10 months prompted referral for neurological evaluation. Head size, weight and length were on the 3rd centile. There was axial hypotonia with inability to sit unsupported. There were intact social responses, babbling, transferring objects and a fine pincer grasp. Hearing responses were reduced and sensorineural deafness was subsequently confirmed.

INVESTIGATIONS

*Brain MRI* showed diffuse high signal abnormality on the T2-weighted and T2 FLAIR sequences involving the periventricular and subcortical regions anteriorly and posteriorly in addition to the white matter of the temporal lobes bilaterally with cyst formation in the anterior temporal lobes.

*CMV* was isolated from urine and CSF. CMV DNA and IgM antibody to CMV was detected in eluate of the blood spot from the neonatal Guthrie card.

COMMENT

Several unnecessary metabolic investigations were carried out in this child pending the confirmation of congenital CMV infection based on retrospective examination of the Guthrie card. At 2½ years, 3 months post-cochlear implant, neurodevelopment is normal.

### 2.10.2 White matter lesions and deafness

A 13-year-old girl was referred from a cochlear implant programme with a history of sensorineural deafness detected at the age of 9 months. There was gradual deterioration over the first few years and she was confirmed deaf at school entry. Birth was at term without any complications or neonatal events. As part of an evaluation for cochlear implant brain MRI was performed which showed multiple high signal abnormalities in the deep white matter in the periventricular and centrum semiovale regions both anteriorly and posteriorly. These were low signal on T1-weighted FLAIR sequences. MRS was normal. The question of a progressive leukodystrophy, possibly mitochondrial, was raised. There were no other abnormal neurological signs.

INVESTIGATIONS

*Brain CT* showed no evidence of calcification.

*Metabolic tests* of blood, urine and CSF were negative.

Eluate of the blood spot from the neonatal Guthrie card showed CMV DNA and IgM antibody to CMV consistent with congenital CMV infection.

COMMENT

The magnetic resonance features of congenital CMV infection have been well defined by van der Knaap and colleagues. CMV infection is much more frequent than neurodegenerative or syndromic causes of deafness with white matter changes.

### 2.10.3 Status epilepticus

A 6-year-old, previously healthy boy presented following an episode of staring, drooling of saliva and unresponsiveness lasting minutes. There was a 3-day history of lethargy, abdominal pain, headache and fever. He remained seizure-free for 30 hours and then began having right-sided clonic seizures with lip smacking and secondary generalization.

He was flushed and pyrexial with mild oral dyskinesia and right-sided facial weakness. The seizures were controlled with phenytoin.

INVESTIGATIONS

There was transient thrombocytopenia and neutropenia with mildly elevated transaminases on admission.

*EEG* showed slowing of the background with seizures originating from the left centrotemporal region.

*Brain MRI* showed two tiny areas of high signal on T2-weighted images in the subcortical white matter anteriorly.

*CSF* – Protein was above the 95th centile at 424mg/L, while cells were 24/cm$^3$ (98% mononuclear).

*HHV6* DNA was detected in CSF on admission. Viral titres in blood and CSF for a broad range of other viruses were negative.

COURSE

Following a brief remission of several weeks the seizures recurred and have persisted since then despite multiple antiepileptic drugs. Imaging and EEG findings were essentially unchanged 18 months later.

COMMENT

The presentation was similar to but not as severe as that described in DESC (devastating encephalopathy in school-age children) or FIRES (febrile infection-responsive epileptic encephalopathies of school age). HHV6 infection of the nervous system has been associated with later severe epilepsy. A preexisting *SCN1A* mutation which might have predisposed to refractory epilepsy was excluded. The role of HHV6 virus in mesial temporal sclerosis remains to be clarified.

### *2.10.4 Deadly falls*

An 18-year-old had been jerking frequently for 4 months, having to support himself with his hands to avoid falling over completely. His academic performance had declined. On examination he had repetitive spasms of 1 second duration followed by loss of tone for 0.5s.

INVESTIGATIONS

*Video-EEG* showed periodic large-amplitude slow-wave complexes coinciding with the spasms.

*CSF* – Protein normal, negative microscopy and culture. Oligoclonal band positive.

*Serum measles antibody titre* by complement fixation assay = 1:320.

*CSF measles antibody titre* by complement fixation assay = 1:64.

COURSE

He received appropriate treatment but his condition deteriorated and he was later found dead.

COMMENT

In much of the world where measles is rife, SSPE is not rare, and is suggested at once by CSF oligoclonal bands. In this case the boy had had measles in the first year of life, *before* his scheduled measles immunization. Very high population immunization rates (currently with the measles, mumps and rubella vaccine – MMR) are necessary to prevent this devastating disease.

## Further reading

Bonthius DJ, Wright R, Tseng B, et al. (2007) Congenital lymphocytic choriomeningitis virus infection: spectrum of disease. *Ann Neurol* **62**: 347–355.

Caselli E, Di Luca D. (2007) Molecular biology and clinical associations of Roseoloviruses human herpesvirus 6 and human herpesvirus 7. *New Microbiol* **30**: 173–187.

Dale RC, Webster R, Gill D. (2007) Contemporary encephalitis lethargica presenting with agitated catatonia, stereotypy, and dystonia–parkinsonism. *Mov Disord* **22**: 2281–2284.

Fotheringham J, Donati D, Akhyani N. (2007) Association of human herpesvirus-6B with mesial temporal lobe epilepsy. *PLoS Med* **4**: e180.

Mikaeloff Y, Jambaque I, Hertz-Pannier L, et al. (2006) Devastating epileptic encephalopathy in school-aged children (DESC): a pseudo encephalitis. *Epilepsy Res* **69**: 67–79.

van Baalen A, Stephani U, Kluger G, et al. (2008) FIRES: febrile infection responsive epileptic (FIRE) encephalopathies of school age. *Brain Dev* **31**: 91.

van der Knaap MS, Vermeulen G, Barkhof F, et al. (2004) Pattern of white matter abnormalities at MR imaging: use of polymerase chain reaction testing of Guthrie cards to link pattern with congenital cytomegalovirus infection. *Radiology* **230**: 529–536.

# Chapter 2.11
## Haematology

This chapter highlights the significance of routine and special haematological tests in the diagnosis of neurological disorders. Other aspects of haematology have been discussed in Chapter 2.9.

### Haemoglobin
Easily treatable iron deficiency anaemia has been reported to be a predisposing factor to various common paroxysmal events of early childhood such as infantile syncopes and febrile seizures. It is also a risk factor for childhood ischaemic stroke (arterial and venous).

More subtly, low iron stores (low serum ferritin) seem to be a feature of those with neurally mediated syncope.

Rarely, anaemia may be of more specific relevance as in vitamin $B_{12}$ deficiency, certain metabolic disorders and lead encephalopathy.

### Blood film (smear)
We have already referred to the character of white cell inclusions in Chapter 2.9. Red cell macrocytosis is usually though not always found in vitamin $B_{12}$ deficiency. Acanthocytes in *PANK2* disorder and echinocytes in GLUT1 deficiency-associated paroxysmal exertional dyskinesia were also mentioned in Chapter 2.9.

Although evidence of haemolytic anaemia may suggest rare hereditary defects of red cell enzymes, beware rare neurological associations such as Aicardi–Goutières syndrome in the neonate and Wilson disease in the older child and adolescent.

Basophilic stippling is well known as a clue to lead encephalopathy.

In the appropriate clinical setting, the appearance of malaria trophozoites may give a clue to the cause of fever and seizures.

### Full blood count

In addition to well-known causes, neutrophil leukocytosis may be seen with acute brain illness of many causes including viral and autoimmune disorders and destructive lesions, and platelets increase as an acute phase reactant (e.g. in acute disseminated encephalomyelitis).

Reduction in all (pancytopenia) or isolated (thrombocytopenia, leukopenia) blood indices may be a feature of many neurological situations:

- Drugs (such as carbamazepine, valproate, ethosuximide)
- Infection (including congenital infection and HIV)
- Aicardi–Goutières syndrome (thrombocytopenia)
- Neonatal alloimmune thrombocytopenia (porencephaly, optic hypoplasia)
- Metabolic diseases (organic acidaemias and congenital disorders of glycosylation)
- Chromosomal instability disorder (e.g. ataxia–pancytopenia syndrome)
- Cerebroretinal microangiopathy with calcification and cysts (CRMCC), otherwise called 'Coats plus'
- Familial haemophagocytic lymphohistiocytosis.

### Sickle-cell disease and sickle cell traits

In many countries children of African or Afro-Caribbean origin are screened for sickle cell disease. In affected individuals presymptomatic screening for cerebrovascular disease using transcranial Doppler ultrasound is now the standard of care as prophylactic blood transfusion in those with high blood flow velocities in the circle of Willis protects against arterial ischaemic stroke.

### General tests of bleeding and clotting

Although it may sometimes be difficult to tell whether a neurological disorder results from haemorrhage or thrombosis it is best to discuss these mechanisms separately.

### Bleeding disorders (coagulopathies)

In most cases coagulation screening tests (prothrombin time and partial thromboplastin time) and if required assays of clotting factors and platelet count and function will make the diagnosis.

Less common presentations include the following:

- *Neonatal alloimmune thrombocytopenia (NAITP)*
  The neonatal thrombocytopenia is obvious, but the neurological impairments (such as porencephaly and optic hypopolasia) need to be carefully sought.

- *Late haemorrhagic disease of the newborn infant*
  The disaster of cerebral haemorrhage at the age of about 5 weeks is almost always preventable by neonatal vitamin K.

If there is a suggestion of a coagulopathy a haematologist should be consulted, as factor deficiencies such as haemophilia might present with haemorrhage.

## Clotting disorders (thrombophilias)

*Arterial ischaemic stroke*
The prevalence of prothrombotic states is variable in different populations but generally lower than in venous thrombosis; whilst the presence of a procoagulant state does not affect acute management, protein C deficiency and thrombophilia in otherwise healthy children have been associated with recurrence.

*Cerebral venous sinus thrombosis*
The prevalence of thrombophilia is higher in children with cerebral venous thrombosis than in those with arterial ischaemic stroke. Though identification of a procoagulant state does not affect acute management, such a diagnosis may be relevant for the child's future healthcare, for example in relation to prophylactic anticoagulation during immobile periods or use of the oral contraceptive pill. The presence of the prothrombin 20210A mutation has been associated with a higher rate of recurrence.

*Haemostatic factor abnormality as a neurodiagnostic clue*
In *congenital defects of glycosylation*, deficiencies of factors IX and antithrombin III may be additional diagnostic pointers.

## Clinical vignettes

### 2.11.1 Optic hypoplasia explained
A 10-year-old boy with bilateral optic hypoplasia and mild spastic diplegia who was unable to stand on one leg for more than a second had always been thought to have septo-optic dysplasia, although brain imaging had never been undertaken. A sibling had died aged 2 hours with 'hydrocephalus'. The neonatal period of the present child had been complicated by thrombocytopenia which had not been further investigated.

INVESTIGATIONS
*EEG* – Normal.

*ERG* – Normal.

*VEP* – Reproducible visual evoked responses could not be obtained.

*Brain CT* – Normal septum pellucidum. Low density posterior to right trigone, consistent with old porus.

*Platelet studies* – The boy's platelets were phospholipase 1 (PLA1) positive, while his mother's were PLA1 negative. She had a strong anti-PLA1 antibody with a titre of 1/16 in her serum, and the boy's platelets were incompatible with his mother's serum.

COMMENT
The parents were glad to have a diagnosis of NAITP, albeit 10 years late.

### 2.11.2 'Congenital infection' explained
A boy was born at 35 weeks gestation weighing 3kg, head circumference 36.9cm. The infant had variable feeding. There was hepatosplenomegaly. Anaemia (Hb 7.7g/dL) and thrombocytopenia (platelet count $6 \times 10^9$/L) was noted. There was a single clonic seizure which settled with phenobarbitone. He was transfused with blood, platelets and fresh frozen plasma. His optic discs were pale and small.

INVESTIGATIONS
Testing of blood and urine for congenital infection was negative.

COURSE
A shunt was inserted at 6 months. There was no neurodevelopment and the boy died at 8 months of age. An autopsy showed evidence of hydrocephalus with pseudopolymicrogyria of temporal and occipital lobes and extensive cortical thinning of the frontoparietal cortex. There was inflammatory change presumed secondary to severe intrauterine intraventricular haemorrhage.

A brother born 1 year later was noted to have petechiae at birth and marked thrombocytopenia. The diagnosis of NAITP was confirmed by antibody and genetic testing.

COMMENT
The finding of the unexplained hepatosplenomegaly, petechiae, thrombocytopenia and destructive brain lesion raised the possibility of a prenatal infection which was excluded on conventional testing. 'Congenital infection' without a confirmed infection begs for a specific diagnosis, whether NAITP or Aicardi–Goutières syndrome.

## Further reading

Anderson G, Smith VV, Malone M, Sebire NJ. (2005) Blood film examination for vacuolated lymphocytes in the diagnosis of metabolic disorders; retrospective experience of more than 2,500 cases from a single centre. *J Clin Pathol* **58**: 1305–1310.

Dale ST, Coleman LT. (2002) Neonatal alloimmune thrombocytopenia: antenatal and postnatal imaging findings in the pediatric brain. *AJNR Am J Neuroradiol* **23**: 1457–1465.

Davidson JE, McWilliam RC, Evans TJ, Stephenson JBP. (1989) Porencephaly and optic hypoplasia in neonatal isoimmune thrombocytopenia. *Arch Dis Child* **64**: 858–860.

Ganesan V, Prengler M, McShane MA, et al. (2003) Investigation of risk factors in children with arterial ischemic stroke. *Ann Neurol* **53**: 167–173.

Ganesan V, Prengler M, Wade A, et al. (2006) Clinical and radiological recurrence after childhood arterial ischemic stroke. *Circulation* **114**: 2170–2177.

Jarjour IT, Jarjour LK. (2008) Low iron storage in children and adolescents with neurally mediated syncope. *J Pediatr* **153**: 40–44.

Kenet G, Kirkham F, Niederstadt T, et al. (2007) Risk factors for recurrent venous thromboembolism in the European collaborative paediatric database on cerebral venous thrombosis: a multicentre cohort study. *Lancet* **6**: 595–603.

Walker RH, Jung HH, Dobson-Stone C, et al. (2007) Neurologic phenotypes associated with acanthocytosis. *Neurology* **68**: 92–98.

# Chapter 2.12
## Immunology

An increasing number of neurological disorders of children are being shown to have an immune basis, and immunological investigations may be helpful in the diagnosis of several.

The immune system may be divided into the innate and the acquired or adaptive, and in each immunological system immunity may be defective (reduced) or excessive (overactive). The innate immune system is the primitive system that protects against pathogens before immunological learning has developed. The acquired or adaptive immune system (the immune system best known to paediatricians and paediatric neurologists!) selects clones of immunologically competent cells to target specific antigens and so develops immunological memory.

### Innate immune system

#### Deficient innate immunity
A defect in one of the toll-like receptors (TLR3) may be a risk factor for sporadic *herpes simplex 1 encephalitis* (test not clinically available at time of writing).

#### Excessive innate immunity
Excessive innate immunity in the form of innate autoimmunity occurs in all the identified varieties of Aicardi–Goutières syndrome, recognized clinically by a congenital infection-like picture and often later chilblains (40–50%), with raised CSF (and often serum) interferon-alpha (IFN-α) (or tubuloreticular inclusions in cells and tissues) and by direct genetic testing.

## Acquired (adaptive) immune system

*Deficient acquired (adaptive) immunity*

B-CELL DEFICIENCY
An important point about hypo- or agammaglobulinaemia is that viruses may remain chronically in the nervous system.

T-CELL DEFICIENCIES
Ataxia–telangiectasia (in which many types of movement disorders may be manifest) has raised serum alpha-fetoprotein as a marker, as has ataxia–oculomotor apraxia type 2.

Purine nucleoside phosphorylase deficiency with dysequilibrium–diplegia has low serum uric acid as a marker.

*Excessive acquired (adaptive) immunity*

ACQUIRED AUTOIMMUNE DISORDERS
We list the main examples, together with the primary immunological investigation in each case.

- *Systemic lupus erythematosus (SLE)* – anti-double stranded DNA and anti-nuclear cell nucleosome antibodies.

- *Hashimoto encephalopathy* – anti-thyroperoxidase (anti-TPO) antibodies.

- *Limbic encephalitis* – anti-potassium channel antibodies (VGKC-Ab and others).

- *Encephalitis with 'psychiatric' features, oral dyskinesia and autonomic dysfunction* – anti-NMDA-receptor antibodies (if positive in a girl, search for ovarian teratoma by pelvic ultrasound).

- *Sydenham chorea* – antistreptolysin O (ASO) titre and anti-DNAase B.

- *PANDAS (paediatric autoimmune neuropsychiatric disorders associated with streptococcal infections)* – anti-basal ganglia antibodies (validity uncertain).

- *Paraneoplastic hypothalamic syndromes* – search for occult neural crest tumour.

- *Opsoclonus–myoclonus* – search for occult neural crest tumour (seek anti-Hu and anti-Ri).

- *Narcolepsy–cataplexy* – low CSF hypocretin.

- *Transverse myelitis* – antibodies against aquaporin 4 [AQP4/NMO-IgG are increased in neuromyelitis/neuromyelitis-optica (NMO) but the clinical spectrum is widening] (see Chapter 3.16).

- *Acute polyneuropathy (Guillain–Barré syndrome and variants)* – anti-ganglioside antibodies could be looked for but are not usually helpful in diagnosis. Culture of *Campylobacter jejuni* does not assist in diagnosis.

- *Myasthenia gravis* – 80% are said to be positive for acetylcholine-receptor or anti-muscle-specific receptor tyrosine kinase (MuSK) antibodies.

- *Miller–Fisher syndrome and Bickerstaff encephalitis* –these previously 'split' conditions should now be 'lumped' as the same condition. Anti-GQ1b IgG antibody is usually found.

*Note:* Myasthenia gravis is a prime example of an autoimmune channelopathy, whereas the congenital myasthenic syndromes (CMS) are (mostly) genetic channelopathies. If a child with apparent myasthenia gravis does not have antibodies it is wise to assume that instead there is an undiagnosed CMS and seek genetic confirmation.

Although *Rasmussen encephalitis* has sometimes been assocated with anti-GluR3 antibodies, current evidence is that these are neither pathogenic nor diagnostic.

Disorders such as multiple sclerosis with oligoclonal bands in the CSF almost certainly involve autoimmunity. A condition with oligoclonal bands previously described as immune-mediated chorea encephalopathy syndrome arguably might be the same as the anti-NMDA receptor encephalitis referred to above.

Other disorders such as coeliac disease (anti-gliadin) with neurological complications and neuro-Behçet disease (anti-cardiolipin) have a probable immunological basis.

A recently recognized presumed paraneoplastic disorder is *cerebellar leukoencephalopathy most likely histiocytosis-related*. Evidence of histiocytosis is usually indirect, but the cerebellar white matter signal change on MRI is striking.

### Alloimmune disorders
In alloimmune disorders it is the immune system of another individual (commonly the mother) that attacks antigens in the host.

NEONATAL ALLOIMMUNE THROMBOCYTOPENIC PURPURA (NAITP)
NAITP has been discussed in Chapter 2.11.

NEONATAL SYSTEMIC LUPUS ERYTHEMATOSUS
Neonatal SLE occasionally leads to neurological problems such as partial (focal) seizures and basal ganglia calcification.

ARTHROGRYPOSIS FROM ANTI-ACETYLCHOLINE RECEPTOR ANTIBODIES
Fetal akinesia may result from asymptomatic maternal myasthenia gravis.

## Clinical vignettes

### 2.12.1 Stroke-like with antibodies
A 14-year-old girl with a background history of treated hypothyroidism and seronegative arthritis presented with an acute hemiplegia and aphasia which was

preceded by a 'generalized tonic–clonic seizure'. There had been a prodrome of poor concentration, malaise and memory lapses over the previous five days.

INVESTIGATIONS (1)
*EEG* showed slowing of the background predominantly in the left temporal region.

*Imaging studies* – MRI, SPECT and catheter cerebral angiography were normal as was Doppler ultrasound of carotids and echocardiography.

Tests for inborn errors of metabolism, SLE and thrombophilias were negative.

COURSE (1)
The patient made a full recovery over the next 72 hours and was commenced on aspirin.

Five months later she presented with a generalized tonic–clonic seizure preceded by a prodrome of sore throat, malaise, word finding difficulties, myoclonus and forgetfulness. Apart from hyperreflexia there were no abnormal neurological signs.

INVESTIGATIONS (2)
*Thyroid function tests* were abnormal with elevated TSH and normal T4 and free T4.

*Antimicrosomal antibody titre and anti-thyroperoxidase antibodies (anti-TPO)* were markedly elevated.

*CSF protein* was elevated at 703mg/L.

COURSE (2)
She was commenced on oral prednisolone, making a complete recovery.

COMMENT
Hashimoto encephalopathy, disorders of glycosylation (CDG1a), familial hemiplegic migraine, alternating hemiplegia of childhood and sometimes epilepsies may present with hemiplegia without any changes on MRI. In Hashimoto encephalopathy the child is often euthyroid and need not have a clinical history of thyroid disease.

### 2.12.2 Congenital 'SLE'
In a consanguineous first-cousin marriage Pakistani family, two brothers had a similar history of congenital encephalopathy.

*First brother:* This boy's birthweight at 38 weeks gestation was 2.6kg with head circumference on the 50th centile. At his 6 weeks assessment he had 'nystagmus', no visual fixation and hypertonia. He made no developmental progress. Cortical blindness, myoclonic jerks, spastic quadriplegia and progressive microcephaly were noted.

INVESTIGATIONS (1)
*EEG* was reported as "support[ing] a generalized seizure disorder."

*Brain CT* at age 4 months showed periventicular and basal ganglia spotty calcifications with cerebral atrophy.

*CSF* was not obtained as consent for lumbar pucture was refused.

*TORCH screen* was negative, as were liver function tests and many other genetic and biochemical studies.

COURSE (1)
Skin lesions were first noted at age 8 months and by 21 months involved all his toes together with his fingers and ears and the tip of his nose. The rash was described as "well circumscribed, scaly, erythematous plaques" with swelling, and a clinical diagnosis of cutaneous lupus was made.

INVESTIGATIONS (2)
*Skin biopsy* confirmed the clinical diagnosis and thick granular deposits of IgM were seen on direct immunofluorescence of the basement membrane zone.

Anti-dsDNA was 2050 IU/mL (normal 0–100) aged 2 years, with low C3 of 38mg/dL (50–90) and increased IgG anticardiolipin antibody at 23.2 IU/mL (0–9).

COURSE (2)
He remained unwell with progression of the skin lesions.

INVESTIGATIONS (3)
By age 4 years his erythrocyte sedimentation rate was 134, anti-dsDNA was 2350 IU/mL (0–100), ANF (antinuclear factor) titre was positive at 1:132 and anti-Ro, anti-La and anti-RNP were all positive.

COURSE (3)
He had streptococcal septicaemia and then renal failure with hypertension and haematuria. He died in his fifth year from pneumococcal septicaemia.

*Second brother:* This boy was born by emergency caesarean section at 32 weeks gestation, 3 years after his brother. His birthweight (1.14kg), length and head circumference (26.5cm) were all below the 3rd centile. He had jaundice and purpura on the first day with hepatosplenomegaly.

INVESTIGATIONS (1)
*Brain ultrasound* showed thalamic calcification.

*Abdominal ultrasound* showed hepatosplenomegaly.

*Platelet count* was low at $20 \times 10^9$/L.

Unconjugated hyperbilirubinaemia and elevated liver enzymes were not explained by multiple other investigations.

COURSE (1)
By age 5 months he had developed myoclonic jerks. There had been no developmental progress and he had progressive microcephaly, cortical blindness and generalized spasticity.

INVESTIGATIONS (2)
*EEG* was reported as indicating "a generalized seizure disorder."

*Brain CT* showed widespread intracranial calcification identical to that in his elder brother.

COURSE (2)
He developed a rash that was the same as in his brother but confined to his fingers and toes.

INVESTIGATIONS (3)
Antinuclear factor was negative, but anti-dsDNA antibodies were elevated at 633 IU/mL (0–100).

COURSE (3)
He died aged 13 months of pneumococcal pneumonia. Later, the parents had an unaffected daughter.

COMMENT
These siblings were very puzzling at the time (Dale et al. 2000). On the one hand, they fulfilled clinical and investigational (especially immunological) criteria for the autoimmune disease SLE. On the other hand, the first brother had features consistent with Aicardi–Goutières syndrome and the second brother had the picture of a supposedly separate condition known variously as pseudo-TORCH, microcephaly–intracranial calcification syndrome and 'autosomal recessive congenital intrauterine infection-like syndrome'. It is only very recently that it has been recognized that all these conditions are the same – and best called Aicardi–Goutières syndrome – with underlying defects in the disposal of nucleic acid breakdown products (including dsDNA) such that both congenital infection and SLE are convincingly mimicked. Desirable investigations in a future case would be CSF IFN-α and DNA for Aicardi–Goutières syndrome gene analysis.

### 2.12.3 Sleepy, sluggish and falling with laughter
This girl presented at age 3 years. Since the age of 2 years and 4 months her parents had noted sleepiness and sluggish movements. The duration of night-time and daytime sleep became longer, up to 15 hours a day, and all her symptoms became more prominent in the evening. At that time she also developed constipation.

At the time of presentation her sleep was very deep. She did not wake up on her own and it was quite difficult to rouse her. She often immediately fell asleep again and could sleep for prolonged periods.

When awake she could unexpectedly lose her muscle tone and fall down. Sometimes it was apparent that she would laugh out of context and lose her tone at the time of such laughter.

She appeared very weak and had ptosis more prominent on the left and muscular hypotonia. Fatigue on sitting, walking and speaking was very prominent, but chewing and swallowing were not affected.

Myoclonias were also seen during sleep and when awake, when moving or at rest.

Nevertheless, the parents noticed that the girl did not lose interest in toys nor for studying new things during the course of the disease.

INVESTIGATIONS (1)
*EEG* – Normal.

*EMG* – Myasthenic reaction of Lambert–Eaton type with 27% incremental response on repetitive nerve stimulation.

*Brain MRI* – Normal.

*ECG* – Normal.

*Routine haematology and biochemistry* were normal.

COURSE (1)
During her stay in hospital her state became worse – she hardly moved at all and stayed in bed very weak; periodically there was tachycardia and tachypnoea.

INVESTIGATIONS (2)
*Chest radiograph* suggested an intrathoracic lesion.

*MRI* of the mediastinum revealed a tumour of sympathetic ganglia size 65 × 19mm in the left costovertebral junction at the level of D5–D9, that showed patchy enhancement and was presumed to be a ganglioneurinoma.

COURSE (2)
She underwent surgery (histology = ganglioneuroblastoma) and three courses of chemotherapy and improved slowly thereafter. On follow up she was doing well, developmentally normal; the weakness, narcolepsy and cataplexy had not recurred.

COMMENT
Opsoclonus–myoclonus is the best known autoimmune manifestation of an occult neural crest tumour. Paraneoplastic hypothalamic syndromes have been much less frequently reported. In this case the neural-crest tumour led to Lambert–Eaton myasthenia, autonomic dysfunction, narcolepsy, cataplexy and myoclonus, and was discovered by looking for it in an expected site of origin.

### 2.12.4 Encephalitis with dyskinesia
A 6½-year-old girl presented following a generalized clonic seizure lasting 40 minutes. There was a prodrome of 48 hours in which she was off her food and 'not herself', during which she had an episode of incontinence and abnormal posturing of the left limbs.

Following admission to hospital a fluctuating left hemiparesis was noted, with dystonic posturing and without Babinski sign (then or later). She had a withdrawn affect but was fully alert.

INVESTIGATIONS (1)

*EEG* showed slowing of the background particularly on the right side.

*MRI/MRA* 1 week apart were normal as was catheter cerebral angiography.

*CSF protein* rose from 209mg/L to 395mg/L, while lymphocyte count rose from 24/cm³ to 47/cm³ over 6 days.

COURSE (1)

Over the following week her condition deteriorated, she became agitated and aggressive with bizarre language and poor responsiveness. She had hallucinations, disruption of sleep pattern (for 6 weeks she rarely slept), plucking and pinching herself and pulling out her hair. Intermittently there was akinesia with eyes open, alternating with very marked limb and orofacial hyperkinesia. There were occasional oculogyric crises. For some time she was mute. There was autonomic instability as evidenced by fluctuating heart rate (up to 140/minute) and variability in temperature, but she was only hypoxic (oxygen saturation down to 60%) on two occasions. She had at least one further convulsive epileptic seizure.

INVESTIGATIONS (2)

(**bold** = abnormal, reference ranges in parenthesess)

*CSF* on day 15 contained the following:

- cells – 0
- protein 273mg/L
- albumin 120mg/L
- IgG 25mg/L
- **oligoclonal bands positive**
- **neopterin 169nmol/L (7–65)**
- **BH$_4$ (tetrahydrobiopterin) 41nmol/L (9–39)**
- dihydrobiopterin 8.4nmol/L (0.4–13.9)
- homovanillic acid 308nmol/L (71–565)
- 5-HIAA 154nmol/L (58–220)
- 5-MTHF 52nmol/L (72–172)
- **INF-α 12 IU/mL (<2)**

*Serum* (at same time as CSF):

- albumin 38g/L
- IgG 7.8g/L
- **INF-α 5 IU/mL (<2)**

*IgG index* (see Chapter 2.7): **1.06** (0.2–0.7)

Viral titres in blood and CSF together with virus cultures from multiple sites were all negative despite exhaustive searches at international laboratories. There was no evidence of *Mycoplasma pneumoniae* infection (but antibody testing unreliable).

Comprehensive autoimmune testing, especially for SLE, was negative.

COURSE (2)
The acute phase lasted approximately 6 weeks. Thereafter there was gradual improvement. Nine months later there was no motor deficit but affect and behaviour had not returned to pre-illness state and there were residual short term memory and language difficulties.

INVESTIGATIONS (3)
*Pelvic ultrasound* (done after clinical diagnosis of anti-NMDA-receptor encephalitis) did not reveal an ovarian teratoma.

*Anti-NMDA receptor antibodies (on stored plasma)* – Strongly positive.

COMMENT
Elevated CSF (and sometimes serum) IFN-α is well known to occur in (1) certain viral infections such as herpes simplex, rubella and HIV, (2) in SLE, and (3) in Aicardi–Goutières syndrome. In this young girl the finding of elevated IFN-α suggested that despite negative virological studies there must have been a viral aetiology and so was most helpful in management of this devastating encephalopathy.

However, since then the clinical picture of anti-NMDA receptor encephalitis has been published and in retrospect we thought this must be the diagnosis, now confirmed by the finding of anti-NMDA receptor antibodies in stored specimens.

### Further reading

Byrne OC, Zuberi SM, Madigan CA, King MD. (2000) Hashimoto's thyroiditis—a rare but treatable cause of encephalopathy in children. *Eur J Paediatr Neurol* 4: 279–282.

Dale RC, Tang SP, Heckmatt JZ, Tatnall FM. (2000) Familial systemic lupus erythematosus and congenital infection-like syndrome. *Neuropediatrics* 31: 155–158.

Dale RC, Church AJ, Surtees RA, et al. (2004) Encephalitis lethargica syndrome: 20 new cases and evidence of basal ganglia autoimmunity. *Brain* 127: 21–33.

Dalmau J, Rosenfeld MR. (2008) Paraneoplastic syndromes of the CNS. *Lancet Neurol* 7: 327–340.

Dalmau J, Gleichman AJ, Hughes EG. (2008) Anti-NMDA-receptor encephalitis: case series and analysis of the effects of antibodies. *Lancet Neurol* 7: 1091–1098.

Dalton P, Deacon R, Blamire A, et al. (2003) Maternal neuronal antibodies associated with autism and a language disorder. *Ann Neurol* 53: 533–537.

Graus F, Saiz A. (2008) Limbic encephalitis: an expanding concept. *Neurology* 70: 500–501.

Iizuka T, Sakai F, Ide T. (2008) Anti-NMDA receptor encephalitis in Japan: long-term outcome without tumor removal. *Neurology* 70: 504–511.

Ito M, Kuwabara S, Odaka M, Misawa S, et al. (2008) Bickerstaff's brainstem encephalitis and Fisher syndrome form a continuous spectrum: clinical analysis of 581 cases. *J Neurol* **255**: 674–682.

Jarius S, Aboul-Enein F, Waters P, et al. (2008) Antibody to aquaporin-4 in the long-term course of neuromyelitis optica. *Brain* **131**: 3072–3080.

McKeon A, Lennon VA, Lotze T, et al. (2008) CNS aquaporin-4 autoimmunity in children. *Neurology* **71**: 93–100.

Maródi L, Notarangelo LD. (2007) Immunological and genetic bases of new primary immunodeficiencies. *Nat Rev Immunol* **7**: 851–861.

Mocellin R, Walterfang M, Velakoulis D. (2007) Hashimoto's encephalopathy : epidemiology, pathogenesis and management. *CNS Drugs* **21**: 799–811.

Nunn K, Ouvrier R, Sprague T, et al. (1997) Idiopathic hypothalamic dysfunction: a paraneoplastic syndrome? *J Child Neurol* **12**: 276–281.

Rigby RE, Leitch A, Jackson AP. (2008) Nucleic acid-mediated inflammatory diseases. *Bioessays* **30**: 833–842.

Stephenson JBP. (2008) Aicardi–Goutières syndrome (AGS). *Eur J Paediatr Neurol* **12**: 355–358.

Singer HS, Gause C, Morris C, Lopez P. (2008) Tourette Syndrome Study Group. Serial immune markers do not correlate with clinical exacerbations in pediatric autoimmune neuropsychiatric disorders associated with streptococcal infections. *Pediatrics* **121**: 1198–1205.

Tan KM, Lennon VA, Klein CJ, et al. (2008) Clinical spectrum of voltage-gated potassium channel autoimmunity. *Neurology* **70**: 1883–1890.

Taanman JW, Rahman S, Pagnamenta AT, et al. (2009) Analysis of mutant DNA polymerase gamma in patients with mitochondrial DNA depletion. *Hum Mutat* **30**: 248–254.

van der Knaap MS, Arts WF, Garbern JY, et al. (2008) Cerebellar leukoencephalopathy most likely histiocytosis-related. *Neurology* **71**: 1361–1367.

Zhang S, Jouanguy E, Ugolini S, et al. (2007) TLR3 deficiency in patients with herpes simplex encephalitis. *Science* **317**: 1522–1527.

# Chapter 2.13
## Genetic Investigations

### Resources

The genetic revolution is under way and is massively accelerating. Keeping abreast of discoveries and developments is well nigh impossible. However, computers and web-based resources assist literature searches, the choice of appropriate genetic investigations and, most importantly, instantaneous consults with knowledgeable and experienced colleagues (subject, of course, to medical consent and confidentiality rules).

SimulConsult (www.simulconsult.com) is a high-quality clinical diagnostic system that is under continuous improvement. It is free of charge to all medical practitioners and may be used by clinical geneticists as well as paediatricians, paediatric neurologists, child psychiatrists and others in the field.

All practitioners will be familiar with PubMed, the enormous literature database of the National Institutes of Health (www.ncbi.nlm.nih.gov/sites/entrez). Indexing here is not always precise and comprehensive, and patience may be necessary to find all the appropriate articles. Online Mendelian Inheritance in Man (OMIM, http://www.ncbi.nlm.nih.gov/sites/entrez?db=omim) might be more helpful to geneticists than to paediatric neurologists or neuropaediatricians.

To discover the genetic investigations that are available a major resource is the GeneTests website (www.genetests.org). This is an international resource, funded by the National Institutes of Health, that is particularly helpful when a genetic investigation is carried out in only a few laboratories worldwide. It includes clinical genetic reviews on over 1000 conditions, in addition to general educational material on genetic testing. There is also information about gene tests that may be available through patient participation in research, as opposed to tests that are carried out on a commercial, service basis.

Although it is not a genetic investigation in the usual sense, the Allen Brain Atlas (www.brain-map.org) is a wonderful source for practitioners at any stage of their development and is an exciting tool for students of any age with curiosity about the expression of genes in the brain. At the time of writing it is the mouse brain – not too different from the human.

Such genetic investigations aim to provide a diagnosis but from the family point of view it is the explanation that is important. Having a name for a condition or a syndrome is supportive and with the more common conditions such as Rett syndrome a parent organization may be particularly helpful.

## Avoidance of other tests
Determining that the neonatal-onset epileptic syndrome is due to 1p36 deletion avoids a battery of unnecessary metabolic investigations. Congenital myotonic dystrophy, Prader–Willi syndrome and Aicardi–Goutières syndrome are other conditions in which confirmation of a clinical diagnosis avoids numerous unnecessary tests.

## Management
Detecting a mutation in *SCN1A* when Dravet syndrome (severe myoclonic epilepsy in infancy) is suspected will help in the management of that epilepsy, as will detection of the maternally inherited deletion in Angelman syndrome.

Although the spectrum of phenotypes resulting from mitochondrial disorders due to mutations in the *POLG1* (polymerase gamma A) gene is increasingly broad, the knowledge that such a *POLG1* mutation is present may greatly assist sensitive terminal management in intractable epilepsia partialis continua.

## Prognosis
The genetic diagnosis allows more accurate prognosis in a great many disorders such as Prader–Willi syndrome, ring chromosome 20, ataxia–telangiectasia and most of the muscular dystrophies and congenital myopathies. In the case of Friedreich ataxia the size of the trinucleotide repeat may assist in the prediction of the long-term prognosis.

## Recurrence
Commonly a genetic diagnosis allows reassurance that the condition will not recur in future pregnancies, such as in 1p36 deletion.

## Family members
In X-linked disorders such as Duchenne muscular dystrophy and fragile X syndrome, the genetic findings have enormous implications for siblings and extended families.

### Range of genetic investigations
Before summarizing the present fluid position, some remarks are in order. The clinician seeing a young patient with unusual features may find a clue to a new basic molecular mechanism. Families, particularly parents, may in due course be comforted if their child eventually contributes to the sum of human knowledge. Exceptions and unusual features not 'in the book' or in SimulConsult need close attention.

As a single gene test for a single disorder may be very expensive, one is duty bound to try to come to a single clinical diagnosis and avoid embarking on a molecular genetic 'fishing trip'. If one is sufficiently clinically convinced of a diagnosis, then a negative gene test result does not necessarily rule that diagnosis out: firstly, there is a small chance of test error or failure to detect a mutation that is truly present; secondly, the pervasive phenomenon of genetic heterogeneity means many, many conditions are caused by mutations in more than one gene, known and unknown. Having stated this, a positive gene result can be necessary when a rare genetic diagnosis is made that carries implications for the family and relatives. For example, type 1 or von Recklinghausen neurofibromatosis is usually clinically evident in adults and young affected relatives, so it rarely needs to be confirmed by a DNA test, whereas the genetically separate type 2 neurofibromatosis (central or acoustic neuroma syndrome) carries such serious complications that it is nearly always confirmed by DNA testing. If prenatal diagnosis of a serious or fatal genetic disorder such as infantile neuronal ceroid lipofuscinosis (INCL) might in the future be an issue for a family then detailed knowledge of the molecular pathology in the living affected child permits speedy and accurate testing early on in a future pregnancy (if the family is willing to consider termination).

We will briefly discuss the genetic tests in present use in the context of neurological investigation.

#### Karyotyping ('chromosomes', G-banding)
Numerous syndromic diagnoses and dysmorphic features lead to karyotype analysis.

In epilepsy, detectable chromosomal abnormalities are found not only in those with dysmorphism and learning difficulties but also in those with atypical epilepsy semiology and EEG features (see Chapter 3.12). When seeking ring chromosomes, in particular ring chromosome 20, it is important to remember that because of mosaicism there might be only 0.5% of mitoses with ring 20 so that 200 mitoses may need to be counted.

In the past one did not know how to proceed when there was an apparent balanced translocation or how to detect submicroscopic deletions in the presence of a de novo clinical phenotype. Now one of the methods below may be utilized.

#### FISH and MLPA for subtelomeric deletions and duplications
FISH (fluorescent in situ hybridization) analysis is a well-known method of seeking microdeletions and duplications near the ends of chromosomes and in certain 'hot-spot' interstitial regions: Prader–Willi, Williams and Smith–Magenis syndromes are three

good examples. Submicroscopic deletions and duplications near the end of the chromosomes (subtelomeric) are present in 2–5% of children with dysmorphism and learning disability: the 1p36 deletion syndrome mentioned above is one of the more frequent such conditions.

MLPA (multiplex ligation-dependent probe amplification) is a robust method of detecting minute microdeletions or duplications of genetic material encompassing several or more genes. This technique employs selected DNA probes that are grouped together in different 'kits' specifically manufactured to analyse selected chromosome regions. MLPA has also been used to detect very small deletions and duplications of genetic material that occur *within* genes (exon deletion and duplication) that might not be detected by conventional DNA sequencing techniques. For example, with Dravet syndrome (*SCN1A*), hereditary spastic paraplegia (*SPAST*) and many other neurological conditions, MLPA adds to the mutation detection yield. Targeted MLPA is particularly useful in revealing duplications of the *MECP2* gene in boys.

*Array comparative genomic hybridization*
This new technique, although expensive and technically demanding, is becoming more widely available and is now being applied to detect microdeletions and microduplications of genetic material in up to 15% of children with learning disability, dysmorphism, growth retardation and microcephaly who were previously undiagnosed. Some children with autism spectrum disorder and learning disability are diagnosed in this way, e.g. with chromosome 3q29 deletion.

*Single gene mutation analysis*
As indicated earlier, single gene mutation analysis, typically by DNA sequencing, is often quite expensive, especially when the gene is large and/or the sequence data are difficult to analyse. In certain clinical scenarios, especially where there is a sufficiently striking or distinctive presentation, such as the possibility of neonatal Aicardi–Goutières syndrome, specific analysis of the suspected gene (*TREX1*) may be sufficiently straightforward to be requested directly.

## Importance of detailed clinical evaluation
The complexity of genetic evaluation seems overwhelming but in large part this is due to the rather crude clinical analyses that were common in the past. A prime example is what is called 'learning disability'. This is such a vague and all-encompassing term that it is no surprise to find huge lists of different genes supposedly responsible. Fine analysis of the behavioural phenotypes should allow more directed genetic analysis in the future. Finally, even with an expanding arsenal of genetic tests, it is a clinical skill, the ability to elicit and interpret the family history, that underpins genetic diagnosis in families.

## Clinical genetics services
In many regions clinical genetics services are available as a resource for family studies, prenatal diagnosis, dysmorphology assessment and advice on laboratory techniques.

## Clinical vignettes

### 2.13.1 Keep trying

A 12-year-old boy was referred for management of epilepsy which began at the age of 8 years. He had been diagnosed with developmental delay at age 2 years. At 6 years facial dysmorphism was noted.

INVESTIGATIONS (1)

*Brain CT* – Normal.

*Karyotype* – Normal.

*Thyroid function, plasma and urine amino acids, and urine organic acids* were all normal.

COURSE (1)

Various syndromes were considered. Then at 8 years epilepsy began, consisting of nocturnal tonic–clonic seizures, startle-induced events and absences. He had severe learning disability but was independently mobile despite being grossly overweight. He had facial dysmorphism recognized in retrospect as including horizontal eyebrows with narrow distance between upper lid and eyebrow.

INVESTIGATIONS (2)

EEG showed multifocal and generalized discharges while awake and asleep.

*Brain MRI* – Normal.

*Karyotype* was again normal.

The availability of *subtelomeric studies* prompted a search for 1p36 deletion, which was confirmed.

COMMENT

Explaining the cause of this child's severe epilepsy, learning and behavioural difficulties was immensely valuable as many incorrect diagnoses had been previously proposed.

### 2.13.2 Learning disability with hyperventilation explained

A 4-year-old boy was referred for investigation of developmental delay with epilepsy (generalized tonic–clonic seizures and drop attacks). There were no perinatal problems and developmental milestones were all delayed. At 4 years he was not walking independently. Head circumference was above the 3rd centile. There was severe learning disability. Bruxism with occasional hyperventilation was noted, and there were dysmorphic features in the form of a slightly coarse face, big ears, wide mouth, short stature and small feet.

INVESTIGATIONS (1)

*Brain MRI* – Normal.

*Karyotype, MECP2 analysis, Angelman methylation analysis, UBE 3A analysis, fragile X and Coffin–Lowry testing* were all negative.

*Thyroid function, plasma NH4, lactate, creatine kinase, plasma and urine amino acids, and urine organic acids* were all normal.

COURSE
Epilepsy control improved over the first decade, while hyperventilation became more prominent with episodes of apnoea and cyanosis. There was no finger clubbing. The hyperventilation prompted further genetic testing.

INVESTIGATIONS (2)
*Video–audio* demonstrated the sight and sound of his hyperventilation.

*Genetics* – Testing for the mutation of the transcription factor 4 gene (*TCF4*) in 18q21.2 was positive, confirming the clinical diagnosis of Pitt–Hopkins syndrome.

COMMENT
Hyperventilation is seen and heard as a prominent feature in Rett syndrome and Pitt–Hopkins syndrome (in Joubert syndrome it is tachypnoea rather than hyperpnoea). In Pitt–Hopkins syndrome overbreathing may not appear until after the age of 3 years, while in Rett syndrome this may abate in the second decade of life.

## Further reading

Ariani F, Hayek G, Rondinella D, et al. (2008) FOXG1 is responsible for the congenital variant of Rett syndrome. *Am J Hum Genet* **83**: 89–93.

Coutelier M, Andries S, Ghariani S, et al. (2008) Neuroserpin mutation causes electrical status epilepticus of slow-wave sleep. *Neurology* **71**: 64–66.

Engelsen BA, Tzoulis C, Karlsen B, et al. (2008) POLG1 mutations cause a syndromic epilepsy with occipital lobe predilection. *Brain* **131**: 818–828.

Gilfillan GD, Selmer KK, Roxrud I, et al. (2008) SLC9A6 mutations cause X-linked mental retardation, microcephaly, epilepsy, and ataxia, a phenotype mimicking Angelman syndrome. *Am J Hum Genet* **82**: 1003–1010.

Guerrini R, Moro F, Kato M, et al. (2007) Expansion of the first PolyA tract of ARX causes infantile spasms and status dystonicus. *Neurology* **69**: 427–433.

Hakonen AH, Isohanni P, Paetau A, et al. (2007) Recessive Twinkle mutations in early onset encephalopathy with mtDNA depletion. *Brain* **130**: 3032–3040.

Kato M, Saitoh S, Kamei A, et al. (2007) A longer polyalanine expansion mutation in the ARX gene causes early infantile epileptic encephalopathy with suppression–burst pattern (Ohtahara syndrome). *Am J Hum Genet* **81**: 361–366.

Lugtenberg D, Kleefstra T, Oudakker AR, et al. (2009) Structural variation in Xq28: MECP2 duplications in 1% of patients with unexplained XLMR and in 2% of male patients with severe encephalopathy. *Eur J Hum Genet* **17**: 444–493.

Macleod S, Mallik A, Tolmie JL, et al. (2005) Electro-clinical phenotypes of chromosome disorders associated with epilepsy in the absence of dysmorphism. *Brain Dev* **27**: 118–124.

Marini C, Mei D, Temudo T, et al. (2007) Idiopathic epilepsies with seizures precipitated by fever and SCN1A abnormalities. *Epilepsia* **48**: 1678–1685.

Raymond FL. (2006) X linked mental retardation: a clinical guide. *J Med Genet* **43**: 193–200.

Rogers RC, Stevenson RE, Simensen RJ, et al. (2008) Finding new etiologies of mental retardation and hypotonia: X marks the spot. *Dev Med Child Neurol* **50**: 104–111.

Tzoulis C, Engelsen BA, Telstad W, et al. (2006) The spectrum of clinical disease caused by the A467T and W748S POLG mutations: a study of 26 cases. *Brain* **129**: 1685–1692.

Valente EM, Ferraris A, Dallapiccola B. (2008) Genetic testing for paediatric neurological disorders. *Lancet Neurol* **7**: 1113–1126.

Wong LJ, Naviaux RK, Brunetti-Pierri N. (2008) Molecular and clinical genetics of mitochondrial diseases due to POLG mutations. *Hum Mutat* **29**: E150–E172.

Zweier C, Peippo MM, Hoyer J, et al. (2007) Haploinsufficiency of TCF4 causes syndromal mental retardation with intermittent hyperventilation (Pitt–Hopkins syndrome). *Am J Hum Genet* **80**: 994–1001.

# Chapter 2.14
## Biochemistry

Chemistry is the basis of life so that the importance of biochemical errors is no surprise. The range of biochemical investigations is almost overwhelming but in this chapter we try to simplify.

We will say something about the philosophy and dangers of the 'screening' approach. While it is inevitable that groups of biochemical tests may be undertaken together as a screening instrument, one danger is that one will stop thinking about the precise diagnosis and imagine that the 'metabolic screen' has excluded a detectable metabolic explanation for the neurological disorder. The second danger is that if a large enough number of separate biochemical tests is included in the screen then one of them may be 'abnormal' on grounds of chance alone.

Biochemical investigations may detect disorders reversible by specific treatment (Chapter 3.23), or more often irreversible disorders of great family significance. Since many of the disorders are progressive, the initial decision about whether to do tests or what tests to do may be a very important and difficult one. A key question is, "Is the condition static or progressive?" If the answer is "don't know" then investigations may have to proceed as if the disorder were progressive. In this chapter we will deal with most of the biochemical tests currently in use in the diagnosis of neurological disorders of children. CSF biochemistry was discussed to some extent in Chapter 2.7 but we will reiterate some important points.

## Urine biochemistry

### Simple urine tests
Aside from the universal urine dip stick (and note that the presence of ketones in the urine of a neonate hints at organic acidaemia), the only simple urine test that is done

universally is the sulphite test for sulphite oxidase and molybdenum cofactor deficiencies. The sulphite test must always be done on completely fresh urine. Even then there are false negatives.

A number of other simple investigations may be done as an extra but may be the sole test available in countries with limited resources. These include ferric chloride for PKU (phenylketonuria), DPNH (dinitrophenylhydrazine) test for MSUD (maple syrup urine disease), cyanide nitroprusside test for homocystinuria and the Benedict test (copper sulphate – galactosaemia). A serious problem is that all of these tests may give both false-negative and false-positive results.

The Bratton–Marshall test for succinylpurines is described as 'simple' but requires a laboratory! (See Tables 2.14.1 Urine biochemistry and 2.14.3 CSF biochemistry.)

*Laboratory urine tests*
We list the main laboratory investigations in Table 2.14.1 without reference to the technique used (chromatography or tandem mass spectrometry, etc.).

It is worth emphasizing two points. First, any disorder which impairs the function of the renal tubular cells will lead to increased excretion of a number of chemicals including amino acids. Second, if the urinary creatinine output is low because of a central defect in creatine synthesis (as in GAMT deficiency) then – if amino acids, organic acids and glycosaminoglycans are estimated in terms of creatinine – a falsely abnormal result may occur.

## Blood biochemistry
Table 2.14.2 lists in alphabetical order the biochemical tests on serum or plasma which may be helpful in neurological investigations. The format is the same as for Table 2.14.1 (see above).

## CSF biochemistry
Table 2.14.3 lists CSF biochemical constituents, once again in the same format, but it is even more important than with urine and blood studies to *think* and *discuss* before embarking on such investigations. This is the stage at which local, national and international consultation may facilitate diagnosis.

The diagnosis of monoamine neurotransmitter disorders is often difficult and usually requires CSF studies (Table 2.14.4). In the first 2 years of life such studies will precede trial of levodopa but in older children levodopa trial is reasonable in the first instance. In either case careful thought and discussion with the supraregional laboratory are in order before the carefully orchestrated lumbar puncture for the specialized CSF analyses.

[continues p. 175]

Table 2.14.1 Urine biochemistry

| Test | Indications | Precautions | Interpretation |
|---|---|---|---|
| α-AASA (α-amino–adipic semialdehyde) | Neonatal epileptic seizures (usually with suppression–burst), or later pyridoxine–responsive epilepsy | No need to obtain urine before giving pyridoxine or pyridoxal phosphate. May be only slightly raised. Do pipecolic acid also in plasma | Pyridoxine–dependent epilepsy (PDE) due to α-AASA-dehydrogenase deficiency (see also Clinical Vignette 2.16.1) |
| Acylcarnitines (plasma more useful) | Acute metabolic encephalopathy (plasma better) | Excretion ↑↑ by carnitine load (100mg/kg) except when enzyme defect confined to brain. May be difficult to interpret | Specific acylcarnitines indicate particular disorders, e.g. octanoyl carnitine in MCAD deficiency, glutaryl carnitine in glutaric acidura type 1 (GA1) |
| Amino acids | Learning disability, acute encephalopathy, intermittent ataxia, various syndromes including Lowe | 24-h sample not necessary. If unusual amino acid being sought (e.g. S-sulphocysteine in sulphite oxidase deficiency) discuss with laboratory | Relate to dietary input. Significance of minor deviations from 'normal' uncertain. Abnormalities in amino–acidopathy, organic acidaemias, sulphite oxidase deficiency, renal tubular leak (including mitochondrial disorders, Wilson disease). 'False' aminoaciduria in GAMT deficiency |
| Bile acids | Suspect peroxisomopathy | Arrange with reference laboratory in advance. Random sample – freeze immediately | Abnormal bile acids excreted in many peroxisomal disorders (especially single enzyme defects as D-bifunctional protein deficiency). Output declines with age so ± negative after early infancy |

Table 2.14.1 continued

| Test | Indications | Precautions | Interpretation |
|------|-------------|-------------|----------------|
| Copper | Acquired movement disorder, acquired behaviour disorder ± abnormal liver function | 24-h urine. Meticulous attention to ensure copper-free containers and to prevent copper contamination | Elevation = Wilson disease (false negative in 5%) |
| Creatine/creatinine ratio | Boys with learning disability | False positives possible if diet high in creatine (meat, oily fish) | ↑ in creatine transporter deficiency |
| GAG (glycosaminoglycans, mucopolysaccharides – see also Oligosaccharides) | Learning disability ± coarse features, corneal clouding, dysostosis. Speech deterioration. Behavioural difficulties, especially aggression in Sanfilippo disease | 24-h collection for heparan sulphate if Sanfilippo likely and initial test for GAG is negative (and specific gene mutation analysis is not possible) | Mucopolysaccharidoses will be detected, especially heparan sulphate in Sanfilippo disease. Excess possible in Lowe and Zellweger syndromes and in peroxisomopathies. False increase in GAMT deficiency |
| | Regression at any age | Wise to check leukocyte beta-galactosidase | Keratan sulphate ± increased in all forms of GM1 gangliosidosis |
| Guanidinoacetate (GAA) | Language delay, early epilepsy, movement disorder | H-MRS for creatine peak desirable | ↑ in GAMT deficiency. ↓ in AGAT deficiency |
| VMA (HMMA), HVA (catecholamines) | Acute or subacute cerebellar ataxia/myoclonus/opsoclonus | Special diet no longer usually indicated; 24-h urine preferred (whole body imaging more reliable) | Increase is consistent with occult neuroblastoma, but result is commonly normal when opsoclonus/myoclonus or other movement disorder is caused by neural crest tumour |

Table 2.14.1 continued

| Test | Indications | Precautions | Interpretation |
|---|---|---|---|
| VMA (HMMA), HVA (catecholamines) | Early dystonia with oculogyric crises | Avoid levodopa beforehand | ↓ in sepiapterin reductase deficiency |
| | Neonatal hypothermia/failure to thrive | Hair may be normal | ↑ HVA/VMA ratio in Menkes disease (>4.0) |
| Myoglobin | Toddler-age encephalopathy with elevated creatine kinase | Random sample | Rhabdomyolysis primary or secondary. Too many causes to list but include carnitine transport defects, fatty acid disorder that will need organic acid analysis and acylcarnitines and possibly muscle biopsy for diagnosis |
| Oligosaccharides | Learning disability ± coarse features, corneal clouding, dysostosis. May be dysmorphic neonate, hydrops. Myoclonus epilepsy | Random sample adequate | Mucolipidoses detected in particular |
| Organic acids (easily recognizable organic acidaemias are not discussed) | Developmental delay, learning disability, 'cerebral palsy', macrocephaly, dystonia, chorea, encephalopathy (± epileptic seizures), regression, myelopathy. Rarely of value in 'pure' epilepsy | Freeze urine immediately. Test during acute illness in a condition with episodes of encephalopathy (such as GA1). False positive with medium-chain triglyceride oil. False ↑ in GAMT deficiency | Specific patterns of acids may suggest diagnoses: glutaric (GA1); glutaric, ethylmalonic, adipic (GA2); L-2-hydroxyglutaric (L-2-hydroxyglutaric aciduria); N-acetylaspartic (Canavan disease); 4-hydroxybutyric (SSADH deficiency); methylmalonic (cobalamin disorders) |

Table 2.14.1 continued

| Test | Indications | Precautions | Interpretation |
|---|---|---|---|
| Orotic acid | Ill neonate... Vomiting–headache–impaired consciousness complex. 'Stroke'. ↑ ammonia | Random sample. Interpretation should be by metabolic expert | If ↑ = ornithine transcarbamylase deficiency, hyperornithinaemia–hyperammonaemia–homocitrullinuria (HHH) syndrome, and other rare pyrimidine synthesis defects. If in doubt, repeat after protein load under expert supervision |
| Oxalic acid | Dysmorphism, developmental delay, hypotonia | Add HCl as preservative | Peroxisomopathies |
| Phosphate | Suspected mitochondrial disorder | Plasma phosphate necessary for formula | Reduced phosphate reabsorption = tubular dysfunction |
| Porphyrins | Acquired motor neuropathy ± convulsive seizures ± abdominal colic (at puberty) | Random sample, then 24-h urine | Excess excretion leads to specific tests for acute intermittent porphyria |
| Pteridines | Delay, seizures, dystonia ± fluctuation | Phenylalanine may be only mildly ↑ in plasma | Biopterin % of pterins: ↓ biopterin synthesis defects (most commonly PTPS deficiency). ↑ DHPR deficiency |
| Sialic acid (free) | Features of infantile free sialic acid storage disease (see literature for further details) | Single urine. Screen for oligosaccharides will not detect free sialic acid | All patients show vacuolated lymphocytes. 10- to 20-fold increase in sialic acid storage disease. 100-fold increase in sialuria |

Table 2.14.1 continued

| Test | Indications | Precautions | Interpretation |
|------|-------------|-------------|----------------|
| Sulphatides | Suspect metachromatic leukodystropy (MLD) | Urinary sediment. Important to test if arylsulphatase A (ARSA) low in case pseudodeficiency | ↑ in all cases of MLD including those with normal ARSA but activator protein (saposin-B) deficiency |
| Sulphite | Neonatal encephalopathy | Stix test must be done *immediately* on freshly passed urine. Bag urine not suitable. Repeat as often as necessary if diagnosis strongly suspected (but may be true negatives) | May be positive in molybdenum cofactor deficiency or sulphite oxidase deficiency. Quantitative determination of sulphite by anion column chromatography is necessary |
| Thiosulphate | As for urine sulphite | Reliable in urine stored at room temperature up to 72h | Positive in sulphate oxidase deficiency and molybdenum cofactor deficiency |
| Uracil | Childhood encephalopathy | Blood ammonia ± urine orotic acid may be normal | ↑ in late-onset ornithine transcarbamylase (OTC) deficiency |
| Urate | Early seizures ± opisthotonus. Early acquired movement disorder with motor delay and high or high–normal plasma urate. Ataxic cerebral palsy ('dysequilibrium–diplegia') | 24h urine preferable. Urine urate is more sensitive than plasma urate estimation | ↑ output = Lesch–Nyhan syndrome or similar disorder. ↓ excretion = deficiency of molybdenum cofactor or purine nucleoside phosphorylase |

Table 2.14.2 Blood biochemistry

| Test | Indications | Precautions | Interpretation |
|---|---|---|---|
| α-AASA | Neonatal epileptic seizures (usually with burst–suppression) and any unexplained refractory epilepsy up to the age of 2 years at onset | | Supports a diagnosis of pyridoxine-dependent epilepsy (PDE) due to α-AASA-dehydrogenase deficiency |
| Acylcarnitines | Acute metabolic encephalopathy. Acute myopathy, rhabdomyolysis. Unexplained hyperCKaemia | | Specific acylcarnitines indicate particular disorders, e.g. octanoyl carnitine in MCAD deficiency, glutaryl carnitine in GA1, propionyl carnitine in cobalamin disorders |
| Albumin | Suspect multisystem disorder (mitochondrial peroxisomal, congenital defect of glycosylation) | Discussion with laboratory may be necessary on techniques of albumin estimation | ↓ albumin may be the earliest clue to liver involvement in mitochondrial disorders such as with *POLG1* mutations |
| | Part of investigation of CSF in immunological abnormality | | Allows calculations of CSF/serum albumin index, IgG albumin ratio and IgG index |
| Alpha-1 antitrypsin | Late neonatal intracranial haemorrhage | | ↓ may be alpha-1-antitrypsin deficiency with PiZZ or PiSZ phenotype. ('Clotting screen' abnormal) |

Table 2.14.2 continued

| Test | Indications | Precautions | Interpretation |
|------|-------------|-------------|----------------|
| Alpha-fetoprotein | Ataxic 'cerebral palsy'. Any type of movement disorder in early childhood. 'Oculomotor apraxia' (saccadic impairment) | | ↑ in ataxia–telangiectasia, ataxia–oculomotor apraxia 2 (AOA2) and DGUOK deficiency (hepatocerebral form of mtDNA depletion) |
| Amino acids | Learning disability. Hypotonia. Early-onset epileptic seizures including spasms. Acute encephalopathy. Intermittent ataxia. Acquired or progressive dystonia (NB consider $BH_4$ deficiency). Arterial ischaemic stroke | Deproteinize plasma promptly if homocystinuria is a possibility (see also homocysteine). Negative in homocystinuria after small dose of ingested pyridoxine. Not helpful for serine synthesis defects – need CSF | Aminoacidopathies (e.g. PKU, homocystinuria, glycine encephalopathy). Clue to early diagnosis of pyridoxal phosphate-responsive epilepsy and mitochondrial disorders. ↑ alanine may indicate chronic pyruvate accumulation |
| Ammonia (see also Ischaemic forearm test at end of this chapter) | Neonatal seizures ± vomiting. Acute encephalopathy. Vomiting–headache–impaired consciousness complex. 'Stroke'. Intermittent ataxia | May be fasting or postprandial or at time of acute illness. Can be venous or arterial but with minimum disturbance. Separate immediately | Normal arterial level is higher than venous. ↑ in urea cycle defects. Some organic acidurias. Reye syndrome, sodium valproate therapy, decompensated fatty acid disorders, illness with shock |
| Bile acids | Peroxisomal phenotype – see text | | ↑ in various peroxisomopathies |

Table 2.14.2 continued

| Test | Indications | Precautions | Interpretation |
|---|---|---|---|
| Biotinidase | Neurological deterioration ± myelopathy ± skin rash ± alopecia. Remission on biotin trial (see Chapter 2.16) | Serum (assay not affected by coincident biotin therapy). Expected organic aciduria may be subtle | ↓ in biotinidase deficiency |
| Ceruloplasmin (copper oxidase) | Early seizures, hypotonia, steely hair<br><br>Movement and/or behaviour disorder 5 years or older | | ↓ in Menkes disease (unreliable in first weeks)<br><br>↓ in Wilson disease (not always) |
| Calcium | Neonatal seizures. Unexplained seizures ± photophobia, learning disability. Acquired dyskinesia. Basal ganglia calcification<br><br>Developmental delay ± elfin face | | ↓ in hypocalcaemia, true and pseudo-hypoparathyroidism, DiGeorge syndrome<br><br>↑ in idiopathic hypercalcaemia, Williams syndrome |
| Carnitine | Acute unexplained encephalopathy. Coma on valproate. Lipid and other acute myopathies | | ↓↓ in primary carnitine transport defect. ↓ in various fatty acid oxidation disorders. (Valproate may be associated with carnitine depletion) |

Table 2.14.2 continued

| Test | Indications | Precautions | Interpretation |
|---|---|---|---|
| Cholestanol | Learning disability, juvenile cataracts, limb pains | | ↑ in cerebrotendinous xanthomatosis |
| Cholesterol | Developmental delay with retinopathy and sensorineural deafness. Skeletal dysplasias. Ataxia especially with oculomotor apraxia. Spinocerebellar ataxia | Fasting | ↓ in peroxisomal deficiency, Smith–Lemli–Opitz syndrome and other defects of cholesterol biosynthesis, and abetalipoproteinaemia. ↑ in ataxia–oculomotor apraxia type 1 (AOA1) |
| Copper | Steely hair, early seizures | Ensure apparatus is completely copper free and avoid copper contamination | ↓ in Menkes disease (unreliable in first weeks) |
| | Movement disorder ± behaviour disorder age 5 years or over | | ↓ in Wilson disease (not always) |
| CoQ10 | Suspect mitochondrial disorder | White cells necessary | ↓ in ubiquinone deficiency |

Table 2.14.2 continued

| Test | Indications | Precautions | Interpretation |
|---|---|---|---|
| Creatine kinase | Expressive speech delay, toe walking, acquired muscle weakness in a boy. Neonatal and infantile weakness in boys and girls | Test with minimal disturbance, preferably not after exercise or biopsy. HyperCKaemia is sometimes unexplained but many causes | ↑↑ in Duchenne and Becker muscular dystrophies ± ↑ in manifesting carriers. ↑ in other dystrophies, esp. α-sarcoglycan and caveolin3 (CAV3) mutations. ↑ or ↑↑ in VLCAD, LCHAD, MADD/GA2, CPTII, myophosphorylase and myoadenylate deaminase deficiencies, ryanidine receptor (RYR) mutations and other malignant hyperthermias, usually provoked. ↑ extreme exertion, dyskinesia, low T4, mitochondrial. ↑ in congenital muscular dystrophy (often), myositis (often) |
| Creatinine | Learning disability, epileptic seizures and movement disorder | | ± ↓ in GAMT and AGAT deficiency |
| DHAP-AT | Peroxisomal phenotype | | ↓ in all cases of reduced peroxisome number |
| 7-dehydrocholesterol | Suggestive dysmorphism | | ↑ in Smith–Lemli–Opitz syndrome |
| Electrolytes (sodium/ potassium chloride/ bicarbonate) | (Any acute illness.) Paroxysmal weakness | | Potassium abnormalities in various periodic paralyses |

Table 2.14.2 continued

| Test | Indications | Precautions | Interpretation |
|---|---|---|---|
| Endocrine (cortisol, insulin etc.) | Hypoglycaemia, may be epileptic seizures | | Low cortisol may indicate reduced ACTH responsiveness |
| Ferritin (↓ iron deficiency) | 'Seizures' | | ↓ neurally mediated syncope |
| | Unpleasant urge to move legs, relieved by sleep | | ↓ restless leg syndrome |
| | 'Infection' | | ↑ familial haemophagocytic lymphohistiocytosis |
| Glucose | Reduced consciousness level. Epileptic seizures | In fasting test do blood levels immediately before lumbar puncture | Various hypoglycaemic situations. Normal blood glucose with ↓ CSF glucose may indicate GLUT1 deficiency |
| GTP cyclohydrolase-1 (GCH1) | Dopa-responsive dystonia and infantile dyskinesia/parkinsonism with oculogyric crises | Estimated in mononuclear cells from peripheral blood – discuss with lab | ↓ in Segawa disease and in autosomal recessive GCH1 deficiency |
| Hexosaminidase A and B (free) | Wide neurological phenotype | Serum or plasma, ± 'low' in normal children | ↓ in Sandhoff disease or juvenile Sandhoff disease |
| Homocysteine (total plasma homocysteine) | Neonatal hypoxic–ischaemic encephalopathy without convincing history | More sensitive than urine sulphite test | ↑ sulphite oxidase deficiency |

Table 2.14.2 continued

| Test | Indications | Precautions | Interpretation |
|---|---|---|---|
| Homocysteine (total plasma homocysteine) | Arterial ischaemic stroke. 'Psychiatric' myelopathy | B$_{12}$ may be normal in genetic cobalamin defects | ↑ in homocystinuria, MTHFR deficiency, cobalamin disorders |
| Lactate (see also Ischaemic forearm test at end of this chapter) | Acute encephalopathy (± ↑ anion gap). Suspect mitochondrial disorder. Intermittent ataxia/ movement disorder. Organic aciduria. Hypoglycaemia | Minimal disturbance of child (ideally collect sample 30min after placing i.v. catheter) and immediate processing of specimen. May be random or 1h before or 1h after feed | ↑ in a wide range of disorders, in particular mitochondrial respiratory chain deficiencies |
| Lysosomal enzymes | Various dysmorphisms, coarse facies, hepatosplenomegaly, developmental regression | Know what is being tested for. Beware inferences from 'heterozygous' levels and pseudo-deficiencies. Pay attention to substrate used and note that activator protein deficiency may cause typical disease with normal enzyme levels | Specific enzyme deficiency confirms specific targeted diagnosis, e.g. Krabbe disease, metachromatic leukodystrophy, etc. |

Table 2.14.2 continued

| Test | Indications | Precautions | Interpretation |
|---|---|---|---|
| Magnesium | Neonatal seizures | | ↓ in disturbances of magnesium metabolism |
| Manganese | Movement disorder, polycythaemia, liver cirrhosis. Brain MRI: manganese in basal ganglia | | ↑↑ in novel very rare treatable autosomal recessive disorder |
| Phosphate | Tetany, occasional epileptic seizure. Basal ganglia ± white matter calcification | Urine study required when renal tubular function is being tested | ↑ in hypoparathyroidism |
| Phytanic acid | Peroxisomal phenotype. Demyelinating neuropathy | Diet dependent | ↑ in various peroxisomopathies including Refsum disease |
| Pipecolic acid | Neonatal or later onset epilepsy responsive to either pyridoxine (PDE) or pyridoxal phosphate | No need to stop pyridoxine treatment | ↑ in PDE with α-amino adipic semialdehyde dehydrogenase deficiency |
| | Peroxisomal-type dysmorphism | | ↑ in peroxisomal and related metabolic disorders including GA2 |
| Prolactin | Unexplained 'convulsions' | Timing important | ↑ after both epileptic seizures and syncopes but not after psychological events |

Table 2.14.2 continued

| Test | Indications | Precautions | Interpretation |
|---|---|---|---|
| Prolactin | Investigation of dopamine-related disorders | | ↑ in dopamine deficiency disorders |
| Pyruvate | As for blood lactate | Preferably 1h after a meal. Unstable: transfer within 30s to 8% perchlorate on ice | ↑ in defects of pyruvate dehydrogenase |
| Thiamine | Acquired neurological deficit such as oculomotor impairments and ataxia with bizarre history | | Low in Wernicke encephalopathy |
| Thyroid function tests | Typical hypothyroid phenotype | | ↓ = hypothyroidism (including in Down syndrome and CDG1a) |
| | Hashimoto encephalopathy | Anti-thyroperoxidase +ve | May be euthyroid |
| | Hereditary chorea | | ± ↓ with thyroid transcription factor (TITF-1) mutation |
| Free T3 (FT3) | X-linked learning disability with dystonic 'cerebral palsy' ± eye movement defect ± delayed myelination | | ↑ free T3 due to monocarboxylate transporter 8 (*MCT8*) gene mutation (T4 often ↓) |

Table 2.14.2 continued

| Test | Indications | Precautions | Interpretation |
|------|-------------|-------------|----------------|
| Transaminases | 'Congenital infection-like' | Negative virology | ↑ Aicardi–Goutières syndrome |
| | Intractable partial seizures ± myoclonus ± acute encephalopathy | | ↑ Alpers (*POLG1*) |
| | Incidental finding | NB transaminases may come from muscle as well as liver | ↑ Muscular dystrophies |
| | Developmental delay with hypotonia | | ↑ in other mitochondrial disorders and CDG |
| Transferrin (isoelectric focusing for sialotransferrin) | Delay, hypotonia, cerebellar hypoplasia/atrophy | Choose your laboratory. False negatives for CDG not uncommon especially in neonates and early childhood. False positives in galactosaemia and hereditary fructose intolerance | Abnormal in CDG especially type 1a |
| Urate | Early acquired movement disorder with motor delay | Urine urate is more reliable (better sensitivity) | ↑ in Lesch–Nyhan or similar disorder |

Table 2.14.2 continued

| Test | Indications | Precautions | Interpretation |
|---|---|---|---|
| Urate | Dysequilibrium–diplegia | | ↓↓ in purine nucleoside phosphorylase deficiency |
| | Neonatal epilepsy with cerebral destructive lesions | | ↓ in molybdenum cofactor deficiency (is normal in isolated sulphite oxidase deficiency) |
| Urea | Atypical headache often with recurrent impairment of consciousness. 'Stroke' | | ↓ plasma urea may indicate urea cycle disorder including heterozygous (OTC) deficiency.<br>↑ in renal failure and gastrointestinal bleeds, any cause |
| Very long–chain fatty acids (VLCFAs) | Suspect peroxisomopathy | Even though D-bifunctional protein (DBP) deficiency affects the VLCFA pathway, DBP deficiency cannot be exluded by normal plasma VLCFA: fibroblast studies needed | ↑ in most peroxisomal disorders including all global peroxisomal deficiencies |
| Vitamin A | School-age regression | | ↑ in adrenoleukodystrophy (ALD) |
| | Loss of vision in autism | | ↓ with deficient diet |

Table 2.14.2 continued

| Test | Indications | Precautions | Interpretation |
|---|---|---|---|
| Vitamin B$_{12}$ | Developmental delay in a purely breast-fed infant ± seizures ± movement disorders | | ↓ when mother on a vegan (or even a vegetarian) diet. Movement disorder may ↑ after B$_{12}$ treatment of deficiency. Macrocytosis is not always present |
| Vitamin E | Developmental delay, with retinal defect and sensorineural deafness, spinocerebellar ataxia ± retinitis pigmentosa | | ↓ in some peroxisomal disorders, abetalipoproteinaemia, selective vitamin E malabsorption |

Abbreviations: CPTII = carnitine palmitoyl transferase II; DHAP-AT = dihydroxyacetone phosphate acyltransferase; LCHAD = long–chain 3-hydroxyacyl–coenzyme A deficiency; MADD/GA2 = multiple acyl-coenzyme A dehydrogenase deficiency/glutaric aciduria type 2; VLCAD = very-long-chain acyl-coenzyme A deficiency.

Table 2.14.3 CSF biochemistry

| Test | Indications | Precautions | Interpretation |
|---|---|---|---|
| Albumin | Routine | | ↑ in blood–brain or blood–CSF barrier, disruption and inflammatory polyneuropathy. May not be ↑ in mitochondrial Guillain–Barré syndrome-like neuropathy. May be ↑ in central demyelination |

Table 2.14.3 continued

| Test | Indications | Precautions | Interpretation |
|------|-------------|-------------|----------------|
| Amino acids | Neonatal hiccups in ill baby (hiccups common in normal newborn infants) | Obtain paired samples of plasma and CSF | ↑ glycine and ↑ CSF/plasma glycine ratio in glycine encephalopathy |
| | Neonatal seizures/ encephalopathy/stiff baby/ microcephaly | Obtain paired samples of plasma and CSF | ↓ serine and glycine in serine synthesis disorders |
| | Suspect mitochondrial disorder | Obtain paired samples of plasma and CSF | Alanine and proline ± ↑ in mitochondrial disorders |
| | Headache, vomiting | Obtain paired samples of plasma and CSF | Glutamine ↑ in OTC deficiency |
| Asialotransferrin (% of total transferrin) (= τ or tau protein) | Pleomorphic central white matter disorder with onset from neonatal to late adolescence. Ataxia (often progressive spastic ataxia) ± dementia ± optic atrophy ± peripheral neuropathy ± macrocephaly ± coma. Deterioration with febrile illness or after head bump or fright | Test not yet validated in neonates and first year of life. Blood transferrin should be normal | ↓ (<8%) in eIF2B-related disorder (includes vanishing white matter but not exclusively so) |

Table 2.14.3 continued

| Test | Indications | Precautions | Interpretation |
|---|---|---|---|
| Biogenic amines (monoamine metabolites) (always analyse both amines and pterins together) | Infantile hypertonia with oculogyric crises and autonomic features. Infantile immobility and bradykinesia. 'Cerebral palsy'/delay ± oculogyric crises (NB easily misdiagnosed as absence epileptic seizures) and normal brain MRI. Acquired movement disorder not typical of known conditions. Acquired gait disturbance when features atypical for Segawa disease (cognitive delay, parkinsonism, oculogyric crises) argue against immediate levodopa trial | Organize in advance with supraregional laboratory. Freeze samples immediately at bedside on dry ice antioxidant mixture. If blood admixed, spin at once and transfer clear CSF to new tubes before freezing. Do not give levodopa within 1 week before | Patterns of dopamine, 5-HIAA and HVA vary in different monoamine neurotransmitter disorders – see also Pterins below |
| Creatine | Global delay, expressive language impairment, early-onset 'generalized' epilepsy, movement disorder (mixed, may be dystonic/ballistic) | Needs to be evaluated by in vitro H-MRS for lack of creatine peak (frozen immediately – discuss with lab in advance) | ↓ in GAMT and AGAT deficiencies and in creatine transporter defect (*SLC6A8*) |

Table 2.14.3 continued

| Test | Indications | Precautions | Interpretation |
|---|---|---|---|
| GABA | In very exceptional cases of hyper- or hypotonia | Organize with supraregional laboratory. *Not likely to be a helpful investigation* | ↑ in GABA-transaminase deficiency and ↑ in succinic semialdehyde dehydrogenase deficiency. ↓ in some cases of hyperekplexia but not helpful in diagnosis |
| Glucose | Epileptic seizures, developmental delay, ataxia, movement disorder, evolving microcephaly | Always take blood for plasma glucose immediately before a lumbar puncture | Numerous inflammatory and other cellular causes of ↓ glucose. Hypoglycaemia. ↓ absolute level of CSF glucose and CSF/blood glucose ratio indicates GLUT1 deficiency |
| Guanidinoacetate | Severe learning disability, epilepsy, movement disorder (often ballistic) | Urine usually | ↑ in creatine synthesis disorder, will need proton brain MRS |
| Lactate | Suspect mitochondrial disorder | Blood for lactate before lumbar puncture | ↑ value suggests a mitochondrial disorder |
| 5-MTHF | Decreasing head growth with agitation, delay, sleep disturbance in infancy followed by developmental arrest or regression with later dyskinesia, ataxia, pyramidal signs, epileptic seizures, and on brain MRI white matter signal change | May not be a primary disorder. Homocysteine will be increased | ↓ in cerebral folate deficiency. ↓ in 5-MTHF reductase deficiency (a form of homocystinuria) |

Table 2.14.3 continued

| Test | Indications | Precautions | Interpretation |
|---|---|---|---|
| Myelin basic protein | Suspect acute demyelination | Sensitivity and specificity not established | ↑ in acute demyelination in multiple sclerosis, ADEM, neuromyelitis/neuromyelitis optica |
| Neopterin | Suspect GTP-CH deficiency | Measure with other pterins and biogenic amines | ↓ in GTP-CH deficiency |
| | Suspect inflammatory CNS disorder, infective or autoimmune, incl. Aicardi–Goutières syndrome | More sensitive than CSF pleocytosis; short half-life | ↑ in inflammatory CNS disorders (including Aicardi–Goutières syndrome) |
| Poliols | Unexplained leukodystrophy | Can also be done in urine | ↑ in ribose-5-phosphate isomerase deficiency |
| Pterins (always analyse both amines and pterins together; see also Neopterin) | As for biogenic amines (always analyse both amines and pterins together) | As for biogenic amines: discuss with supraregional laboratory. Sepiapterin may need separate analysis (see below) | As for biogenic amines. ↓ neopterin (and others) in various monoamine disorders |
| | Congenital infection-like picture | | ↑ neopterin in inflammation when T-lymphocytes or macrophages involved; autoimmunity; Aicardi–Goutières syndrome |

Table 2.14.3 continued

| Test | Indications | Precautions | Interpretation |
|---|---|---|---|
| Pyridoxal 5'-phosphate (PLP) | Intractable neonatal epileptic seizures. *Possibly* other neurological phenotypes | Do pyridoxal phosphate trial first (Chapter 2.16) | ↓ in PNPO deficiency |
| Sepiapterin | Developmental delay with atypical features, especially bulbar symptoms, oculogyric crises, diurnal variation | May be missed on standard pterin study | Sepiapterin reductase deficiency |
| Succinylpurines | Learning disability, autism. As for urine succinylpurines | Freeze specimen for Bratton–Marshall test | ↑ ADSL deficiency<br>↑ AICA-ribosiduria |

Table 2.14.4 CSF pterins and monoamines

| Enzyme deficiency | BH$_4$ | BH$_2$ | Neo-pterin | Sepia-pterin | HVA | 5HIAA | 3OMD |
|---|---|---|---|---|---|---|---|
| AD GTP-CH | ↓ | N | ↓ | | ±↓ | ±↓ | N |
| AR GTP-CH | ↓ | N | ↓ | | ↓ | ↓ | N |
| Sepiapterin reductase | ±↓ | ↑ | N | ↑ | ↓ | ↓ | N |
| Tyrosine hydroxylase | N | N | N | | ↓ | N | N |
| AADC | N | N | N | | ↓ | ↓ | ↑ |

Abbreviations: AADC = aromatic L-amino acid decarboxylase; AD = autosomal dominant; AR = autosomal recessive; BH$_2$ = 7,8-dihydrobiopterin; BH$_4$ = tetrahydrobiopterin; GTP-CH = guanosine triphosphate cyclohydrolase; 5HIAA = 5-hydroxyindole acetic acid; HVA = homovanillic acid; N = within reference range for age and laboratory; 3OMD = 3-O-methyldopa.

## Organelle-related investigations

Some remarks follow on organelle-related biochemical investigations and when biochemical tests are indicated.

### Lysosomal disorders

Lysosomal enzyme deficiencies may be sought in serum or plasma, in leukocytes (white cell pellet) or in cultured fibroblasts.

Although it is evident that there is great variation in the severity of the neurological disorders which may result from a severe lysosomal enzyme deficiency, extreme caution is necessary when partial deficiency is found, particularly 'within the heterozygous range', since in some of these disorders the prevalence of heterozygosity is quite high in the normal population.

The term 'pseudodeficiency' is used in lysosomal storage diseases to denote the situation in which individuals show greatly reduced enzyme activity but remain clinically healthy. Pseudodeficiencies have been reported for several lysosomal hydrolases. Pseudodeficiency is particularly important in relation to arylsulphatase A (ARSA), which is the enzyme classically deficient in metachromatic leukodystrophy (MLD). In pseudo-MLD, patients will not have the appropriate clinical features, and although they have ARSA levels of 10–15% of the normal mean, they do not have excess urinary sulphatides or toluidine blue staining metachromatic granules in urine (second morning specimen).

Genetic testing for the genes involved is often possible.

Considerations of sensitivity and specificity should prevent, for example, the diagnosis of MLD in a child with primary generalized epilepsy or isolated dystonia with heterozygous levels of ARSA. These clinical presentations would be inappropriate indications for assay of this enzyme, but having obtained a low result the clinician may feel bound to pursue the diagnosis by culturing fibroblasts and searching for sulphatide in urinary sediment and in sural nerve biopsy. Such temptations should be strongly resisted.

A further consideration is activator protein deficiency, best known in the case of MLD. The catabolism of sulphatide requires both the enzyme ARSA and a specific sphingolipid activator protein, saposin-B, encoded by the prosaposin gene (*PSAP*). ARSA activity is deficient in the classical forms of MLD, but a substantial proportion of cases of MLD are due to saposin-B deficiency with mutations in the *PSAP* gene and thus have normal ARSA but markedly increased urinary excretion of sulphatides.

### Mitochondrial disorders

With the explosion of knowledge about disorders of the mitochondria, definitive investigations have become more complex and specialized. However, clinical clues can point towards a mitochondrial disorder and fairly simple tests support the diagnosis sufficiently to proceed to specific investigations of mitochondrial function.

To a certain extent there is a relationship between the type of disease and the site of metabolic defect along the pathway from the inner mitochondrial membrane to the termination of the respiratory chain, but there is considerable heterogeneity and for simplicity we will tend to lump rather than split.

It has long been known that most of the genes responsible for mitochondrial function are nuclear rather than mitochondrial genes, and recently some of these nuclear genes have become much more accessible to analysis. The most important of these is *POLG* or *POLG1*, that is, mitochondrial DNA polymerase-gamma A. A major way by which mutations in *POLG1* affect mitochondrial function is by inducing mitochondrial depletion. Such mitochondrial depletion may be either generalized or organ specific. Other genes of recent interest include *Twinkle*, *DGUOK* and the gene for thymidine kinase 2.

CLINICAL CLUES TO MITOCHONDRIAL DISORDERS (most common genes in parentheses)
- Myopathy with fatigue (various mt tRNA mutations).

- 'Progressive neuronal degeneration of childhood' – Alpers disease – with hemiclonic and focal myoclonic seizures often with epilepsia partialis continua, associated with developmental regression and cerebral atrophy ± terminal liver failure (*POLG1*).

- Leigh disease: regression with hypotonia, oculomotor and respiratory disturbances, with symmetrical lesions on imaging in basal ganglia, thalami, substantia nigra, red nuclei, cerebellum and commonly also in periaqueductal grey matter and spinal cord, and often COX (COX = cytochrome c oxidase = complex IV of the respiratory chain) deficiency in muscle (genetically heterogeneous: many mitochondrial mutations, especially *ATPase6* and genes for tRNA, nuclear genes, especially *SURF1* – codes for assembly factor for COX – and genes for Complex I, but only rarely *POLG1*).

- Leigh-like syndrome: similar to Leigh but oculomotor and respiratory impairment usually absent, more variable neurology (genes as in Leigh).

- Episodic, static or progressive ataxia ± other neurological deficits ± cerebellar lactate peak on H-MRS (*POLG1*, mtDNA depletion, ubiquinone deficiency).

- Chronic encephalomyopathy of childhood; fatigue, pigmentary retinopathy, oculomotor disturbance, sensorineural deafness, ataxia, pyramidal signs, regression, including NARP (mtDNA *T8993G* or *C* in complex V = *ATPase6*).

- Kearns–Sayre syndrome: ptosis and ophthalmoplegia, pigmentary retinopathy, heart block, short stature (large mitochondrial rearrangements).

- Pearson syndrome: infantile-onset pancreatic disorder, sideroblastic anaemia, later Kearns–Sayer (large mitochondrial deletion).

- MELAS – mitochondrial myopathy, encephalopathy, lactic acidosis and stroke-like episodes: severe migraines, partial epileptic seizures, hemipareses, and cerebral lesions on imaging which superficially look as if they were ischaemic but do not correspond to known vascular territories (mtDNA *A3243G* or *T3271C*).

- MERRF – myoclonic epilepsy with ragged red fibres: myoclonic epileptic seizures with repetitive myoclonus and progressive ataxia and regression in late childhood (mtDNA *A8344G*).

- MNGIE – mitochondrial neurogastrointestinal encephalomyopathy (nDNA thymidine phosphorylase).

- LHON – Leber hereditary optic neuropathy (mtDNA *G3460A*, *G11778A*, *T14484C* in complex I subunits).

- Movement disorders and various semiologies including paroxysmal dystonia (PDH deficiency, but also mt tRNA and LHON mutations).

- Guillain–Barré type acute polyneuropathy with atypical features including normal CSF protein but increased lactate, with or without recurrence (E1α mutations in PDH complex).

- Infantile spinocerebellar ataxia with axonal neuropathy (perhaps *Twinkle* and *twinky*).

- Nonspecific combination of static or progressive neurodevelopmental disorder with paroxysmal events such as epileptic seizures and migraine, and evidence of more than one component of the nervous system (*POLG1* especially).

INVESTIGATION RESULTS FOUND IN MITOCHONDRIAL DISORDERS
Because these disorders of oxidative phosphorylation (OXPHOS) result in impaired

aerobic energy metabolism, primary indicators are increased blood and CSF lactates. However, normal lactates do not exclude a mitochondrial disorder, especially in *POLG1*.

Combinations of the following investigations (listed in chapter order as in this book) may give clues, depending on the systems involved:

- EEG polyspikes mini-bursts on rhythmic slow activity

- Slow nerve conduction velocity

- CT: calcification of the basal ganglia

- MRI: altered signal in basal ganglia structures (especially globus pallidus), substantia nigra, red nuclei, periaqueductal grey matter, alterations in white matter of centrum semiovale cerebellum

- Neuronal migration disorder in some, e.g. perisylvian polymicrogyria

- MR spectroscopy

  – Lacate peak on proton MRS in basal ganglia

  – Lactate peak on H-MRS in cerebellum – especially when ataxia

- CSF: increased protein (increased albumin).

- ECG: cardiac conduction defect including heart block and Wolff–Parkinson–White syndrome

- Haematology: marrow suppression

- Blood biochemistry

  – Low albumin

  – Increased alanine and proline

  – Raised transaminases

- Urine biochemistry

  – Generalized aminoaciduria

  – Impaired phosphate reabsorption

  – Krebs cycle organic acids (e.g. fumarate, succinate).

SPECIAL MITOCHONDRIAL INVESTIGATIONS
The combination of clinical and investigation results may point not only to a mitochondrial disorder but also to a specific phenotype. Phenotypes such as MELAS, MERRF or Kearns–Sayre relate to a defect of the mitochondrial genome, whereas phenotypes such as Alpers–Huttenlocher would point towards a nuclear mitochondrial gene, in particular polymerase gamma (*POLG1*) or the mitochondrial DNA helicase *Twinkle*.

If the clinical picture points to a deficiency in pyruvate dehydrogenase (PDH) such as neonatal encephalopathy with lactic acidosis and absent, hypoplastic or dysplastic corpus callosum or in the older child progressive dystonia with altered signal in globus pallidus on imaging, PDH activity may be measured in cultured skin fibroblasts.

While the clinical phenotype suggesting mitochondrial depletion will have pointed towards studies of *POLG1* and *Twinkle* as indicated above, or when there is a less defined but persuasive suggestion of mitochondrial dysfunction, then the next stage is study of muscle and possibly liver.

Histological examination of muscle biopsy may show ragged red fibres on Gomori stain, lipid droplets and abnormal staining for cytochrome c oxidase. Mitochondria may be abnormal on electronmicroscopy. Functional studies of all components of the mitochondrial respiratory chain will be undertaken on fresh specimens. Liver biopsy with functional studies may be needed when the muscle biopsy studies are negative despite pointers to a mitochondrial disorder.

While until recently it has been recommended that CoQ10 be estimated in fresh muscle, white cell (or fibroblast) CoQ10 may be a better way of determining ubiquinone deficiency.

MITOCHONDRIAL 'CONFUSION'
Diagnostic confusion is not infrequent between mitochondrial disorders and other conditions. There may be 'pseudo-' or secondary mitochondrial deficiencies, but also true mitochondrial disorders may masquerade as for instance monoamine neurotransmitter conditions.

### Peroxisomal disorders
Peroxisomes are spherical 1μm diameter organelles with a multitude of oxidative and other enzymes packed within a single-layered membrane (http://www.peroxisomedb. org). To simplify, we will concentrate discussion on the following:

[1] 'global' peroxisomal disorders with impaired peroxisomal biogenesis (fewer or even no peroxisomes), together with those single peroxisomal enzyme defects that induce a similar phenotype (in particular, D-bifunctional protein deficiency)

[2] adrenoleukodystrophy, due to an X-linked defect of the peroxisomal *ABCD1* gene that codes for the peroxisomal membrane protein ABCD1, a member of the ATP-binding cassette transporters.

While estimation of very long chain fatty acids (VLCFA) may detect many peroxisomal disorders there is no 'metabolic screen' that will detect them all. Some wider clinical clues to the peroxisomopathies under discussion follow.

CLINICAL CLUES TO PEROXISOMAL DISORDERS
[1]
- Neonatal hypotonia (especially extreme hypotonia of the neck)
- Neonatal seizures (refractory or phenytoin-responsive in a hypotonic baby)

- Neonatal unresponsiveness (except reflex crying)
- Non-development
- Retinal blindness ('Leber amaurosis')
- Sensorineural deafness
- Gross dysmorphic features of Zellweger syndrome type (high forehead, flat face, simian creases, simple genitalia)
- Mild dysmorphism (large fontanelle with open metopic suture, absent ear lobules)
- Leukodystrophy, neuronal migration defects especially perisylvian polymicrogyria
- Hepatomegaly (± hepatic insufficiency)
- Developmental delay with malabsorption features, retinopathy and sensorineural deafness
- Development delay with seizures and areflexia (peripheral neuropathy).

[2]
- School-age regression in a boy with previously normal development (± Addison disease)
- Spastic paraplegia in older females.

INVESTIGATION RESULTS FOUND IN PEROXISOMAL DISORDERS
*In neonatal and early manifesting peroxisomal disorders:*
- EEG trains of repetitive spikes shifting from side to side
- Slow nerve conduction (± EMG denervation)
- Low or absent ERG
- Brainstem auditory evoked potentials (BAEP) – gross abnormalities
  - High threshold
  - Delayed wave V latency
  - Lack of response
- MRI evidence of migration disorder
- MRI white matter altered signal
- Patellar or other chondral calcification
- Bone age retardation
- Echogenic renal cortex on ultrasound
- Increased CSF protein
- Liver biopsy: hepatic fibrosis
- Clotting defect of hepatic type

- Increased AST and ALT

- Low cholesterol

- Low vitamin E

- Increased phytanic acid

- Increased pipecolic acid

- Urinary excretion: amino acids, glycosaminoglycans, dicarboxylic acids.

*In the regressing school child:*

- Visual evoked potential (VEP) – latency increase

- BAEP increased latency of wave V

- MRI increased signal in posterior central white matter on T2 images usually but not always.

SPECIAL PEROXISOMAL INVESTIGATIONS
Once sufficient clinical and investigational clues have been assembled, special tests for peroxisomal disorders may be sought at specialized laboratories. These primarily test

1. The size of the peroxisomal compartment – simply, are peroxisomes missing and all functions depressed?

2. The integrity of the peroxisomal beta-oxidation pathway, which metabolizes VLCFAs and also, in part, bile acids.

The tests of most direct help are as follows.

*VLCFAs in plasma*
VLCFAs are increased in all disorders with absent or grossly diminished peroxisomes, and in *most* disorders of the VLCFA metabolic pathway (but not in all defects of isolated peroxisomal enzymes). This is the only test necessary for confirmation of the diagnosis of adrenoleukodystrophy in the regressing schoolchild.

*VLCFAs in fibroblasts*
If a peroxisomopathy is suspected – as when there is characteristic dysmorphism, non-development and retinal and sensorineural hearing defects, then normal plasma studies (including normal plasma VLCFA) do not exclude D-bifunctional protein (DBP) deficiency. In this clinical situation, request full fibroblast studies including fibroblast C26:0 beta-oxidation rate and VLCFA ratios.

*Bile acids.* Abnormal bile acids are found in the urine, plasma and duodenal juice in infants with a lack of peroxisomes, and in those with peroxisomal DBP deficiency.

*Dihydroxyacetone phosphate acyl transferase (DHAP-AT).* This is estimated in fibroblasts (and in platelets). It is reduced in all cases of general lack of peroxisomes.

*Liver biopsy with special studies.* It is possible to demonstrate lack of peroxisomes by special histochemistry and electronmicroscopy, and enlarged peroxisomes in biochemical lesions of the beta-oxidation pathway, but such studies are no longer essential for diagnosis. Immunoblot methods allow determination of the individual beta-oxidation enzymes, but as these enzymes may be totally inactive despite demonstrable protein, it cannot at present be said that liver biopsy is a necessary investigation.

### Golgi and endoplasmic reticulum disorders (congenital defects of glycosylation)

Attaching sugar molecules to proteins or lipids (glycosylation) is mediated by the Golgi apparatus or complex and by the endoplastic reticulum and is necessary for numerous biochemical functions. Defects may be divided into what one might call soluble and structural abnormalities.

The 'soluble' congenital defects of glycosylation (CDG) – predominantly defects of N-glycosylation – are many and increasing in number but by far the most important is CDG1a. We will not deal here with the 'structural' defects of O-glycosylation as these at present comprise congenital and later onset muscular dystrophies that are investigated by completely different methods.

CLINICAL CLUES TO CDG

The symptomatology may be highly variable even within the same family but some of the following features may be seen:

- Facial and hand dysmorphism often mild

- Fat pads, particularly on the buttocks

- Flat or inverted nipples (inverted nipples are more common in those without CDG!)

- Slow cognitive development

- Slow motor development

- Strabismus

- Feeding difficulties

- Stroke-like episodes (hemipareses)

- Epileptic seizures (not as an isolated phenomenon)

- Retinopathy

- Hepatomegaly or disorder of liver function

- Cardiomyopathy

- Palpable kidneys

- Endocrine defects, e.g. hypothyroidism, hyperinsulinism, hypergonadotrophic hypogonadism (in females)

- Miscellaneous defects, skeleton, etc.

Neurological phenotypes similar to those well recognized in mitochondrial disorders may be seen, and it is wise to ensure that congenital defects of glycosylation have been excluded before one proceeds to invasive investigation for mitochondrial disorders.

INVESTIGATION RESULTS IN CDG
Isoelectric focusing (IEF) for transferrins (sialotransferrins) is the major primary diagnostic investigation. The clinical spectrum of CDG is so wide that transferrin IEF must always be done when the diagnosis is a possibility.

Other investigations that may be abnormal in CDG and may give clues towards the diagnosis are as follows:

• EEG during stroke-like episodes showing repetitive spike complexes contralateral to the hemiparesis

• Slow nerve conduction

• Cerebellar atrophy or pontocerebellar atrophy and particularly progressive cerebellar atrophy

• CSF protein increase

• Coagulation abnormality, in particular decreased factor IX and antithrombin III, protein C and protein S

• Abnormal liver function tests, especially increased transaminases.

The precise biochemical defect causing the CDG can be elucidated by performing leukocyte or fibroblast enzyme assays and then by DNA mutation studies in cases where the clinical phenotype points towards a specific enzymatic deficiency. Where this is not the case, powerful tandem mass spectrometry techniques can be utilized to provide information on the glycoprotein in question, hence providing a clue towards the precise enzymatic block.

## Miscellaneous tests of body chemistry
We append some notes on biochemical investigations that do not depend on single urine, blood or CSF analyses.

### Fibroblast culture studies
The storage of cultured fibroblasts, like the retention of DNA samples, is one of the prerequisites for later genetic diagnosis of unexplained disorders. Some types of fibroblast study are particularly important.

PYRUVATE DEHYDROGENASE (PDH)
Clinically heterogeneous, including neonatal hypotonia and epileptic seizures, Leigh and Leigh-like syndromes, episodic ataxia and paroxysmal dystonia. Lactates may be normal. Basal ganglia abnormality (especially globus pallidus) may be a clue.

FATTY ACID OXIDATION
Also clinically heterogeneous but urinary organic acid and plasma carnitine and acylcarnitine studies will prompt this evaluation.

VERY LONG CHAIN FATTY ACID STUDIES
Usually done in peroxisomopathies, but essential for diagnosis of DBP deficiency when plasma studies are normal.

CHOLESTEROL ESTER TRAFFICKING
Employed for definitive diagnosis of Niemann–Pick type C phenotype.

### Phenylalanine load
This is a method for stressing the pterin system, but may be unreliable. It was developed as a biochemical marker for pterin synthesis defects associated with dopamine-responsive dystonia, especially GTP-CH deficiency. A dose of 100mg/kg of phenylalanine is used. A phenylalanine/tyrosine ratio >7.5 is suggestive, but not diagnostic, of a pterin synthesis defect. The phenylalanine must rise above 600µmol/L for the test to be valid. This test has low sensitivity and specificity.

### Ischaemic forearm test
This test measures basal and post-exercise venous lactate and ammonia levels. The blood lactate is measured after the fist has been clenched repeatedly for 1 minute with the arm made ischaemic using a sphygmomanometer. Samples are taken at –10 minutes (pre-exercise) and at 0, 1, 3, 5, 10 and 20 minutes following release of the cuff.

A normal response is characterized by a lactate increase of 3–5 fold over baseline with a peak at 1–3 minutes post-exercise, while ammonia increases 5–10 fold over the same time. An absent or inadequate (less than 1.5-fold) increase in lactate is seen in myophosphorylase, phosphofructokinase and distal glycolytic enzyme deficiencies. A normal lactate response with impaired ammonia production is characteristic of myoadenylate deaminase deficiency.

A non-ischaemic test involving maximal intermittent hand-grip exercise for 1 minute has been shown to have the same diagnostic power for McArdle disease as the ischaemic test and is better tolerated in children.

## Clinical vignettes

### 2.14.1 Explosive 'onset' of neurological disease
The onset of multifocal myoclonus in this boy at age 10 months was certainly explosive, although his intelligent parents had noticed that beforehand he was floppy with delayed gross motor development and poor truncal control, with a diagnosis of dysequilibrium. While with his parents in a shopping centre he suddenly developed jerks in both legs and arms and sudden loss of head control making him extremely floppy and generally quite unresponsive. On arrival in the intensive care unit he had multifocal high-

amplitude myoclonic jerks, generalized hypotonia and respiratory insufficiency, such that he was intubated and ventilated.

INVESTIGATIONS (1)

*EEG* – No normal background, multifocal discharges including asynchronous bilateral periodic polyphasic complexes commonly associated with limb myoclonus. Recording included runs of slow waves with multiple spikes on the upstroke of each wave, suggestive of Alpers disease.

*Nerve conduction* – Left common peroneal 38.5m/s (normal).

*EMG* – No spontaneous activity except bursts during jerks.

*Brain CT* – Normal.

*CSF protein* = 1.2g/L, no cells; repeat 0.86g/L.

*CSF lactate* = 2.4mmol/L; repeat 0.8mmol/L (normal 1.2–1.9).

*Blood lactate* = 0.9mmol/L.

*Virology* – Negative.

*Liver function tests and coagulation factors* – Normal.

*Liver biopsy* – Normal.

COURSE (1)

His jerks improved and after 1 week he was breathing air without aid.

INVESTIGATIONS (2)

*EEG* – Slow background; repeat: within normal limits.

*CSF* – Protein = 1.1g/L, IgG = 0.08g/L.

*VEP* – Significant delay (N1 88ms, P1 112ms, N2 163ms).

COURSE (2)

Intensity and frequency of jerking varied, sometimes noted to involve diaphragm and abdominal muscles. Though profoundly hypotonic and weak he remained interactive, fixing and following and smiling.

INVESTIGATIONS (3)

*EEG* – Mixed frequency background but no discharges during jerks.

*Brain CT* – Increased size of basal cisterns, ventricular system and extra-axial spaces; grey matter had slightly low density, especially in frontal and parietal regions.

*CSF* – Protein = 0.9 g/L; IgG/albumin ratio = 0.32 (0.26–0.66); no oligoclonal bands; lactate = 2.4mmol/L, pyruvate = 99μmol/L; plasma lactate = 0.9mmol/L.

COURSE (3)

He was allowed home, tube-fed by his parents. He had 3 weeks with no jerks seen but then twitching recurred and worsened. After 47 days at home he was readmitted having constant twitching and no longer regaining full consciousness.

INVESTIGATIONS (4)
*EEG* – Very typical Alpers disease appearance with clustered polyspikes on crest of each slow wave.

*Brain CT* – Further increase in atrophy.

*AST (aspartate transaminase)* = 115u/L.

COURSE (4)
He died in his parents' arms at the age of 14 months and they allowed detailed post-mortem examination within 2 hours of death.

INVESTIGATIONS (5)
*Brain pathology* – The main findings included very striking atrophy of the superior vermis with loss of Purkinje and granule cells while the lower half of the vermis had normal cytology; foci of neuronal loss in thalami, cerebral cortex (including posterior part of sylvian fissure and sulci over the upper part of the parietal convexity) and in the hippocampi, including recent cell loss in the hippocampi.

*Liver histology* – Mild centrilobular steatosis.

*Muscle histology* – 17% COX-negative fibres.

*MtDNA:nDNA ratios* were low in several tissues (7% liver, 23% muscle, 25% kidney, 37% brain, 80% heart). Fibroblast mtDNA was 19–27% (control 39–193).

*TFAM (mitochondrial transcription factor, mtTFA)* was reduced 2–4 fold in most tissues.

COURSE (5)
The family kept in contact with the hospital and were praised for their very generous contribution to fundamental research. They knew of the 25% recurrence risk but also that so far prenatal diagnosis was not possible.

INVESTIGATIONS (6)
Fifteen years after the boy's death he was found to have been a compound heterozygote for pathogenic mutations in *POLG1* [c.2740A>C (p.T914P) and c.3286C>T (p.R1096C)].

COURSE (6)
The parents hugely appreciated the meticulous work that had allowed demonstration of the basis of their son's mitochondrial depletion disorder, and the detailed genetic advice now available to them.

COMMENT
In the end the immense emotional investment of the parents was rewarded by academic studies of the highest order. Thanks to such research, the neurological investigation of

the not uncommon Alpers disease phenotype is now quick and 'simple', going directly from the EEG rhythmic high-amplitude delta with superimposed polyspikes to *POLG1*.

However, if a similar infant were to present today before the myoclonus onset, and with only disequilibrium from cerebellar vermis involvement, there is not enough evidence to say whether H-MRS of the cerebellum for a lactate peak or CSF protein (and lactate) or *POLG1* analysis would be the first step after brain MRI.

### 2.14.2 Elusive peroxisomopathy

More than one child was affected in this consanguineous family, in which the father believed it was a poison in his wife that was responsible. Most information is available on the boy now described, whose sister had earlier died age 5 months.

He weighed 2.76kg when born at term in 1986. He was mildly dysmorphic with a 'flat' face and huge metopic extension of his anterior fontanelle. He showed extreme axial hypotonia from birth (when he was aged 2 months the description was: "startling neck hypotonia as if his head was not actually connected to his trunk except by a scarf"). Eye movements were jerky but optic fundi were always normal with no visible retinopathy. He made no developmental progress. Twitchy epileptic seizures began aged 6 hours.

INVESTIGATIONS (1)

*EEG* – Unremarkable: no interictal spike discharges (later, occasional spikes).

*Motor nerve conduction velocity* – Within normal limits (21.5m/s at 1 month).

*EMG* – Normal.

*ERG* – Photopic b wave 4µV, scotopic b wave 7µV (~1/30th normal amplitude).

*BAEP* – No waves detected on either side.

*Brain imaging (ultrasound, CT, MRI)* – Unremarkable.

*Bone radiographs* – Normal.

*Ultrasound kidneys* – Cortex relatively echogenic.

*CSF protein* = 0.9g/L on day 15.

*ECG* – Normal.

*Haematology routine* – Normal.

*Biochemistry* – Routine screenings including amino acids and organic acids: normal.

*Short synachthen test* – Cortisol increase from 406 to 1235nmol/L.

*Special peroxisomal studies:*

- *Plasma VLCFAs* – Grossly elevated (C26 3.4µg/mL, C24:C22 ratio 1.68, C26:C22 ratio 0.262)

- *Platelet and fibroblast DHAP-AT activity* – Normal

- *Plasma phytanic acid* – Not detected

- *Bile acids* – fast atom bombardment mass spectrometry (FAB-MS) of urine gave a peak at m/z (mass per charge) 572 suggesting taurine-conjugated tetrahydroxy C27 bile acid; capillary GC-MS of plasma showed dihydroxyprostanic acid (DCA) and trihydroxyprostanic acid (THHCA) but no C29 dicarboxylic acid

- Liver biopsy: abundant structurally normal peroxisomes up to 1µm in diameter (<0.5µm).

Course (1)
He remained extremely hypotonic, fed poorly and had frequent short clonic and tonic epileptic seizures. Age 5 months he had a prolonged run of epileptic infantile spasms. At 6 months although there was zero nuchal tone, his limbs began to be rigid. Subtle tapetoretinal degeneration with 'salt and pepper' appearance and some vessel attenuation was first seen age 7 months. He died age 10 months.

Investigations (2)
Limited general necropsy revealed no specific abnormalities.

*Neuropathology* – No developmental abnormalities were detected in the brain; in particular there was no neuronal migration disorder, with normal architecture of all the components of the brainstem, cerebrum and cerebellum. Occasional globoid cells were seen in white matter (Fig. 2.14.1). Loss of neurons in the thalamus and brainstem (with total absence in some areas) were of the type usually associated with hypoxia. There was no neuronal loss in the cerebellum.

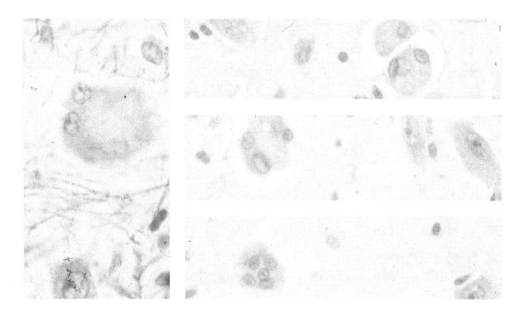

Figure 2.14.1 Example of globoid cell in white matter of infant with D–bifunctional protein deficiency.

COURSE (2)
Two months after this boy's death another affected son was born.

INVESTIGATIONS (3)
Cultured fibroblasts were examined by immunoblotting and enzymatic methods: peroxisomal bifunctional protein was present, but lacked enzymatic activity.

COMMENT
This vignette illustrates both the severe phenotype of a peroxisomopathy – profound axial hypotonia associated with severe impairments of both ERG and BAEP – and the complexity of the necessary investigations. Although our patient was 'pseudo-Zellweger' – having features similar to infants without peroxisomes – yet he had abundant (albeit large) peroxisomes in his biopsied liver. Investigators were misled at the time by a contemporary publication suggesting that peroxisomal thiolase deficiency led to 'pseudo-Zellweger', whereas reinvestigation 16 years later (Ferdinandusse et al. 2002) has shown that the defect in that reported patient was in D-bifunctional protein, as in our own patient. 20 years later it may be simpler to go to gene analysis of *HSD17B4*, much as one goes to *PEX1* when the evidence points to a defect in peroxisomal biogenesis.

### 2.14.3 Pseudo-peroxisomopathy
The first of two sisters was born in 1990.

*First sister:* She smiled at age 2 months, was feeding normally at 2½ months, and at 3 months was turning to voices and watching people, but she never had good muscle tone or normal head control. At age 3½ months she was admitted with altered behaviour, having stopped smiling, and poor feeding, with brief episodes of hypothermia and hypoglycaemia. She had a 'peroxisomal' look: her forehead was prominent and bossed, her anterior fontanelle large with a long metopic extension, her eyes deep-set, her mouth tent-shaped and her palate high. Head circumference at 43.5cm was over the 98th centile, but height was below the 3rd centile. There was (acquired) retinal blindness (on fundoscopy pigment clumping and thinning of the retinal pigment epithelium), profound nuchal hypotonia and diaphragmatic respiration. Hepatomegaly was gross, with large palpable kidneys.

INVESTIGATIONS (1)
*EEG* – Normal.

*Nerve conduction velocity (posterior tibial)* = 20m/s.

*ERG (gold foil)* – 90μV but amplitude decrease with dark adaptation.

*Flash VEP* – Normal.

*CSF* – Protein = 1.78g/L; glucose = 5.2mmol/L.

*Brain CT* – Moderate dilatation of ventricular system and prominent gyral pattern.

*Bone radiography* – No joint calcification, bone age 3 months = chronological age.

*Ultrasound abdomen* – Liver and kidneys enlarged.

*ECG* – Normal.

*Karyotype* – Normal female.

*Urine amino acids* – Moderate generalized aminoaciduria, no excess pipecolic acid.

*Urine organic acids* – Gross dicarboxylic aciduria, including – in mg/g creatinine – ethylmalonic 55, glutaric 1040, adipic 1605, 2-hydroxyglutaric 145, suberic 185 [GC-MS (gas chromatography–mass spectroscopy) ≡ 'mild' MADD].

*Urine bile acids by FAB-MS* – No C27 bile acids, normal infant bile acid pattern.

*Blood* – pH 7.17, base excess –12.

*Plasma:*

- *amino acids* – Generalized hypoaminoacidaemia; pipecolate 346μmol/L (gross elevation).
- *free carnitine* = 10μmol/L (normal 19–60), total 49μmol/L (normal 30–73).
- *cholesterol* = 5.2 mmol/L; vitamin E = 30.0μmol/L; phytanic acid not detected.
- *bile acids:* no C27 bile acids.

*Serum VLCFAs* – C26/22 ratio 0.017 (normal control 0–0.03).

*Platelet DHAP-AT* – Normal.

*Duodenal aspirate* – Normal infant bile acid pattern, no C27 bile acids.

*Fibroblast [9.10(n)-³H] myristic acid oxidation* – 0.71pmol/min/mg protein (normal controls 10.0–28.2, GA2 severe form 0.30, 0.90).

COURSE (1)
She died 2 days after admission.

INVESTIGATIONS (2)
*Post-mortem examination* the same day showed

- brain weight 680g, wide sulci
- liver histology: severe fatty change with vesicles and large fat droplets
- kidneys: no cysts; severe cloudy swelling with marked vesicular change in tubular epithelial cells; *no* glomerular basement membrane thickening.

COURSE (2)
It rapidly became apparent that despite her dysmorphology, neurology and hyperpipecolic acidaemia, she had glutaric aciduria type 2 (GA2) rather than a primary peroxisomopathy.

INVESTIGATIONS (3)
Fibroblast ability to dehydrogenate and decarboxylate glutaryl-CoA without added

artificial electron acceptor (with intact electron transport chain), but very low myristic acid oxidation rate, was in keeping with MADD.

*Second sister:* In a second pregnancy after high amniotic fluid glutarate was detected the mother was started on riboflavin 20mg/d throughout the last trimester. When a baby girl was born in 1993 riboflavin 50mg/d and L-carnitine 100mg/d were started immediately.

On examination aged 12 days this second baby looked very normal (as had her sister at the same age) but had slightly large-looking head (circumference 37.7cm – 98th centile), a prominent metopic suture and a degree of axial hypotonia. She was alert with visual fixation and followed well with her eyes.

At age 6 weeks visual fixation and following were still good, and she had enough head control to keep her head horizontal when held prone. Head circumference was 39.9cm, just above the 98th centile; the parents' head sizes were 1 SD and 2 SD below the mean.

INVESTIGATIONS (1)
*Karyotype* – Normal female.

*Pipecolic acid* not detected in plasma or urine.

*Urine organic acids* – Pattern as in elder sister – in mg/g creatinine: ethylmalonic 320; glutaric 710; adipic 340; L-hydroxyglutaric 330; suberic 185 – all these values being very high.

COURSE (1)
Later feeding became very difficult and she was finally floppy (totally hypotonic) and unresponsive, with an increasingly large liver. She died age 3 months.

COMMENT
Technical difficulties and the state of medical science at that time prevented full evaluation of the presumed multiple coenzyme-A dehydrogenase deficiency (MADD) or GA2. The high plasma pipecolic acid in the first sister was a novel finding that seemed to support the initial view that this was a peroxisomopathy. It is now known that pipecolic acid is also increased (though to a much lesser degree) in pyridoxine-dependent epilepsy with mutations in the *ALDH7A1* gene which encodes antiquitin.

*2.14.4 'Psychogenic' peculiar gait*
An 11-year-old girl presented with psychotic symptoms starting several weeks after a stressful event in school. She initially refused to go to school, and parents reported that she ate very little for about a month. Upon reenrolment in a different school after about a month at home, she became anxious, then confused, with apparent hallucinations, and seemed unable to walk without help. She accomplished activities of daily living very slowly and only with continuous direction. By the time of hospital admission and neurological consultation, 2 months after onset, she was disorientated with memory loss and a very unusual gait which the paediatric team and the child psychiatrists

thought was psychogenic. Her parents also thought the entire problem was due to the stress of returning to school and were amenable to psychiatric intervention. She had intermittent incontinence, both nocturnal and apparent urge incontinence during the day. She had episodes of apparent unresponsiveness to questions, without convulsive activity and without EEG changes.

On detailed neurological examination she was found to have normal cranial nerves and fundi. Strength was most likely normal, but she was hard to formally examine. Tendon jerks were very brisk at the knees with crossed adductors and clonus. She was intermittently noted to have ankle clonus, and bilateral extensor plantar (Babinski) response. Passive muscle tone was not spastic. Her gait was wide-based, very irregular and odd. She could not stand with feet together nor tandem walk, but gait varied almost moment to moment, such that without the reflex changes one might have agreed that it was psychogenic. Sensory examination was inconsistent and thought to be unreliable, but she fairly consistently did not seem to have normal position sense in the feet. She could not stand with feet together, eyes open or closed.

INVESTIGATIONS (1)
*EEG* was abnormal due to bifrontal slowing, not epileptiform.

*Brain MRI* – Normal.

*Full spine MRI* – There was symmetrical, confluent abnormal signal in the posterior columns of the spinal cord extending from C2 to C7. The posterior spinal columns demonstrated abnormal low signal on T1-weighted sequences and increased signal on T2-weighted sequences bilaterally. There was mild cord expansion and subtle diffuse enhancement of the same region. There was a small syrinx extending from C6–C7/T1. The maximum diameter of the syrinx was 3–4mm. The syrinx was not felt to be related to posterior column abnormality. The nerve roots of the cauda equina and the filum terminale were normal in size and position. The vertebral bodies and intervertebral disk spaces were well maintained.

COURSE (1)
It was now obvious this was more than psychiatric!

INVESTIGATIONS (2)
*Blood:*

- Complete blood count was unremarkable except for haemoglobin of 11.0g/dL; mean corpuscular volume was normal at 88fL

- cobalamin (vitamin $B_{12}$) level was normal (566pg/mL); folic acid level was also normal (22.9ng/mL)

- plasma total homocysteine was markedly elevated at 270μmol/mL (normal up to 10.3).

*Urine organic acids* – Methylmalonic acid 1520mmol/mol creatinine (normal <5).

COURSE (2)
She was placed on a very low protein diet. She received initially daily, then twice weekly injections of hydroxycobalamin. Despite continued elevation of methylmalonic acid and homocysteine, all neurological and psychiatric findings completely reversed. Follow-up full-spine MRI showed improvement in the findings.

COMMENT
'Psychiatric' disorders may have neurological explanations (Chapter 3.11). Close cooperation between child psychiatrists and paediatric neurologists may reduce the chance of missing rare treatable disorders (Chapter 3.23) such as the cobalamin C disorder in the girl in this vignette.

### 2.14.5 It takes time and persistence
A 9-week-old girl was referred because of failure to thrive from birth with fever, loose stools and intermittent vomiting in association with head lag and arching. Her head circumference was on the 50th centile but weight well below the 2nd centile. There was dystonic posturing of the neck and limbs, rotatory nystagmus and pigmentary retinopathy.

INVESTIGATIONS (1)
*ERG* – Absent response.

*Platelet count* – Elevated on admission, normal thereafter.

*EEG, VEP, brain CT and MRI, CSF (cells, microbiology, protein, glucose, lactate, amino acids), barium swallow and barium enema, sigmoidoscopy and rectal biopsy, TORCH, HIV, bone marrow aspirate, immunoglobulins, karyotype, amino acids (plasma and urine), ammonia, cholesterol, creatinine, electrolytes and urea, lactate, transaminases, urine sugars and organic acids, lysosomal enzymes* – Normal or negative.

*DHAP-AT in plasma* – Normal.

*VLCFAs in plasma* – Normal.

COURSE (1)
She began to thrive on a chicken-based feed followed by a cow's milk protein-free diet. At 14 months she was sitting unsupported, beginning to crawl, reaching, transferring objects and beginning to imitate. Sensorineural deafness was confirmed and mild pigmentary retinopathy persisted.

INVESTIGATIONS (2) (14mo–5y)
*Transaminases* – Mildly elevated (<100).

*Platelet DHAP-AT activity* was low, 0.74nmol/h per mg protein (control 1.20–4.70); several borderline 'normal' results were reported.

*Fibroblast DHAP-AT activity* = 0.20nmol/h per mg protein (control 3.46–5.41).

*Plasma VLCFAs* showed an increase in C26:C22 ratio at 0.23 or 0.043 (control 0.01–0.037).

*Fibroblast VLCFAs* showed an abnormal profile with an increase in C26:C22 ratio similar to plasma.

*Plasma bile acids* showed the presence of trihydrocoprostanic and dihydrocoprostanic acid and other intermediates in keeping with a defect in bile acid synthesis.

*Plasma phytanic acid* = 57mg/L (control 0.00–3.0).

COURSE (2)
The above findings were interpreted as consistent with a mild generalized peroxisomal defect.

At 18 years she has moderate learning disability, minimal ataxia, sensorineural deafness, pigmentary retinopathy and enamel hypoplasia. She is independent in all daily self-help skills.

INVESTIGATIONS (3)
*Brain MRI* showed patchy increase in signal in the deep white matter bilaterally and in the anterior thalami, corpus callosum and cerebellar white matter.

*Mutation analysis* showed that she was homozygous for the common 2528G>A mutation of the *PEX1* gene.

COMMENT
This girl had an unusually mild phenotype of a Zellweger-type generalized peroxisomal disorder. The diagnosis was delayed because of several borderline results possibly related to the intercurrent poor nutrition.

The pigmentary retinopathy and sensorineural deafness were the clues to an underlying peroxisomopathy, and the vignette illustrates that early negative results need not deflect one from pursuing a suspected diagnosis.

### 2.14.6 Arching in infancy
A boy, the first of three children born to first-cousin parents, had normal development until the age of 11 months. In the course of a fever he began arching with stiffening of the limbs, flexion of the wrists and inversion of the feet. There was eye rolling and distress without apparent loss of consciousness. The episodes lasted up to 3 hours and occurred several times daily. In between events examination was normal.

INVESTIGATIONS (1)
*EEG* – Mild slowing of the background activity.

*ERG/VEP/BAEP* – Normal.

*Brain MRI* – Abnormal high T2 and low T1 signal in the globus pallidus bilaterally.

*Haematology* – ? acanthocytes seen.

*Blood* – Ammonia, transaminases, creatine kinase, lactate, amino acids, lysosomal enzymes and lipoproteins all normal.

*CSF* – Lactate, protein, glucose, cell count and microscopy all normal.

Course (1)
A specific cause for the paroxysmal events was not found. The possibility of Hallervorden–Spatz disease was raised but the imaging features were considered atypical. There was no response to therapeutic trials of levodopa, benzhexol or carbamazepine. Developmental progress slowed down but new skills were acquired all along.

Investigations (2) (age 6½ years)
*EEG* showed slowing of the background without any spike discharges.

*Brain MRI* showed similar changes to those seen on the initial scan at age 18 months. There was no change in the appearance and extent of the signal abnormality.

*Blood film* – Normal (*no* acanthocytes).

*Genetics* – PANK2 mutation analysis negative.

*Blood* – Urea, electrolytes, acid base status, creatine kinase, ammonia, uric acid, lactate, transaminases, $B_{12}$, ceruloplasmin, copper, carnitine and acylcarnitine, VLCFAs, transferrin isoforms, biotinidase were normal.

*Urine* – Amino acids and organic acids were normal.

*CSF* – Glucose (including CSF/blood glucose ratio), protein, lactate, amino acids and amine metabolites were normal.

*Muscle histology, electronmicroscopy and respiratory chain enzyme analysis* were normal.

*Fibroblast PDH activity* was reduced at 0.35nmol/mg protein/min (normal controls 0.7–1.1).

*Molecular analysis* showed that the patient was homozygous for a missense mutation in the *DLAT* gene encoding dihydrolipoamide acetyltransferase, the E2 core component of the PDH complex. His parents were heterozygous for this mutation. Functional complementation studies confirmed that the mutation was the cause of the PDH deficiency. At 11 years the episodic dystonia rarely occurs. A ketogenic diet was not implemented for family reasons. He is thriving and making good progress on lipoic acid and thiamine supplementation.

Comment
This patient had the relatively rare presentation of PDH deficiency, namely paroxysmal dystonia. The CSF lactate was unexpectedly normal but the MRI changes strongly suggested a metabolic basis.

## Further reading

Basheer SN, Waters PJ, Lam CW. (2007) Isolated sulfite oxidase deficiency in the newborn: lactic acidaemia and leukoencephalopathy. *Neuropediatrics* **38**: 38–41.

Debray FG, Lambert M, Mitchell GA. (2008) Disorders of mitochondrial function. *Curr Opin Pediatr* **20**: 471–482.

Deconinck N, Messaaoui A, Ziereisen F, et al. (2008) Metachromatic leukodystrophy without arylsulfatase A deficiency: a new case of saposin-B deficiency. *Eur J Paediatr Neurol* 12: 46–50.

de Koning TJ, Klomp LW. (2004) Serine-deficiency syndromes. *Curr Opin Neurol* 17: 197–204.

DiMauro S, Schon EA. (2008) Mitochondrial disorders in the nervous system. *Annu Rev Neurosci* 31: 91–123.

Djukic A. (2007) Folate-responsive neurologic diseases. *Pediatr Neurol* 37: 387–397.

Erol I, Alehan F, Gümüs A. (2007) West syndrome in an infant with vitamin B12 deficiency in the absence of macrocytic anaemia. *Dev Med Child Neurol* 49: 774–776.

Ferdinandusse S, van Grunsven EG, Oostheim W, et al. (2002) Reinvestigation of peroxisomal 3-ketoacyl-CoA thiolase deficiency: identification of the true defect at the level of d-bifunctional protein. *Am J Hum Genet* 70: 1589–1593.

Ferdinandusse S, Denis S, Mooyer PA, et al. (2006) Clinical and biochemical spectrum of D-bifunctional protein deficiency. *Ann Neurol* 59: 92–104.

Grattan-Smith PJ, Wilcken B, Procopis PG, et al. (1997) The neurological syndrome of infantile cobalamin deficiency: developmental regression and involuntary movements. *Mov Disord* 12: 39–46.

Grossi S, Regis S, Rosano C, et al. (2008) Molecular analysis of ARSA and PSAP genes in twenty-one Italian patients with metachromatic leukodystrophy: identification and functional characterization of 11 novel ARSA alleles. *Hum Mutat* 29: E220–E230.

Grünewald S. (2007) Congenital disorders of glycosylation: rapidly enlarging group of (neuro)metabolic disorders. *Early Hum Dev* 83: 825–830.

Haas D, Kelley RI, Hoffmann GF. (2001) Inherited disorders of cholesterol biosynthesis. *Neuropediatrics* 32: 113–122.

Hass RH, Parikh S, Falk MJ, et al. (2007) Mitochondrial disease: a practical approach for primary care physicians. *Pediatrics* 120: 1326–1333.

Haas RH, Parikh S, Falk MJ, et al. (2008) The in-depth evaluation of suspected mitochondrial disease. *Mol Genet Metab* 94: 16–37.

Hart CE, Race V, Achouri Y, et al. (2007) Phosphoserine aminotransferase deficiency: a novel disorder of the serine biosynthesis pathway. *Am J Hum Genet* 80: 931–937.

Horstmann M, Neumaier-Probst E, Lukacs Z, et al. (2003) Infantile cobalamin deficiency with cerebral lactate accumulation and sustained choline depletion. *Neuropediatrics* 34: 261–264.

Huck JH, Verhoeven NM, van Hagen JM, et al. (2004) Clinical presentations of patients with polyol abnormalities. *Neuropediatrics* 35: 167–173.

Jaeken J, Matthijs G. (2007) Congenital disorders of glycosylation: a rapidly expanding disease family. *Annu Rev Genomics Hum Genet* 8: 261–278.

Jurecka A, Zikanova M, Tylki-Szymanska A, et al. (2008) Clinical, biochemical and molecular findings in seven Polish patients with adenylosuccinate lyase deficiency. *Mol Genet Metab* 94: 435–442.

Jones CM, Smith M, Henderson MJ. (2006) Reference data for cerebrospinal fluid and the utility of amino acid measurement for the diagnosis of inborn errors of metabolism. *Ann Clin Biochem* 43: 63–66.

Khayat M, Korman SH, Frankel P, et al. (2008) PNPO deficiency: an under diagnosed inborn error of pyridoxine metabolism. *Mol Genet Metab* 94: 431–434.

Klepper J, Leiendecker B. (2007) GLUT1 deficiency syndrome – 2007 update. *Dev Med Child Neurol* 49: 707–716.

Koch H. (1998) Dipsticks and convulsions. *Lancet* 352: 1824.

Kure S, Korman SH, Kanno J, et al. (2006) Rapid diagnosis of glycine encephalopathy by 13C-glycine breath test. *Ann Neurol* 59: 862–866.

Lang TF, Parr JR, Matthews EE, et al. (2008) Practical difficulties in the diagnosis of transient non-ketotic hyperglycinaemia. *Dev Med Child Neurol* **50**: 157–159.

Lundy CT, Ward P, Doherty GM, et al. (2007) Should creatine kinase be checked in all boys presenting with speech delay? *Arch Dis Child* **92**: 647–649.

Maj MC, Cameron JM, Robinson BH. (2006) Pyruvate dehydrogenase phosphatase deficiency: orphan disease or an under–diagnosed condition? *Mol Cell Endocrinol* **25**: 1–9.

Matsuo M, Tasaki R, Kodama H, Hamasaki Y. (2005) Screening for Menkes disease using the urine HVA/VMA ratio. *J Inherit Metab Dis* **28**: 89–93.

Mercimek-Mahmutoglu S, Stoeckler-Ipsiroglu S, Adami A, et al. (2006) GAMT deficiency: features, treatment, and outcome in an inborn error of creatine synthesis. *Neurology* **67**: 480–484.

Montero R, Sánchez-Alcázar JA, Briones P, et al. (2008) Analysis of coenzyme Q10 in muscle and fibroblasts for the diagnosis of CoQ10 deficiency syndromes. *Clin Biochem* **41**: 697–700.

Moretti P, Sahoo T, Hyland K, et al. (2005) Cerebral folate deficiency with developmental delay, autism, and response to folinic acid. *Neurology* **64**: 1088–1090.

Ormazabal A, Oppenheim M, Serrano M, et al. (2008) Pyridoxal 5´-phosphate values in cerebrospinal fluid: reference values and diagnosis of PNPO deficiency in paediatric patients. *Mol Genet Metab* **94**: 173–177.

Papadimitriou A, Dumitrescu AM, Papavasiliou A, et al. (2008) A novel monocarboxylate transporter 8 gene mutation as a cause of severe neonatal hypotonia and developmental delay. *Pediatrics* **121**: 199–202.

Ramaekers VT, Blau N. (2004) Cerebral folate deficiency. *Dev Med Child Neurol* **46**: 843–851.

Rass U, Ahel I, West SC. (2007) Defective DNA repair and neurodegenerative disease. *Cell* **130**: 991–1004.

Rötig A, Mollet J, Rio M, et al. (2007) Infantile and pediatric quinone deficiency diseases. *Mitochondrion* **7**: S112–121.

Saunders-Pullman R, Blau N, Hyland K, et al. (2004) Phenylalanine loading as a diagnostic test for DRD: interpreting the utility of the test. *Mol Genet Metab* **83**: 207–212.

Smith W, Kishnani PS, Lee B, et al. (2005) Urea cycle disorders: clinical presentation outside the newborn period. *Crit Care Clin* **21**: S9–S17.

Strassburg HM, Koch J, Mayr J. (2006) Acute flaccid paralysis as initial symptom in 4 patients with novel E1alpha mutations of the pyruvate dehydrogenase complex. *Neuropediatrics* **37**: 137–141.

Verbeek MM, Blom AM, Wevers RA, et al. (2008) Technical and biochemical factors affecting cerebrospinal fluid 5-MTHF, biopterin and neopterin concentrations. *Mol Genet Metab* **95**: 127–132.

Vanderver A, Hathout Y, Maletkovic J, et al. (2008) Sensitivity and specificity of decreased CSF asialotransferrin for eIF2B-related disorder. *Neurology* **70**: 2226–2232.

Vaurs-Barrière C, Deville M, Sarret C, et al. (2009) Pelizaeus–Merzbacher-like disease presentation of MCT8 mutated male subjects. *Ann Neurol* **65**: 114–118.

Wanders RJ, van Roermund CW, Schelen A, et al. (1990) A bifunctional protein with deficient enzymic activity: identification of a new peroxisomal disorder using novel methods to measure the peroxisomal beta-oxidation enzyme activities. *J Inherit Metab Dis* **13**: 375–379.

Wiltshire E, Davidzon G, DiMauro S, et al. (2008) Juvenile Alpers disease. *Arch Neurol* **65**: 121–124.

Wolf NI, Smeitink JA. (2002) Mitochondrial disorders: a proposal for consensus diagnostic criteria in infants and children. *Neurology* **59**: 1402–1405.

Wolf NI, Rahman S, Schmitt B, et al. (2008) Status epilepticus in children with Alpers' disease caused by POLG1 mutations: EEG and MRI features. *Epilepsia* **6**: 1596–1607.

# Chapter 2.15
# Antiepileptic Drug Monitoring

Adequate therapeutic effect without toxicity is often helped by monitoring the concentrations of antiepileptic drugs (AEDs) in body fluids. The wise use of these levels needs more than the data provided in tables of so-called therapeutic ranges. This chapter gives a very brief guide to principles.

*Reference ranges* for AEDs are probabilistic ranges of blood (or saliva) concentration that have been determined in populations, usually adults, as an attempt to guide clinicians. The so-called optimal levels are sometimes called 'normal' but of course this is impossible – the only normal value for any of these drugs is zero.

*Therapeutic range* is not a term to be recommended. A *therapeutic level* can only be determined in an individual. It is the concentration of the drug in body fluids below which epileptic seizures may recur and above which epileptic seizures are prevented. A drug which has these properties is described as level-dependent. The therapeutic level for any drug will certainly vary between one person and another and between one seizure type and another. Thus, if an individual has more than one type of seizure, then for a particular drug the therapeutic level for one seizure may be considerably higher than that for the other.

*Toxic level.* The so-called toxic level for a given drug also varies between individuals. Although it may be at a level suggested in published tables, it may on occasion be considerably lower or higher. If in an individual with a particular type of seizure a toxic level is reached without abolition of the seizures, then no therapeutic level can be obtained. On the other hand if the toxic level for a given drug is higher than usual in a particular individual with an apparently resistant epileptic seizure type, then it may be possible to reach a therapeutic level which is above the usual 'reference range'.

*Level-dependent drugs.* Phenytoin, which has nonlinear kinetics, is the most precisely level-dependent drug, both with respect to its antiepileptic properties and its toxicity, bearing in mind that the therapeutic level and the toxic level will vary from patient to patient and from seizure to seizure. Other drugs in which level measurements may be to some extent useful include phenobarbitone, carbamazepine, ethosuximide, lamotrigine, and sodium valproate.

*Saliva* is a convenient fluid for measurement of phenytoin, lamotrigine and ethosuximide in particular and may be obtained from infancy onwards without the use of citric acid (which has been blamed for errors in drug measurement). Some children, however, actually prefer giving a sample of blood to spitting into a container.

## Co-studies in children on antiepileptic drugs

Drug companies may advise monitoring blood counts and liver function studies in children on antiepileptic therapy but there seems to be no evidence to support such recommendations.

Although sodium valproate may precipitate hepatic decompensation in some children with *POLG1* mutations, there are no easily available investigations to predict who will be affected: when to give or not to give valproate must be a clinical decision.

## Summary

Time and money should not be wasted in monitoring drug levels when this is not helpful. However, when monitoring is necessary the laboratory must be prepared to perform frequent analyses, accept saliva when appropriate, and provide answers within hours rather than days.

## Clinical vignette

### 2.15.1 No therapeutic level possible

An infant began to jerk on the third day of life. Flurries of apparent flexion myoclonus involved one or more limbs, often all four. These runs lasted up to 30 minutes.

INVESTIGATION (1)
*Interictal EEG* – Normal.

COURSE (1)
Epilepsy was diagnosed and phenytoin prescribed. The jerks were refractory and the dose increased.

INVESTIGATION (2)
*Phenytoin levels* exceeded the 'therapeutic range'.

COURSE (2)
The myoclonus became worse but the treatment was continued.

INVESTIGATION (3)
*Brain imaging* at follow-up showed a small cerebellum.

COURSE (3)
On further review it was found that the myoclonus had occurred only in sleep. When phenytoin was discontinued the jerking soon stopped also.

COMMENT
Benign neonatal sleep myoclonus is common and is harmless unless the infant comes under the care of a physician who does not recognize it. If AEDs have any effect it is to make it worse. Although in this case serial imaging studies were not done to distinguish cerebellar atrophy from hypoplasia, phenytoin levels were high and phenytoin is known to have the potential to induce cerebellar atrophy.

If phenytoin is used levels should be monitored very frequently, preferably by saliva, but of course this was not appropriate here. The only neurological investigation that might have helped would have been a home video to show to someone familiar with benign neonatal sleep myoclonus.

## Further reading

Johannessen SI, Patsalos PN, Tomson T, Perucca E. (2008) Therapeutic drug monitoring. In: Engel J, Pedley TA, eds. *Epilepsy. A Comprehensive Textbook. 2nd edn.* Philadelphia: Lippincott, Williams & Wilkins, pp. 1171–1183.

Kozer E, Scolnik D, Agamata WM, et al. (2003) Utility of antiepileptic drug monitoring in the pediatric emergency department. *Ther Drug Monit* 25: 17–21.

Lowry JA, Vandover JC, Degreeff J, Scalzo AJ. (2005) Unusual presentation of iatrogenic phenytoin toxicity in a newborn. *J Med Toxicol* 1: 26–29.

Macleod S, Appleton R. (2007) The new antiepileptic drugs. *Arch Dis Child Educ Pract Ed* 92: 182–188.

Malone SA, Eadie MJ, Addison RS, et al. (2006) Monitoring salivary lamotrigine concentrations. *J Clin Neurosci* 13: 902–907.

Paro-Panjan D, Neubauer D. (2008) Benign neonatal sleep myoclonus: experience from the study of 38 infants. *Eur J Paediatr Neurol* 12: 14–18.

Patsalos PN, Berry DJ, Bourgeois BF, et al. (2008) Antiepileptic drugs—best practice guidelines for therapeutic drug monitoring: a position paper by the subcommission on therapeutic drug monitoring, ILAE Commission on Therapeutic Strategies. *Epilepsia* 49: 1239–1276.

# Chapter 2.16

## Diagnosis by Therapeutic Trial

An important part of neurological investigation is the diagnostic therapeutic trial, especially if a positive response allows sustained improvement. Table 2.16.1 lists some of the more important diagnostic trials in which the administered agent is more or less specific.

A word is in order about the use of levodopa, the effect of which seems 'miraculous' in classical Segawa-type dopa-responsive dystonia. We advise caution and the verification of the CSF monoamine neurotransmitter metabolites (together with all the appropriate pterin studies) in *atypical* cases *before* levodopa is started to avoid incomplete diagnosis.

We had to make a decision on what to include in the table. Quinidine does not make it into the list, although the evidence is compelling that it could be used in this way for the diagnosis of slow channel syndrome, an anticholinesterase inhibitor-resistant form of congenital myasthenia.

Therapeutic trials of antiepileptic drugs (AEDs) are *not* to be recommended as part of the diagnosis of epilepsy and indeed this practice may sometimes be dangerous in the extreme (see Clinical Vignette 2.2.2).

### Clinical vignettes

#### 2.16.1 Polymorphous epilepsy cured
A boy presented aged 14½ months with bout epilepsy (clusters of epileptic seizures with seizure-free interludes). His multiple seizure types included generalized shaking, turning to the right or to the left, myoclonic jerks, some sort of jerking of his hand, going stiff with his head locked round (his parents' description) and stares. His development had been previously normal but his behaviour had regressed. His family history was negative and his parents were not consanguineous.

Table 2.16.1 Therapeutic trials

| Test drug | Indications | Precautions | Interpretation |
|---|---|---|---|
| Acetazolamide | Episodic ataxia with long bouts and eye movement disorder | Daily oral dose (depends on age) | Episodes usually cease in episodic ataxia type 2 (EA2) |
| Biotin | Developmental delay, brainstem and spinal cord lesions, seizures ± rash, encephalopathy, characteristic urine organic acids | Oral 10mg daily for 1 week – continue if symptoms remit | Biotinidase deficiency: confirm by enzyme assay (no need to stop biotin) Biotin transporter defect |
| | Rapid regression, dystonia, akinesis, MRI 'necrosis' in caudate and putamen | Oral 10mg/kg/dose t.i.d. | Biotin-responsive basal ganglia disorder |
| Edrophonium | Floppy neonate, suspected myasthenia | Video procedure. Beware phenotypes suggestive of COLQ, DOK7 or slow-channel syndromes (may exacerbate) | Most myasthenia. Neostigmine 0.1mg/kg i.m.+ atropine allows longer evaluation |

Table 2.16.1 continued

| Test | Indications | Precautions | Interpretation |
|---|---|---|---|
| Folinic acid | Intractable neonatal epileptic seizures | Oral 5mg two doses 6h apart | Folinic acid-responsive seizures (are the same as pyridoxine-dependent epilepsy but not clear if distinct from pyridoxal phosphate-responsive seizures) |
| Levodopa (as co-careldopa) | 'Toe-walking', 'spastic diplegia', dystonia, especially if diurnal variation | Estimate CSF monoamines and pterins before trial if any doubt that it is pure Segawa disease. Start low dose, e.g. 12.5mg/d (with carbidopa). In older children with dystonia give maximum tolerated dose up to 10mg levodopa/kg/d divided into at least four doses for at least 3 months | Disappearance of dystonia indicates Segawa disease. Re other dopa-responsive disorders, see text and Chapter 3.7 |
| Pyridostigmine | Floppy neonate, unexplained apnoea, contractures, suspected myasthenia | Video control desirable. Perform in hospital. Beware phenotypes suggestive of COLQ, DOK7 or slow-channel syndromes (may exacerbate) | Remission indicates myasthenia, most varieties |

Table 2.16.1 continued

| Test | Indications | Precautions | Interpretation |
|---|---|---|---|
| Pyridoxal-5′-phosphate | Neonatal epileptic seizures not due to correctable causes. EEG often suppression–burst | Pyridoxal-5′-phosphate oral 10mg/kg/dose, two doses 2h apart, with or without EEG control (if no response give folinic acid two 5mg doses 6h apart) | Cessation of seizures indicates either pyridoxine dependent epilepsy (PDE) – ↑ α-AASA and pipecolic acid in body fluids – or pyridoxal phosphate-responsive epilepsy – ↓ PNPO in lymphocytes |
| Pyridoxine | Neonatal epileptic seizures including tonic–clonic not due to correctable causes. EEG often suppression–burst | 100mg pyridoxine i.v. while EEG running: have naloxone available in case of opioid reaction | EEG normalization = PDE: confirm by ↑ α-AASA and pipecolic acid in body fluids while continuing oral pyridoxine |
| | Intractable epilepsy (including SCN1A- negative) up to age 3y | 100mg/d oral (not known if oral pyridoxal phosphate should be used in these circumstances) | Cessation of epilepsy indicates late-onset PDE. Confirm by ↑ α-AASA and pipecolic acid in body fluids while continuing oral pyridoxine |

INVESTIGATIONS (1)
Two routine EEGs contained some ongoing 3–4Hz activity postcentrally and some excess EMG activity but with no paroxysmal features. Occasional jerks of the fingers of his left hand were not associated with any definite EEG change.

COURSE (1)
Seizures continued, with bouts of 4–5 seizures at a time.

INVESTIGATIONS (2)
*24-hour EEG age 16 months* included in the parental tape diary: "agitated, restless, moaning, head turning to right, mouth twisting, intermittent jerking of body and limbs, eyes moving in jerks, staring, lips blue, mouth open, right hand twitching." Prolonged runs of alternately lateralized irregular fast spiking were predominant over the right or the left hemisphere intermittently, but the electroclinical correlation was difficult to establish (video was not available).

*Brain MRI (1.5T)* – Normal.

COURSE (2)
Seizures continued despite various AEDs, but head circumference growth was normal and on his father's percentile curve.

INVESTIGATIONS (3)
Pyridoxine 50mg/d was started age 18 months.

COURSE (3)
He became seizure-free immediately, but since lamotrigine was also started at the same time there was a delay in establishing the pyridoxine effect. Age 19 months pyridoxine was stopped and he had a seizure with generalized shaking 18 days later. Pyridoxine was restarted and other AEDs were tailed off completely until he was on pyridoxine alone age 24 months. Four weeks later pyridoxine was stopped for the second time and a seizure recurred 14 days later. Pyridoxine was restarted and he became seizure free again. After a third withdrawal and seizure relapse he was put onto pyridoxine long term with no recurrence of epileptic seizures.

INVESTIGATIONS (4)
*Plasma pipecolic acid* (age 10 years, on pyridoxine 50mg/d) 3.4µmol/L (control, Bok et al. 2007: ≤2.46µmol/L).

*Urine α-aminoadipic semialdehyde (α-AASA)* at age 10 years was 1.3mmol/mol creatinine (control, Bok et al. 2007: ≤1mmol/mol creatinine).

*Mutation analysis* of *antiquitin* gene revealed a missense mutation in exon 6 of one allele, but to date a mutation has not been found in the other allele.

COURSE (4)
He remains seizure free on pyridoxine 100mg/d. Although earlier he had autistic features these resolved and he is now at mainstream school with mild learning disability.

COMMENT

This vignette illustrates some of the difficulties in the investigation and diagnosis of late-onset pyridoxine-dependent epilepsy (PDE). This child with atypical drug-resistant epilepsy and unusual EEG fulfilled the Baxter criteria for definite PDE with prompt response to pyridoxine and relapse on withdrawal (twice – in his case, thrice), but elevations of plasma pipecolic acid and urinary α-AASA were only modest. Pyridoxine trial was here a more robust diagnostic tool than molecular genetics. The prevalence of late-onset PDE is not known nor indeed is the upper age limit for a therapeutic trial of pyridoxine or pyridoxal phosphate.

### 2.16.2 Walking unsteadily to a diagnosis

A girl, the first child of healthy unrelated parents was referred at the age of 4½ years because of an abnormal gait. She walked at 16 months and had normal cognitive and language development. Around the age of 2 years she became unsteady with frequent falls and inversion of both feet, particularly on the right side. The symptoms were progressive and there was poor exercise tolerance. She was thought to have weakness of dorsiflexion with intact tendon reflexes and otherwise normal examination.

INVESTIGATIONS (1)

*EMG and nerve conduction studies* – Normal.

*Brain CT and MRI* – Normal.

*Molecular genetic testing* for HMSN1a, Friedreich ataxia and spinocerebellar ataxia types 1, 2, 3 and 6 – Negative.

*Blood* – Lactate, creatine kinase, cholesterol, triglycerides, liver and thyroid function tests, amino acid lysosomal enzymes, phytanic acid, all normal.

*Urine* – Amino acids and organic acids normal.

COURSE (1)

There was gradual deterioration over the following 3 years with the child requiring a wheelchair for walking any distance. Orthoses were provided for her feet.

INVESTIGATIONS (2)

*Gait analysis* suggested an underlying diplegic pattern

*Fibroblast cytochrome oxidase assay and beta oxidation of fatty acids* – Normal.

COURSE (2)

Between the ages of 7 and 8 years there was marked deterioration in her gait and mobility to the extent that she was unable to sit unsupported or use a walker and required a wheelchair. Her handwriting became illegible.

INVESTIGATIONS (3)

A trial of levodopa 25mg/carbidopa 6.25mg three times daily was administered. There was an immediate response and within 1 week she was considered normal.

COURSE (3)
Following withdrawal of the levodopa/carbidopa for CSF studies there was a dramatic deterioration within days.

INVESTIGATIONS (4)
*CSF neurotransmitters* showed low homovanillic acid at 102nmol/L (233–928) and 5-hydroxyindole acetic acid at 39nmol/L (normal for age 74–345). (It was commented that she had been on levodopa/carbidopa intermittently up to 2 days preceding the lumbar puncture because at the time of the study *age-related* reference intervals were not known for these monoamine metabolites.)

*Phenylalanine loading test* showed no obvious inhibition of conversion of phenylalanine to tyrosine, with maximum phenylalanine/tyrosine ratio of 7.2 at a plasma phenylalanine level of 740µmol/L (normal).

*Molecular genetic analysis* for mutations in the coding sequence of the *GCH1* gene showed her to be a heterozygote for a known pathogenic mutation.

COURSE (4)
Six years later at 14 years she is neurologically unimpaired on low-strength levodopa/carbidopa.

COMMENT
The very slow deterioration seen in this girl is typical for the Segawa-type dopa-responsive dystonia with defective guanosine triphosphate cyclohydrolase (GTP-CH). Diurnal fluctuation was not reported. The three recognized causes of dopa-responsive dystonia are GTP-CH deficiency, tyrosine hydroxylase deficiency and sepiapterin reductase deficiency. GTP-CH 1 (GCH1) deficiency is the most common in the British Isles.

A trial of levodopa is indicated in unexplained gait disorder of this type. While our recommendation is that in *atypical* cases CSF neurotransmitter and pterin studies should be undertaken *before* the levodopa trial, there is an argument for doing the therapeutic trial first, *provided that* the family know that, should the levodopa trial be positive, the drug will be withdrawn and CSF studies done before gene analysis and lifelong treatment recommendations.

## Further reading

Bok LA, Struys E, Willemsen MA, et al. (2007) Pyridoxine-dependent seizures in Dutch patients: diagnosis by elevated urinary alpha-aminoadipic semialdehyde levels. *Arch Dis Child* 92: 687–689.

Gallagher RC, Van Hove JL, Scharer G, et al. (2009) Folinic acid-responsive seizures are identical to pyridoxine-dependent epilepsy. *Ann Neurol* 65: 550–556.

Harper CM, Engel AG. (1998) Quinidine sulfate therapy for the slow-channel congenital myasthenic syndrome. *Ann Neurol* 43: 480–484.

Surtees R, Wolf N. (2007) Treatable neonatal epilepsy. *Arch Dis Child* 92: 659–661.

# Chapter 3.1
## Neonatal Seizures

Paroxysmal events are common in the neonate. It is not always easy to tell if these episodes are epileptic seizures because EEG discharges may not always be seen in epileptic seizures at this age.

### Non-epileptic events

*Benign neonatal sleep myoclonus*
If the physician is not able to observe an episode of this common condition then simple video recording (Chapter 2.1) is the only necessary investigation. If home videocamera or mobile phone filming is not possible, then the parents may be shown video recordings of known examples to confirm, "That's it." Flurries of multiple flexion jerks in long runs are seen in sleep. EEG is not indicated but if ictal EEG is carried out it is most important to avoid misinterpreting rhythmic artefacts as epileptic discharges. Bear in mind that as with other non-epileptic events (see Chapter 3.14) benign neonatal sleep myoclonus may be seen in newborn infants who are not entirely 'normal', and is common in neonatal abstinence syndrome.

*Hyperekplexia*
In a neonate with some combination of tremulousness, stiffness, and cyanotic attacks (with high voltage runs of EMG 'artefact' on ictal EEG and ECG traces – see Fig 1.1) and with head retraction on tapping the tip of the nose and auditory startle, then DNA for analysis in a specialized laboratory is indicated. Most cases are due to mutations in the gene for the alpha subunit of the strychnine-sensitive glycine receptor (*GLRA1*) or in that for GlyT2, the postsynaptic glycine transporter (*SLC6A5*).

*Paroxysmal extreme pain disorder*
Video recording of the paroxysmal autonomic manifestations, in particular the

Harlequin sign, may be helpful to share with others experienced in this disorder. SCN9A mutations may be analysed in a specialized laboratory.

## Seizures (of presumed epileptic mechanism)

Initial investigations by a neonatologist will depend upon the clinical scenario. Cranial ultrasound will detect gross structural lesions. MRI will detect more, including the acute cerebral ischaemia (arterial or venous) most easily seen with diffusion-weighted imaging (DWI). When a cause is not thereby apparent then further investigations will be necessary, often simultaneously performed. What we say below refers to difficult, refractory, unexplained seizures of epileptic type.

### Early investigations for rare treatable disorders (see also Chapter 3.23)

*Pyridoxal phosphate trial (Chapters 2.16, 3.23)*
Cessation of seizures will indicate either pyridoxal phosphate responsiveness or pyridoxine-dependent epilepsy. Confirmation of pyridoxine-dependent epilepsy will be by finding α-AASA in blood and urine, followed by mutation analysis of the *ALDH7A1* (antiquitin) gene. In pyridoxal-5′-phosphate-responsive seizures due to pyridox(am)ine phosphate oxidase (PNPO) deficiency there may be elevated threonine and glycine in plasma and CSF (and possibly reduced CSF homovanillic acid and 5-hydroxyindole acetic acid). CSF pyridoxal-5′-phosphate will also be reduced. Confirmation is by mutation analysis of the *PNPO* gene.

*GLUT1 (glucose transporter 1) deficiency*
To recognize GLUT1 deficiency investigations should be carried out just before a feed is due. Blood is best taken for glucose estimation immediately before CSF glucose is measured. In the absence of infection or haemorrhage, a CSF/plasma glucose ratio <0.5 is strongly suggestive of GLUT1 deficiency. This diagnosis may be confirmed by mutation analysis and/or erythrocyte uptake studies at a specialized laboratory.

*Cerebral creatine disorders*
An absent creatine peak on H-MRS is diagnostic of a creatine deficiency syndrome such as GAMT or AGAT deficiency. (H-MRS may also show increased glycine in glycine encephalopathy and increased lactate in mitochondrial disorders, but therapeutic options in these disorders are limited.)

*Serine biosynthesis disorders*
Disorders of each of the enzymes involved in the serine biosynthesis pathway have been described, of which phosphoserine amino transferase deficiency might be the most potentially treatable. The essential investigation is estimation of the CSF serine and glycine level, after such fasting as can be tolerated (before a feed).

*Investigations for less obvious diagnoses*
A number of investigations may be done in parallel when common conditions have

been dealt with and rare treatable disorders eliminated.

ELECTROENCEPHALOGRAPHY

A normal-for-gestational-age interictal EEG is of little help in diagnosis, and various abnormalities are also nonspecific. Beyond early preterm birth and in the absence of severe asphyxia, a suppression–burst pattern (in which a 'flat' or isoelectric trace is interrupted by brief high-voltage discharges) suggests the following:

1. Glycine encephalopathy

2. Pyridoxine-dependent or pyridoxal phosphate-responsive epilepsy

3. 'Ohtahara syndrome' (inverted commas indicate that an underlying primary diagnosis should still be sought).

Table 3.1.1 summarizes the various known associations of neonatal suppresson–burst EEG.

BRAIN IMAGING

Although many structural malformations, especially cortical dysplasia, are epileptogenic, the finding of structural abnormality on brain imaging does not exclude a metabolic explanation for neonatal seizures. The following imaging features may be clues to metabolic disorders.

- *Basal ganglia/thalamic lesions:*
  mitochondrial disorders, creatine synthesis defects.

- *Cystic encephalomalacia or localized infarction:*
  sulphite oxidase deficiency, mitochondrial disorder.

- *Cerebellar or pontocerebellar hypoplasia:*
  congenital defect of glycosylation/mitochondrial disorder.

- *Cortical dysplasia/neuronal heterotopia:*
  peroxisomopathies, mitochondrial disorders, molybdenum cofactor deficiency.

- *White matter abnormalities:*
  peroxisomal and mitochondrial disorders, organic acidaemias, aminoacidopathies.

- *Agenesis of the corpus callosum:*
  many metabolic disorders, including glycine encephalopathy, pyruvate dehydrogenase and pyruvate decarboxylase deficiency, early-onset mitochondrial OXPHOS (oxidative phosphorylation) disorders.

- *Pericerebral or subdural collections:*
  glutaric aciduria type 1, Menkes disease.

BRAIN H-MRS

We give a separate heading for H-MRS to emphasize that if possible this should be done at the same time as MRI to aid detection of some of the metabolic disorders listed above.

Table 3.1.1 Neonatal burst–suppression EEG

| Condition | Comments |
|---|---|
| Normal preterm birth | Especially <28 weeks |
| Term asphyxia | Common, probably overdiagnosed |
| Overwhelming brain infection | Beta-haemolytic streptococcus |
| Malformations | Especially brainstem |
| *ARX* mutation | Pure neurological disorder. Not all boys. No metabolic clues. Abnormal male genitalia only with lissencephaly or other malformation (corpus callosum agenesis, hydranencephaly) |
| Pyridoxine-dependent epilepsy | Mother may report prenatal seizures, responds to pyridoxine or pyridoxal-5′-phosphate |
| Pyridoxal-5′-phosphate responsive epilepsy | Responds to pyridoxal-5′-phosphate. Biochemical tests later |
| Menkes disease | Low serum copper and ceruloplasmin. Low plasma catecholamines |
| Mitochondrial glutamate *SLC25A22* mutation | Pure neurological disorder. No metabolic clues |
| Epileptic encephalopathy ('Ohtahara syndrome') | Hindbrain abnormalities reported at autopsy |
| Glycine encephalopathy (NKH) | Mother may report prenatal seizures, elevated CSF:plasma glycine ratio |
| Molybdenum cofactor deficiency | Positive fresh urine sulphite test. Low plasma uric acid |
| Isolated sulphite oxidase deficiency | Positive fresh urine, sulphite test. Low plasma total homocysteine |
| Purine synthesis disorder | Succinylpurines: urine, plasma, CSF |

## Biochemical investigations beyond 'metabolic screen'

The philosophy of this book is not to recommend 'screens', but most neonatal units carry out 'full' baseline metabolic investigations:

*Blood:* urea and electrolytes including calcium, magnesium and phosphorus, creatinine, liver function tests, ammonia, uric acid, lactate, amino acids, creatine kinase

*Urine:* amino acids, organic acids and sulphite.

Further investigations are prompted by the clinical features together with results of EEG and brain imaging and the results of basic biochemistry.

*Glycine encephalopathy*
Particularly in the context of suppression–burst EEG, blood and CSF glycine are measured simultaneously. In glycine encephalopathy the CSF:plasma glycine ratio is ≥0.1 (normal ≤0.025).

*Mitochondrial disorder*
Elevation of blood or CSF lactate or the finding of a lactate peak on H-MRS strongly point to a mitochondrial disorder and will lead to specialized mitochondrial studies (Chapter 2.14).

*Peroxisomal disorders*
A clinical phenotype with multisystem involvement plus nonspecific findings of disturbed liver function or calcific stippling on radiography may point to a peroxisomal disorder and measurement of very long chain fatty acids and other peroxisomal markers (see Chapter 2.14).

*Congenital defect of glycosylation (CDG)*
Multisystem involvement, nonspecific abnormalities of liver function, creatine kinase, etc. will prompt measurement of sialotransferrin (Chapter 2.14).

*Molybdenum cofactor deficiency – isolated sulphite oxidase deficiency*
Multicystic encephalomalacia on imaging with or without other brain malformation will prompt estimation of uric acid (low in molybdenum cofactor deficiency) and total plasma homocysteine (low in isolated sulphite oxidase deficiency). For the urine sulphite test to have a chance of being positive the sample must be tested immediately, but true false negatives (and false postives) have been reported, so specific analysis of uric acid and total plasma homocysteine are mandatory.

## Genetic studies

*Chromosomal studies*
Karyotyping would have been carried out in any undiagnosed neurological disorder. Various ring chromosome abnormalities should be sought in unexplained refractory seizures. Special tests for 1p36 (see Chapter 2.13) are worth pursuing.

*Single gene targeted investigations*
Although it may not have a major impact on management, the detection of mutations or submicroscopic deletions or duplications or one of the epilepsy genes may be helpful

to families. Such genes include *KCNQ2* in benign familial neonatal seizures and *SCN2A* in benign neonatal infantile seizures.

*Collagen gene mutations in apparent traumatic brain damage*
The presence of perinatal cerebral haemorrhage ± *porencephaly* may reflect pathogenic mutations in the collagen 4 alpha-1 gene (*COL4A1*). Brain MRI of a parent may show leukoencephalopathy and/or silent microhaemorrhages (need echo-gradient sequence for detection); fundoscopic examination may reveal retinal arteriolar tortuosity.

## Further reading

Bahi-Buisson N, Guttierrez-Delicado E, Soufflet C, et al. (2007) Spectrum of epilepsy in terminal 1p36 deletion syndrome. *Epilepsia* 49: 509–515.

Basheer SN, Waters PJ, Lam CW, et al. (2007) Isolated sulfite oxidase deficiency in the newborn: lactic acidaemia and leukoencephalopathy. *Neuropediatrics* 38: 38–41.

Berkovic SF, Heron SE, Giordano L, et al. (2004) Benign familial neonatal–infantile seizures: characterization of a new sodium channelopathy. *Ann Neurol* 55: 550–557.

Co JP, Elia M, Engel J Jr, et al. (2007) Proposal of algorithm for diagnosis and treatment of neonatal seizures in developing countries. *Epilepsia* 48: 1158–1164.

Djukic A, Lado FA, Shinnar S, et al. (2006) Are early myoclonic encephalopathy (EME) and the Ohtahara syndrome (EIEE) independent of each other? *Epilepsy Res* 70: 68–76.

Held-Egli K, Rüegger C, Das-Kundu S, et al. (2009) Benign neonatal sleep myoclonus in newborn infants of opioid dependent mothers. *Acta Paediatr* 98: 69–73.

Heron SE, Cox K, Grinton BE, et al. (2007) Deletions or duplications in KCNQ2 can cause benign familial neonatal seizures. *J Med Genet* 44: 791–796.

Incorpora G, Pavone P, Ruggieri M, et al. (2008) Neonatal onset of hot water reflex seizures in monozygotic twins subsequently manifesting episodes of alternating hemiplegia. *Epilepsy Res* 78: 225–231.

Kato M, Saitoh S, Kamei A, et al. (2007) A longer polyalanine expansion mutation in the ARX gene causes early infantile epileptic encephalopathy with suppression–burst pattern (Ohtahara syndrome). *Am J Hum Genet* 81: 361–366.

Molinari F, Raas-Rothschild A, Rio M, et al. (2005) Impaired mitochondrial glutamate transport in autosomal recessive neonatal myoclonic epilepsy. *Am J Hum Genet* 76: 334–339.

Nissenkorn A, Michelson M, Ben-Zeev B, et al. (2001) Inborn errors of metabolism: a cause of abnormal brain development. *Neurology* 56: 1265–1272.

Paro-Panjan D, Neubauer D. (2008) Benign neonatal sleep myoclonus: experience from the study of 38 infants. *Eur J Paediatr Neurol* 12: 14–8.

Saitsu H, Kato M, Mizuguchi T, et al. (2008) De novo mutations in the gene encoding STXBP1 (MUNC18-1) cause early infantile epileptic encephalopathy. *Nat Genet* 40: 782–788.

Sirsi D, Nadiminti L, Packard MA, et al. (2007) Apneic seizures: a sign of temporal lobe hemorrhage in full-term neonates. *Pediatr Neurol* 37: 366–370.

Shellhaas RA, Soaita AI, Clancy RR. (2007) Sensitivity of amplitude-integrated electroencephalography for neonatal seizure detection. *Pediatrics* 120: 770–777.

Shimomura K, Hörster F, de Wet H, et al. (2007) A novel mutation causing DEND syndrome: a treatable channelopathy of pancreas and brain. *Neurology* 69: 1342–1349.

Tekgul H, Gauvreau K, Soul J, et al. (2006) The current etiologic profile and neurodevelopment outcome of seizures in term newborn infants. *Pediatrics* 117: 1270–1280.

# Chapter 3.2

# Abnormal Neonatal Neurology

Before discussing targeted investigations in the newborn infant with abnormal neurology it is important to put in a strong word on what is abnormal. In some parts of the world newborn infants are diagnosed with 'abnormal' neurology when they have nothing seriously wrong with them and merely express some of the myriad features of healthy normality. This chapter will focus on genuine abnormalities. Any overlap with the previous chapter on neonatal seizures is intentional.

As elsewhere in this book, if we draw attention to rare disorders it is either because they are treatable or have genetic implications or because it is important for the family to discover the reason for the infant's problems.

### Flat baby

By a flat baby we mean a 'lifeless' baby who requires resuscitation at birth. In such a situation the priorities are of course resuscitation and stabilization but further neurological investigations are indicated when the aetiology is not clearly asphyxia, trauma, infection or poisoning.

Contributory causes include myotonic dystrophy and some congenital myopathies, glycine encephalopathy, mitochondrial derangements, Aicardi–Goutières syndrome and the central hypoventilation syndrome.

### Apnoeic baby

Neonatal paediatricians will be familiar with many causes of apnoea particularly in the preterm infant. Apnoea as a feature of subtle neonatal epileptic seizures is also well known.

*Myasthenia*
We discuss this below but the more places it appears the better. A response to edrophonium or neostigmine or a positive result on stimulation single fibre EMG (stimSFEMG) should clarify, once myasthenia is thought of.

*Hyperekplexia*
Hyperekplexia has been discussed in Chapter 3.1 in relation to paroxysmal tremulousness and stiffness but may present predominantly as episodes of severe apnoea with high-voltage *rhythmic* 8–30 CMAP (compound muscle action potential) superimposed on ictal EEG and ECG traces (see Fig 1.1): if there is auditory startle and head retraction without habituation on tapping the tip of the nose then it is permissible to go straight to analysis of hyperekplexia genes (*GLRA1* and *GlyT2*).

*Brainstem malformations*
What may be found depends on the quality of MRI available.

*Central hypoventilation (Ondine's curse)*
Although apnoea is more likely to occur in sleep with most causes, in congenital hypoventilation it exclusively does so. This disorder of autonomic regulation may be associated with Hirschsprung disease and later neural crest tumours. Polyalanine repeats are found in the paired homeobox gene *PHOX2b*.

# Floppy baby
The clinical distinction should be attempted between non-paralytic hypotonia which tends to be axial hypotonia, and weakness which tends to affect preferentially the head and the limbs.

*Ill floppy baby*
Investigations will include microbiological tests, CSF examination, brain ultrasound (± MRI), blood ammonia and lactate, plasma and urine amino acids and urine organic acids. Dysmorphism will lead to chromosome analysis as well as determining copper, copper oxidase, very long chain fatty acids (VLCFAs) and sialotransferrin status.

*Axial hypotonia without limb weakness*

PRADER–WILLI SYNDROME
Prader–Willi syndrome would be suggested by the need for tube feeding, cat-like cry, sticky saliva, extreme poverty of movement and a combination of axial hypotonia and limb dystonia. FISH (fluorescent in situ hybridization) testing should be conducted for deletion on chromosome 15q13 and, if negative, MLPA (multiplex ligation-dependent probe amplification – see Chapter 2.13).

PEROXISOMAL DISORDERS
Peroxisomal investigations are described in Chapter 2.14.

BRAIN MALFORMATIONS

Brain malformations shown on imaging may be associated with metabolic disorders (see Chapter 3.1).

### Generalized weakness

MYASTHENIA

When maternal myasthenia is present little difficulty arises. In the absence of maternal myasthenia various congenital myasthenic syndromes (CMS) should be considered in any infant with stridor, respiratory (including apnoeic attacks or 'infantile syncope') and feeding difficulties. Eye signs such as ptosis may be minimal or absent and a high index of suspicion of CMS is needed to allow directed investigations.

The intravenous edrophonium (Tensilon) test may not give a clear-cut response, and the use of neostigmine before feeds or a trial of pyridostigmine may be preferable (Chapter 2.16). Trials of such acetylcholinesterase inhibitors may be hazardous in certain kinds of CMS (Table 3.2.1) and should always be performed in hospital with resuscitation facilities on hand and under video surveillance. There are several types of CMS for which molecular genetic tests are available (Table 3.2.1): the number of genes involved is still expanding. Such testing is usually performed at a national myasthenia reference laboratory. Stimulation single fibre EMG (stimSFEMG) may be helpful if a decremental response is detected following repetitive nerve stimulation, and in the diagnosis of CMS has good sensitivity (0.88) and specificity (0.79).

Unlike myasthenia, in *neonatal botulism* the weakness will not develop until the age of 10 days or later. In contrast to myasthenia, there is an incremental response to repetitive nerve stimulation, and microbiological evidence of infection with *Clostridium* will confirm the diagnosis.

CONGENITAL DYSTROPHIES AND MYOPATHIES

Maternal examination and EMG followed by molecular genetic analysis for trinucleotide repeats will confirm congenital myotonic dystrophy. While creatine kinase may be elevated in some congenital myopathies and dystrophies, the confirmatory test is needle biopsy of muscle. A specific myopathy (centronuclear, nemaline, etc.) may be confirmed on muscle biopsy, while, if a congenital dystrophy is found, further immunohistochemical staining (for merosin) in conjunction with brain imaging and ophthalmological evaluation will assist in clarifying the type of congenital dystrophy syndrome.

### Weakness sparing the face

While facial weakness may not be very obvious in some of the above congenital muscular disorders, weakness above the neck is more often absent in the following four conditions.

SPINAL MUSCULAR ATROPHY (SMA OR WERDNIG–HOFFMANN DISEASE)

Molecular genetic testing for the typical *SMN* gene deletion confirms the clinical

Table 3.2.1 Congenital myasthenic syndromes

| Condition (including usual gene/s) | Age at onset | Clinical features | Response to AChE inhibitors |
|---|---|---|---|
| CHAT | Birth or infancy | Bulbar weakness. Episodic apnoea, less with time | ↑ |
| DOK7 | Mostly 2nd year | Often normal motor milestones. Waddling 'limb–girdle' weakness ± ptosis ± respiratory crises. May improve with ephedrine or albuterol | Usually → or ↓. Rarely ↑ briefly |
| COLQ | Birth or later if milder | Severe progressive weakness, scoliosis, chronic respiratory failure, bulbar weakness, ptosis and ophthalmoplegia ± slow light pupil response. May improve with ephedrine or albuterol | Usually → or ↓ |
| Acetylcholine receptor deficiency (CHRNE, CHRNA1, CHRND, CHRNB1) | <2 years; mostly at birth | Choking, feeding difficulties; ptosis in most; ophthalmoplegia; delayed motor milestones | ↑ |
| AChR deficiency (RAPSN) | Birth, infancy and much later | Arthrogryposis frequent in early-onset phenotype. Episodic apnoea: may be relatively well between crises and improve over time | ↑ |
| Slow channel | Variable | Selective weakness ± multiple CMAPs. Quinidine or fluoxetine may help | ↓ |
| Fast channel | <2 years | Ptosis, ocular bulbar and limb weakness | ↑ |

Key: ↑ = improved; ↓ = worse; → = no change.

diagnosis. Findings on EMG and muscle biopsy are nonspecific and mainly allow the exclusion of other disorders pending the results of the molecular genetic studies.

SMARD1
Spinal muscular atrophy with respiratory distress (SMARD) may present with respiratory

failure due to diaphragmatic paralysis. Mutations in the immunoglobulin μ-binding protein gene (*IGHMBP2*) lead to SMARD1, in which there is usually respiratory failure with onset between 6 weeks and 6 months and the presence of diaphragmatic eventration or preterm birth.

CERVICAL CORD DAMAGE

Pre- or intrapartum injury or cervical cord developmental abnormalities are possible. Neonates with intrapartum cervical cord damage will be ill at birth and often with temporary generalized oedema. Congenital Horner syndrome might be seen. Birth asphyxia may coexist and lead to diagnostic confusion. MRI of the cervical cord and nerve routes is the definitive investigation in this situation.

PERIPHERAL NEUROPATHY

Demyelinating peripheral neuropathy is extremely rare in the neonate. Congenital hypomyelinating neuropathy may present with severe hypotonia, feeding and respiratory difficulties and limb deformities. Motor nerve conduction velocity will be profoundly delayed (<5m/s), while CSF protein is elevated. Sural nerve biopsy will show virtual absence of myelin and molecular genetic testing for this disorder will confirm the diagnosis (see http://neuromuscular.wustl.edu/time/hmsn.html).

## Stiff baby

### Hyperekplexia

Stiffness or hypertonia in the newborn infant is usually due to hyperekplexia. Clues on history include startle disease in a parent or the recognition of 'jumps' in the latter part of the pregnancy. The stiffness will be increased on stimulation and diminished or abolished by sleep. Non-habituating head retraction on tapping the tip of the nose and/or auditory startle support the diagnosis. If EEG, ECG and EMG are recorded during an apnoeic episode, high-voltage repetitive and rhythmic CMAP 'spikes' at 8–30Hz are characteristic (see Fig. 1.1). Other investigations are not indicated before proceeding directly to gene analysis focusing on mutations in the gene for the α-1 subunit of the glycine receptor (*GLRA1*) or in the glycine transporter GlyT2. Other genetic associations with neonatal hyperekplexia are very rare.

### Prenatal thalamic injury

Neonatal hypertonia of a degree greater than that found in hyperekplexia is seen after thalamic injury earlier in the pregnancy. A history of maternal cardiac arrest might occasionally be obtained but usually lesions are 'silent'. Investigation is by brain MRI. It may be prudent to test blood and CSF lactate in case this is a manifestation of a mitochondrial disorder.

### Other stiff babies

Not all stiff babies have hyperekplexia or prenatal thalamic injuries. *Swartz–Jampel syndrome* is obvious, but *KCNA1*-related neuromyotonia/myokymia has not been reported at such an early age. *Dentato-olivary dysplasia* might be missed on brain MRI.

Congenital absence of the pyramidal tracts is difficult to diagnose in life. Those with neonatal stiffness and epileptic seizures may have a *serine synthesis deficiency* syndrome but in general have so far not been well characterized, so in this phenotype there is scope for further thoughtful investigations.

## Increased movements

As in other sections in this neonatal chapter it is easy to overdiagnose abnormality and it is exceedingly important not to do so. In particular, some degree of tremulousness or jitteriness is very common in normal healthy newborn infants and in those with hypoglycaemia and hypocalcaemia.

### Jitteriness

Despite what we just said about jitteriness in normal newborn infants, lymphocytic choriomeningitis virus (LCMV) infection is one of the causes – all with LCMV-related jitteriness have cerebellar hypoplasia that will be apparent on imaging.

### Neonatal abstinence syndrome

The diagnosis of drug ingestion by the mother during pregnancy will usually be obvious but if need be urine toxicology should clarify. Around 70% have benign neonatal sleep myoclonus.

### Transient biochemical disturbances

Hypoglycaemia, hypocalcaemia and hypomagnesaemia will be recognized on routine blood examination.

### Urea cycle defects

Investigation will include plasma urea, ammonia, amino acids and urine amino acids and orotic acid.

### GLUT1 deficiency

If symptoms persist and GLUT1 deficiency seems possible, then blood and CSF glucose estimation (blood immediately before lumbar puncture) are indicated.

### Brain malformation, etc.

Persisting symptoms would also prompt brain ultrasound or MRI.

### Aicardi–Goutières syndrome

We discuss this further in a later section, 'Congenital infection-like syndrome'.

## Reduced movement (hypokinesia)

In contrast to the overdiagnosis of jitteriness or hyperkinesia in newborn infants, reduced movements or hypokinesia tend to be under-recognized and diagnosed late.

*Prader–Willi syndrome*
Extreme poverty of movements, axial hypotonia and some degree of limb dystonia, together with a difficult to elicit and peculiar cry with a need for nasogastric feeding characterize Prader–Willi syndrome. No ancillary investigations are indicated before going direct to genetic analysis.

*Myopathies*
Creatine kinase elevation should distinguish congenital muscular dystrophies from connatal spinal muscular atrophy and congenital myopathies. Examination of the mother (including EMG if possible) will allow the provisional diagnosis of congenital myotonic dystrophy, which will be confirmed by finding the trinucleotide repeats. In the weak immobile newborn infant with facial sparing, DNA will be investigated for a deletion in the survival motor neuron gene (*SMN*) on chromosome 5q12–13.

*Brain malformations including chromosome abnormalities*
Brain MRI and chromosome karyotyping should clarify.

*Thalamic infarctions*
As well as being stiff, such infants with prenatal symmetrical thalamic damage may be immobile. Brain MRI will clarify the thalamic lesions. Increased lactate levels and the lack of any antecedent during the pregnancy would point to possible pyruvate dehydrogenase deficiency, which is confirmed by fibroblast enzyme analysis and then testing for the specific mutations.

*Prenatal cerebral infarction*
While there may be hypokinesia (even ipsilateral if a thrombus is in the subclavian artery) this is not necessarily so; in any case, MRI with diffusion weighting will clarify. If there is porencephaly and/or a family history, consider COL4A1 and NAITP (neonatal thrombocytopenia).

*Neurotransmitter disorders*
Athough very rare, neurotransmitter disorders are important because they may be treatable.

In the past, although retrospectively symptoms may have begun in the neonatal period, most patients were not recognized until later in infancy. Features such as lack of movement, autonomic disturbances, oculogyric crises and dystonia will prompt CSF biogenic amine and pterin estimations (see Chapters 3.5, 3.7, 3.21 and 3.23). These studies are best done before levodopa trial (Chapter 2.16).

*Arthrogryposis*
The important point is not to imagine that arthrogryposis multiplex congenita is a diagnosis. Rather, it should be a trigger for further specific diagnostic investigations.

MATERNAL EXAMINATION
Examine and/or investigate for myotonic dystrophy, myasthenia gravis and centronuclear myopathy.

IMAGING
Brain MRI may reveal primary malformation or ventricular dilatation in congenital myotonic dystrophy. Elevated right hemidiaphragm and thin horizontal ribs on chest radiograph suggest congenital myotonic dystrophy.

OTHER INVESTIGATIONS
Depending on the clinical appearances consider now or later creatine kinase, chromosomes, EMG/nerve conduction velocity, brain MRI, muscle biopsy, acetylcholine receptor antibodies (± other antibodies), metabolic tests for mitochondrial and peroxisomal disorders and CDG, and CSF asialotransferrin.

*Congenital infection-like syndrome*
What we mean by congenital infection-like syndrome is a clinical constellation of some or all of the following: a neurologically abnormal infant (feeding difficulty, jitteriness, seizures of some kind), hepatosplenomegaly, abnormal liver function tests, basal ganglia and/or white matter calcification, cerebral white matter abnormalities on MRI.

HIV infection in the mother will usually be already known. TORCH screen is too well known to require detailed description. Cytomegalovirus may be cultured from the urine or other body fluids, and for later retrospective diagnosis the Guthrie card will be stored. The increase in the incidence of syphilis makes this another diagnostic possibility.

AICARDI–GOUTIÈRES SYNDROME
When the clinical picture is of congenital infection as described above but microbiological investigations are negative then Aicardi–Goutières syndrome becomes highly likely (old names such as pseudo-TORCH and microcephaly–intracranial calcification syndrome are now obsolete except for occasional genetic rarities, and what used to be called Cree encephalitis is the same disorder as Aicardi–Goutières syndrome). It is permissible to go straight to genetic analysis for *TREX1* without the need for CSF examination, but if the CSF is examined then Aicardi–Goutières syndrome at this age will usually contain an excess of lymphocytes ($\geq 5/cm^3$) and always an increase in interferon-alpha.

# Dysmorphic neonate
In several parts of the world newborn infants are misdiagnosed as 'abnormal' because of supposed dysmorphism of the fontanelle and such like. True dysmorphism is recognized when either the newborn infant has the same syndromic characteristics as one of the parents or is different in appearance from either of the parents or other members of the family. When dysmorphism is associated with neurological abnormality the yield from investigations (karyotype and brain imaging) is high. If the karyotype is normal but an underlying brain malformation is found, specific genetic investigations may be indicated. Metabolic disorders with brain malformation include the following:

- peroxisomal disorders – elevated VLCFAs

- mitochondrial disorders – elevated plasma and CSF lactate

- carbohydrate deficient glycoprotein disorders – abnormal sialotransferrin
- glutaric aciduria type 2 – abnormal urine organic acids.

## Further reading

Bonthius DJ, Wright R, Tseng B, et al. (2007) Congenital lymphocytic choriomeningitis virus infection: spectrum of disease. *Ann Neurol* **62**: 347–355.

Burke G, Cossins J, Maxwell S, et al. (2004) Distinct phenotypes of congenital acetylcholine receptor deficiency. *Neuromuscul Disord* **14**: 456–464.

Crow YJ, Livingston JH. (2008) Aicardi–Goutières syndrome: an important Mendelian mimic of congenital infection. *Dev Med Child Neurol* **50**: 410–416.

Eicke M, Briner J, Willi U, et al. (1992) Symmetrical thalamic lesions in infants. *Arch Dis Child* **67**: 15–19.

Francisco AMO, Arnon SS. (2007) Clinical mimics of infant botulism. *Pediatrics* **119**: 826–828.

Kinali M, Beeson D, Pitt MC, et al. (2008) Congenital myasthenic syndromes in childhood: diagnostic and management challenges. *J Neuroimmunol* **201–202**: 6–12.

Leijser LM, de Vries LS, Rutherford MA, et al. (2007) Cranial ultrasound in metabolic disorders presenting in the neonatal period: characteristic features and comparison with MR imaging. *AJNR Am J Neuroradiol* **28**: 1223–31.

McSweeney N, Cowan F, Manzur A, et al. (2008) Perinatal dyskinesia as a presenting feature in Prader Willi Syndrome. *Eur J Paediatr Neurol* **13**: 350–355.

Mihaylova V, Müller JS, Vilchez JJ, et al. (2008) Clinical and molecular genetic findings in COLQ-mutant congenital myasthenic syndromes. *Brain* **131**: 747–759.

Parisi JE, Collins GH, Kim RC, et al. (1983) Prenatal symmetrical thalamic degeneration with flexion spasticity at birth. *Ann Neurol* **13**: 94–97.

Pitt M. (2008) Neurophysiological strategies for the diagnosis of disorders of the neuromuscular junction in children. *Dev Med Child Neurol* **50**: 328–333.

Raspall M, Ortega-Aznar A, del Toro M. (2006) Neonatal rigid–akinetic syndrome and dentato-olivary dysplasia. *Pediatr Neurol* **34**: 132–134.

# Chapter 3.3
## Delayed Development

Developmental delay means a slowness in acquiring milestones and may be global (previously called psychomotor) or selective – as in the fields of gross or fine motor development or the development of expressive speech or comprehension of language. Delay implies later than normal acquisition of developmental milestones, but in the first instance it is essential to determine that the developmental delay is abnormal in the neurological sense.

### Bottom-shuffling and other normal motor development variants

This is not a textbook of paediatric neurology, but larger texts often omit this important topic. Although a substantial majority of infants show a developmental pattern that goes from prone lying to prone creeping to crawling to walking, a sizeable minority have a shuffling developmental phenotype. Such infants prefer supine lying, they sit late, when lifted off the floor they flex their hips and extend their knees, their preferred method of floor locomotion is bottom-shuffling (scooting or hitching) and they usually walk late. When this developmental pattern is familial (it seems to be dominantly inherited) then some affected infants will have rapid motor development with no floor locomotion before independent walking. When cognitive development is normal (with appropriate abilities in symbolic play) and there are no abnormalities on general paediatric examination, then no neurological investigations are indicated.

When this bottom-shuffling developmental progression complicates a static encephalopathy that would in a crawling infant give signs of spastic diplegia, then the signs of spasticity may be manifest late. When bottom-shuffling is superimposed on a disorder with cognitive delay such as Rett syndrome, then the usual investigations will be appropriate (*MECP2* in the case of Rett).

Other aspects of developmental delay will be discussed in Chapters 3.4 (Floppy Infant),

3.5 (Wobbly-Eyed Baby), 3.7 ('Cerebral Palsy'), 3.8 (Peculiar Gait), 3.9 (Learning Disability/Mental Retardation), 3.10 (Speech and Language Disorders), 3.11 ('Psychiatric' Disorders) and 3.19 (Weakness and Fatigue).

### Global developmental delay

Global developmental delay has been defined as significant delay in two or more of the developmental domains: motor, speech and language, cognition, emotional and social, and activities of daily living. Not surprisingly, isolated speech and language delay or isolated motor delay exclude the diagnosis, but for less obvious reasons autism spectrum disorders are also excluded (but see Chapter 3.11).

The aims of investigation are to establish causation, perhaps to alter management, to predict prognosis for recurrence risks, to attempt to influence prevention strategies and not to miss treatable disorders (see Chapter 3.23).

Published guidelines have low-level recommendations for investigations in the preschool age group. With no clinical clues whatever the evidence is not strong enough to suggest tests other than chromosome karyotype and fragile X. However, too limited a range of investigations may miss important genetic conditions (Chapter 2.13) and rare – and not so rare – treatable disorders (Chapter 3.23).

As we wrote in the Introduction, this is not a 'cookbook', and as always thought and perception and clinical acumen are needed before deciding what should be looked for.

Consider – *consider, think about* – the following:

*EEG* – a clue to Angelman syndrome (posterior high-voltage 3–4/s sharps with smaller spikes/sharps on passive eye closure) or cortical dysplasia (excess fast activity). Slow background is a feature of *MECP2* duplication in boys.

*Brain MRI* – when safe to do, and with limited expectations! Hypomyelination *might* be suggested (or missed if MRI is performed at too early an age), and further investigations depend on other clinical handles. Recognizing that brain MRI will *not* be requested without proton MRS (H-MRS) at the same time should put a brake on 'reflex' MRI requesting.

*Brain H-MRS* – if it's worth doing MRI it's worth doing H-MRS to look for absent or reduced creatine peak in creatine synthesis disorders, and also lactate in mitochondrial disorders.

*Chromosome karyotype* – including fragile X test.

*Thyroid function tests* – hypothyroidism is too well known to require description, but in males, especially with Pelizaeus–Merzbacher-like disease phenotype, check for ↑ free T3 and ↓ free T4 as clues to *MCT8* mutation.

*Urine biochemistry*

- Stick tests for phenylketonuria, homocystinuria, etc.

- Organic acids (organic aciduria, including mild Canavan disease – Chapter 3.7)

- Heparan sulphate (Sanfilippo)

- Creatine/creatinine ratio (increased in creatine transporter deficiency)

- Guanidinoacetate [increased in guanidinoacetate methyltransferase (GAMT) deficiency, decreased in L-arginine:glycine amidinotransferase (AGAT) deficiency].

*Blood biochemistry*

- Urea (urea cycle defects)

- Creatinine (may be reduced in GAMT deficiency)

- Creatine kinase (of course increased in Duchenne muscular dystrophy but beware hyperCKaemias and test not recommended without clinical suspicion)

- Uric acid (decreased in molybdenum cofactor deficiency)

- Lactate (increased in many mitochondrial disorders)

- Ammonia (increased in urea cycle defect)

- Amino acids (especially for phenylketonuria and homocystinuria and rare case of mild sulphite oxidase deficiency with low total plasma homocysteine)

- Sialotransferrins (as for all the above, only if clinical clues – looking for congenital disorders of glycosylation).

*CSF H-MRS* – Creatine decreased on H-MRS of CSF sample in all creatine synthesis or transporter disorders.

*Maternal biochemistry* – Plasma amino acids (phenylketonuria, hyperphenylalaninaemia).

## Non-development
The explanation of this tragic situation is not always obvious. Brain MRI should clarify if there is

- pan-cortical malformation (lissencephaly)

- pan-cortical destruction (ischaemic or metabolic cystic encephalomalacia)

- thalamic destruction (prenatal maternal cardiac arrest, for instance)

- hypomyelination with increased signal on T2 (Pelizaeus–Merzbacher or Pelizaeus–Merzbacher-like disorder)

- myelin rarefaction with decreased signal on T1 and increased signal on T2 [eukaryotic translation initiation factor 2B (eIF2B)-related disorder, severe form].

*Brain malformations and prenatal brain destruction*
Brain MRI is the primary investigation, but if other features (such as the development of chilblains) hint at Aicardi–Goutières syndrome then brain CT or ultrasound may be more helpful in demonstrating basal ganglia and white matter calcification (chilblains alone will prompt referral for genetic investigations for Aicardi–Goutières syndrome).

In the past only some of those with early infantile epileptic encephalopathy (up to now called Ohtahara syndrome) have been found to have brain malformations when they have come to autopsy. We guess that MRI at high field strength *might* be able to demonstrate more such lesions in the future.

*Chromosomal disorders*
Karyotype will reveal trisomies and other major chromosomal aberrations.

*Biochemical errors*
Classical glycine encephalopathy would have been diagnosed in the neonatal period, as likely will molybdenum cofactor deficiency and sulphite oxidase deficiency. Pyridoxine and pyridoxal phosphate responsive conditions were discussed in Chapter 3.1.

Certain mitochondrial disorders, peroxisomopathies – including D-bifunctional protein deficiency – and congenital defects of glycosylation may have no developmental progress. Chapter 2.14 deals with investigations in depth.

Glutaric aciduria type 2 (GA2) will have a peroxisomal-looking dysmorphism and organic aciduria.

## Lack of responsiveness
Impaired responsiveness to the environment may be characterized in terms of the type of sensory deficit and the impaired processing. We list the disorders and suggested possible investigations.

*Auditory unresponsiveness*
- Deafness
    - Audiology ± brainstem auditory evoked potentials
    - Guthrie card: retrospective diagnosis of congenital cytomegalovirus.
- Language comprehension disorder
    - EEG if regression, for Landau–Kleffner syndrome
    - Karyotype, fragile X test.
- Autism spectrum disorder
    - Avoid EEG if uncomplicated.

*Visual unresponsiveness*

- Low vision

  - Ophthalmological evaluation

  - If possible, ERG and visual evoked potentials (see also Chapter 3.5).

- Cortial visual impairment

  - Periventricular leukomalacia is seen particularly after preterm birth but may also be of prenatal origin in a term-born infant. MRI is indicated.

*Social unresponsiveness*

- Autism spectrum disorder

  - Avoid EEG if uncomplicated.

## Further reading

Ashwal S, Russman BS, Blasco PA, et al. (2004) Practice parameter: diagnostic assessment of the child with cerebral palsy: report of the Quality Standards Subcommittee of the American Academy of Neurology and the Practice Committee of the Child Neurology Society. *Neurology* 62: 851–863.

Clayton PT. (2001) Clinical consequences of defects in peroxisomal b-oxidation. *Biochem Soc Transact* 29: 298–305.

Janson CG, Kolodny EH, Zeng BJ, et al. (2006) Mild-onset presentation of Canavan's disease associated with novel G212A point mutation in aspartoacylase gene. *Ann Neurol* 59: 428–431.

Lugtenberg D, Kleefstra T, Oudakker AR. (2009) Structural variation in Xq28: MECP2 duplications in 1% of patients with unexplained XLMR and in 2% of male patients with severe encephalopathy. *Eur J Hum Genet* 17: 444–453.

McDonald L, Rennie A, Tolmie J, et al. (2006) Investigation of global developmental delay. *Arch Dis Child* 91: 701–705.

Robson P. (1984) Prewalking locomotor movements and their use in predicting standing and walking. *Child Care Health Dev* 10: 317–30.

Wolf NI, Harting I, Boltshauser E, et al. (2005) Leukoencephalopathy with ataxia, hypodontia, and hypomyelination. *Neurology* 64: 1461–1464.

# Chapter 3.4
# Floppy Infant

In this chapter we deal with the investigation of infants and young children whose dominant feature is floppines or hypotonia. Some aspects of the very earliest presentation have been dealt with in Chapter 3.2 (Abnormal Neonatal Neurology). A prime example is Prader–Willi syndrome in which hypotonia steadily declines with age during the first year of life. The most common setting for milder hypotonia is a child with one of the familial variants of normal motor development, in particular the bottom-shuffler. In this situation no investigations are indicated.

In the various conditions with prominent pathological hypotonia, the nature of the disorder may be suspected from the history and non-neurological features, and the site of the lesion from careful clinical and neurological examination. We now discuss these disorders with reference to the site of the lesion, and conclude with a discussion of the investigations in disorders in which several mechanisms are involved.

## Brain

### 'Atonic' cerebral palsy and profound learning disability
This is a common situation, where there is profound axioproximal weakness. Tendon reflexes are present if carefully elicited. Some of these children will have a history of severe hypoxic–ischaemic damage with lesions on MRI demonstrated both in the neonatal period and on follow-up. Chromosome studies are indicated despite the low yield. Targeted multiplex ligation-dependent probe amplification for *MECP2* duplication in boys is worth consideration. Other investigations which may be considered depend upon a level of responsiveness and are discussed elsewhere in the section on 'Unresponsive infant' in Chapter 3.3.

### 'Ataxic cerebral palsy'
The danger of a clinical diagnosis of 'ataxic cerebral palsy' is that one may imagine this

is a consequence of neonatal brain injury rather than being caused by a genetic disorder as is usual, except in some low-birthweight survivors where cerebellar injury is increasingly recognized. Brain MRI is indicated. See particularly Chapter 3.7.

## Spinal cord

The site and extent of spinal cord lesions should be determined by the neurological examination but very extensive indolent spinal cord tumours may prove difficult. Spinal MRI is the investigation of choice.

## Anterior horn cell

### Spinal muscular atrophy

WERDNIG–HOFFMANN DISEASE

The clinical diagnosis is confirmed by molecular genetic studies with the finding of deletions in the *SMN* gene on chromosome 5. Needle EMG may be done to demonstrate denervation in the interval between clinical suspicion and the result of the genetic study.

SPINAL MUSCULAR ATROPHY WITH RESPIRATORY DISTRESS (SMARD)

Autosomal recessive SMARD is heterogeneous. When the clinical history includes manifestations of respiratory failure with onset between 6 weeks and 6 months and the presence of diaphragmatic eventration or preterm birth then SMARD1, caused by a mutation in the immunoglobulin μ-binding protein gene (*IGHMBP2*) is highly probable.

INTERMEDIATE SPINAL MUSCULAR ATROPHY (TYPE 2 SMA)

Investigation involves testing the same gene as in SMA1, that is, *SMN*.

## Peripheral nervous system

### Hereditary neuropathies

HEREDITARY MOTOR AND SENSORY NEUROPATHY (HMSN)

HMSN may very rarely present at this age (as HSMN3). Motor nerve conduction velocity will be very slow with prolonged distal latencies. CSF protein may be increased.

CONGENITAL HYPOMYELINATING NEUROPATHY

In congenital hypomyelinating neuropathy there is profound hypotonia with absent tendon reflexes and weakness. Nerve conduction velocity is extremely slow and on sural nerve biopsy the myelin sheaths are absent or very thin. It is genetically heterogeneous and mutations have been found in *MPZ, EGR2, PMP22* and *MTMR2 (see also* http://neuromuscular.wustl.edu/time/hmsn.html).

RILEY–DAY SYNDROME
Diagnosis should be evident on clinical grounds (insensitivity to pain, lack of tears, smooth tongue, etc.) without further investigations.

## Neuromuscular junction

### Myasthenia
The diagnosis of a congenital myasthenic syndrome (CMS) can be very difficult. The edrophonium (Tensilon) test is most easily interpreted when there is ptosis or ophthalmoplegia. When recurrent apnoea or feeding difficulties accompany generalized weakness it is easier to detect the effect of neostigmine given before feeds, or else to use a pyridostigmine trial (Chapter 2.16). Improvement after acetylcholine esterase inhibitors does not usually occur when CMS is due to *COLQ*, *DOK7* or slow channel syndrome. The clinical state of these infants may indeed be made worse by acetylcholinesterase inhibitors (see Tables 2.16.1 and 3.2.1).

Stimulation single-fibre EMG (stimSFEMG) with repetitive nerve stimulation (Chapter 2.3) will precede discussion with a CMS supraregional reference unit.

### Botulism
See Chapter 3.2.

## Muscle

### Myotonic dystrophy
Most cases will have been diagnosed in the neonatal period (Chapter 3.2). Others will present later with hypotonia and delay. Maternal EMG and molecular testing for a trinucleotide repeat will confirm the diagnosis.

### Congenital muscular dystrophy (CMD)
There are two main categories of CMD: CMD due to merosin deficiency (CMD1A); and CMD in association with brain ± eye abnormalities.

CMD1A DUE TO MEROSIN (LAMININ 2) DEFICIENCY
There will be severe generalized weakness with feeding and respiratory difficulties from birth, normal intelligence, creatine kinase elevated to 1000 units per litre, white matter changes on brain MRI, and a dystrophic picture with absence of merosin on immunohistochemistry of muscle. Molecular genetic studies at a CMD reference laboratory will confirm the diagnosis.

CMD WITH BRAIN ± EYE ABNORMALITIES
Several disorders result from defects in the glycosylation of alpha-dystroglycan, including Walker–Warburg syndrome, muscle–eye–brain disease and Fukuyama congenital muscular dystrophy. Brain MRI and ophthalmological evaluation will assist

in targeting the specific mutation in discussion with the CMD reference unit.

*Infantile myositis*
This rare disorder is treatable by corticosteroids so diagnosis is important. The condition must be differentiated from the more common CMD by the finding of inflammation on targeted muscle biopsy.

*Congenital myopathy*
Clinical clues such as involvement of extraocular muscles or predominance of respiratory and bulbar symptoms will point to a specific condition which will be confirmed on muscle histology followed by molecular genetic testing.

## Tendoskeletal disorders
Neurological examination will be normal in the various conditions which may masquerade as a floppy baby, such as congenital laxity of the ligaments, various forms of Ehlers–Danlos syndrome, hypochondroplasias and osteogenesis imperfecta. Neurological investigations are not indicated.

## Mixed mechanisms
Various combinations of abnormalities of eye, brain, spinal cord, anterior horn cell, nerve, muscle, etc. may be seen.

*Muscle–eye–brain disorders*
Walker–Warburg syndrome (congenital hydrocephalus, agyria and ocular abnormalities) and similar syndromes will be suggested by the clinical findings, ERG, brain MRI and muscle histology, and confirmed by the appropriate molecular genetic test.

*Lowe syndrome*
The dysmorphism with corneal and lens changes should allow recognition of this X-linked disorder caused by a deficiency of phosphatidylinositol 4,5-biphosphate-5-phosphatase activity. Mutation analysis for the *OCRL1* gene on Xq25–26 confirms the diagnosis. When the gene is deleted this may be detectable by fluorescent in situ hybridization.

*Peroxisomopathies*
See section on peroxisomal disorders in Chapter 2.14.

*Pompe disease*
In glycogenosis type 2 hypotonia may be as profound as in the other groups of conditions which involve the brain, anterior horn cell and muscles. The waxy appearance of the skin may suggest the diagnosis, supported by ECG abnormalities including short PR interval, high R waves and T-wave inversion. EMG and muscle biopsy are normally no longer necessary and the assay of acid-glucosidase may be

bypassed by going directly to DNA analysis: mutations are found in the gene for alpha-1,4-glucosidase (*GAA*).

### Mitochondrial disorders

Central nervous system, eye, peripheral nerve and muscle may be involved in various mitochondrial disorders. Findings on investigation are sometimes subtle and inconstant.

Investigational abnormalities include increased blood lactate, renal tubular leak including amino acids, elevated CSF protein (not explicable by demyelinating neuropathy), slow motor and sensory nerve conduction, and a great variety of abnormalities on brain MRI including altered signal in basal ganglia. Proton MRS may show a lactate peak. Muscle biopsy may show ragged red fibres on Gomori trichrome stain. Studies of mitochondrial enzyme (respiratory chain, etc.) activity on muscle may point to a specific defect which may be further clarified by mutation analysis.

Specific phenotypes presenting with dominant hypotonia in the first year include those due to *POLG1* and *SURF1* mutations.

### Congenital defect of glycosylation (CDG)

In the most common form of CDG (CDG1a) the typical phenotype includes hypotonia with abnormal fat distribution (especially fat pads on the buttocks), convergent strabismus, and small cerebellum (± small pons) on MRI. Sialotransferrins are abnormal in most cases.

### Eukaryotic translation initiation factor 2B-related disorder (vanishing white matter, etc.)

Rarely, demyelinating peripheral neuropathy accompanies the central motor disorder in this polymorphic disorder. Brain MRI shows abnormal white matter signal, and CSF asialotransferrin is low.

### Neuroaxonal dystrophy

Although it may be difficult in some cases to show that this is a progressive disorder – early on the child seems to be a 'floppy baby' of unknown cause – it is unequivocally a disorder of a progressive loss of skills and will be discussed further in Chapter 3.22.

### Organic acidaemias

A wide variety of organic acidaemias may present in this way, so that assay of urine organic acids together with blood and urine amino acids is indicated in otherwise unexplained hypotonia.

### Hypothyroidism

Classical hypothyroidism will normally have been detected in the neonatal period but occasionally will present later.

X-linked mutation in the monocarboxylate transporter 8 gene (*MCT8* = *SLC16A2*) results in severe hypotonia and global delay, which may include phenotype of Pelizaeus–Merzbacher-like disease. Thyroid function tests show normal thyroid-stimulating hormone, *high free T3* and often low free T4. The elevated free serum triiodothyronine (FT3) is the marker for this disorder.

*Biotinidase deficiency*
This condition is rare and would be expected to be detected on urine organic acid analysis. Plasma biotinidase may be assayed directly or a biotin trial may be given (Chapter 2.16).

*Glucose transporter 1 deficiency*
Occasionally, epileptic seizures and movement disorders do not predominate and hypotonia and delay are prominent features. Particularly if the CSF has to be examined for any reason, blood glucose should be measured immediately before CSF glucose.

*Purine synthesis disorder*
In adenylosuccinate lyase (adenylosuccinase) deficiency infantile hypotonia may be a feature, possibly with emerging autistic features, before the onset of epileptic seizures.

Examination of urine succinylpurines will show elevation of succinyladenosine and other purine metabolites.

*Poisoning*
Rarely in the context of Munchausen by proxy an infant will be given benzodiazepines in feeds leading to hypotonia and sleepiness. If an EEG is carried out, diffuse fast (beta) activity will be seen. Toxicological investigations are in order.

*Nonspecific disorders*
In many other systemic disorders presenting in infancy such as malabsorption and renal tubular acidosis, hypotonia may be a prominent feature. Investigations will depend on the general clinical examination, but bear in mind that mitochondrial disorders present in this way with failure to thrive while neurological features are still elusive and subtle (Clinical Vignette: Introduction.1).

## Summary
A large proportion of the available neurological investigations are necessary in the total range of children who present as floppy babies. Systematic clinical analysis is therefore necessary to limit the investigations to those most likely to help in curative therapy, interim management and genetic advice.

## Further reading

Guenther UP, Varon R, Schlicke M, et al. (2007) Clinical and mutational profile in spinal muscular atrophy with respiratory distress (SMARD): defining novel phenotypes through hierarchical cluster analysis. *Hum Mutat* **28**: 808–815.

Kinali M, Beeson D, Pitt MC, et al. (2008) Congenital myasthenic syndromes in childhood: diagnostic and management challenges. *J Neuroimmunol* **201–202**: 6–12.

Klein A, Clement E, Mercuri E, et al. (2008) Differential diagnosis of congenital muscular dystrophies. *Eur J Paediatr Neurol* **12**: 371–377.

Mihaylova V, Müller JS, Vilchez JJ, et al. (2008) Clinical and molecular genetic findings in COLQ-mutant congenital myasthenic syndromes. *Brain* **131**: 747–759.

North K. (2008) What's new in congenital myopathies? *Neuromuscul Disord* **18**: 433–442.

Parr JR, Jayawant S. (2007) Childhood myasthenia: clinical subtypes and practical management. *Dev Med Child Neurol* **49**: 629–635.

Peat RA, Smith JM, Compton AG, et al. (2007) Diagnosis and etiology of congenital muscular dystrophy. *Neurology* **71**: 312–321.

Rabie M, Jossiphov J, Nevo Y. (2007) Electromyography (EMG) accuracy compared to muscle biopsy in childhood. *J Child Neurol* **22**: 803–808.

Russman BS. (2008) Spinal muscular atrophy: clinical classification and disease heterogeneity. *J Child Neurol* **22**: 946–951.

Smit LS, Roofthooft D, van Ruissen F. (2008) Congenital hypomyelinating neuropathy, a long term follow-up study in an affected family. *Neuromuscul Disord* **18**: 59–62.

Tidswell T, Pitt MC. (2007) A new analytical method to diagnose congenital myasthenia with stimulated single-fiber electromyography. *Muscle Nerve* **35**: 107–110.

Vanderver A, Hathout Y, Maletkovic J, et al. (2008) Sensitivity and specificity of decreased CSF asialotransferrin for eIF2B-related disorder. *Neurology* **70**: 2226–2232.

Vasta I, Kinali M, Messina S, et al. (2005) Can clinical signs identify newborns with neuromuscular disorders? *J Pediatr* **146**: 73–79.

Wilmshurst JM, Pollard JD, Nicholson G. (2003) Peripheral neuropathies of infancy. *Dev Med Child Neurol* **45**: 408–414.

# Chapter 3.5
## Abnormal Head Size

The need for further investigations in a child with abnormal head size is influenced by the head size of the parents, the head size of the child at birth, the trajectory of head growth on the head circumference chart, and the presence or otherwise of neurodevelopmental disorders or dysmorphic features.

When the head sizes of the parents and of the child are plotted on a 0–18 year head circumference chart, the child's head circumference should not normally be on a higher centile than the parent with the larger head nor smaller than the parent with the smaller head. Dominantly inherited large and small heads occur without additional abnormality.

The size of the head at birth and the trajectory thereafter give some clue as to the process underlying the abnormal head size, in that a change in centile may indicate a progressive process. However, the distinction is not always clear and one may have either an acceleration or a deceleration in head growth with an apparently static disorder or even when there is nothing wrong with the child.

The explanation of the abnormal head size may be deduced from the clinical appearance of the child such that syndrome identification might be followed by chromosome analysis or other investigations depending on the clinical features. The presence of marked neurodevelopmental difficulties will merit further investigation irrespective of the head size, and several of the cerebral malformations can have large, normal or small head circumferences.

### Microcephaly
If microcephaly is defined as a head circumference of more than three standard deviations below the mean, then a good 25% will have autosomal recessive inheritance, so diagnosis is important.

*Small head at birth*
The principal investigations are:

- *3-view skull radiograph.* This will demonstrate extensive synostosis (if this diagnosis cannot be made clinically). Only gross intracranial calcification may be detected.

- *Maternal phenylalanine level* – easily overlooked.

- *Virus cultures.* Throat swab and urine culture for viruses (rubella and cytomegalovirus) obtained within the first two weeks of birth.

- *Guthrie test.* Confirmation of prenatal cytomegalovirus may be obtained by examination of DNA extracted from the neonatal Guthrie card.

- *Karyotype.* This simple evaluation is always worthwhile.

- *Ultrasound brain imaging.* Only gross malformation or destructive changes may be detected, but calcification may be inferred.

- *Brain CT and/or MRI.* In cases where the diagnosis is not certain, brain CT (looking for calcification) and/or MRI may clarify the cause.

- *Metabolic investigations.* Metabolic investigations (including CSF amino acids for serine synthesis disorders, etc.) may be indicated if there are other features such as seizures, hypotonia, failure to thrive, etc. (see Chapter 2.14).

*Microcephaly evolving in infancy*
The precise clinical details will influence the choice of investigations, but some of the following may be necessary:

- *Plasma and urine amino acids* – especially for increased phenylalanine.

- *Plasma total homocysteine* – low in sulphite oxidase deficiency.

- *Urine organic acids* – looking for abnormalities seen in biotinidase deficiency or mitochondrial disorders.

- *Urine sulphite test* – usually positive in isolated sulphite oxidase deficiency.

- *Plasma biotinidase.* Perioral rash or alopecia with pale hair may not be present in this neurologically pleomorphic disorder.

- *Chromosomes* – include prometaphase banding and fluorescent in situ hybridization testing for Angelman syndrome. When the phenotype is suggestive of Angelman syndrome but genetic testing is negative, seek mutations in *SLC9A6*.

- *MECP2 mutation* – will be indicated in the setting of Rett syndrome.

- *EEG* – looking for posterior spike–wave on passive eye closure in Angelman syndrome. The appearance of burst–suppression or hypsarrhythmia will not be expected in the absence of considerable developmental impairment.

- *Brain CT* may show calcification typical of congenital infection or congenital infection-like syndrome (Aicardi–Goutières syndrome).

- *Brain MRI* will demonstrate various malformations or destructive lesions.

- *CSF.* Lymphocytosis or more reliably interferon-alpha (and/or pterins) may indicate Aicardi–Goutières syndrome. Paired fasting blood and CSF glucose analysis will show a low CSF:plasma ratio (<0.5) in GLUT1 deficiency.

*Acquired microcephaly with apparent neurodevelopmental regression*
Both pathologically static and true degenerative disorders may present in this manner.

- *EEG* – may detect hypsarrhythmia which underlies the regression in various malformations. Brain imaging will clarify.

- *MECP2 mutation anlaysis* will confirm the diagnosis of Rett syndrome in a girl. Mutations in other genes may need to be sought.

- *Fasting plasma and CSF amino acid and glucose analysis* will show low CSF serine in serine synthesis disorder, while low CSF:plasma glucose ratio will be seen in GLUT1 deficiency.

- *Protein palmitoyl thioesterase enzyme assay* together with electronmicroscopy of lymphocytes in a buffy coat pellet (looking for granular osmiophilic deposits) followed by *CLN1* mutation analysis will confirm the diagnosis of infantile neuronal ceroid lipofuscinosis (Chapter 3.22).

## Macrocephaly
Macrocephaly should probably be regarded as a head circumference of three or more standard deviations above the mean. Many take the cut-off point as two standard deviations, or even regard a head size of over the 90th centile as large, so that many normal heads are investigated. The most common cause of a 'large' head is familial 'megalencephaly', of no pathological significance.

*Large head at birth*
Brain ultrasound will normally clarify the explanation for the large head in so far as it will indicate which structures or fluid spaces are enlarged. Brain MRI is indicated if unexplained hydrocephalus has been detected. This may reveal holoprosencephaly with giant pericallosal cyst, the latter being amenable to treatment.

It is important to recognize the benign nature of the pericerebral or extracerebral fluid collections that may be detected on imaging the child with a large head.

Toxoplasma titres are indicated in unexplained hydrocephalus.

Hydrocephalus associated with dysmorphism, poor responsiveness from birth and specific ocular findings will suggest the diagnosis of muscle–eye–brain disease or Walker–Warburg syndrome. Investigations may show a flat ERG, lissencephaly with white matter abnormality on MRI and specific mutation in the *POMT1* glycosyltransferase.

*Large head appearing later*
Other clinical features may suggest further investigations. For example, external signs of

neurofibromatosis or tuberous sclerosis may be present in a child with evolving megalencephaly. Evidence of storage disease (corneal clouding, visceromegaly or dysostosis) may direct investigations into one or other lysosomal enzyme deficiency. Delayed bone age will suggest hypothyroidism.

Macrocephaly with or without hypotonia or developmental delay may be a presenting symptom of glutaric aciduria type 1, and failure of opercularization at the sylvian fissures and increased pericerebral fluid may be the earliest signs of this disorder. Urine organic acid analysis will suggest the diagnosis in the majority of cases, but if there is a high clinical suspicion (consanguinity, family history, delay) fibroblast enzyme analysis will be necessary to exclude this disorder.

Aqueductal stenosis with or without a slow growing tumour may lead to accelerated head growth over years and investigation is by brain MRI.

In osteopetrosis the head size is often increased, with wobbly eyes and progressive visual loss. Radiography of a long bone will confirm the diagnosis.

Enlarging head with irritability, crying and loss of interest and vision may be a presenting feature of Canavan disease. MRI will show abnormal signal in the cerebral white matter, with elevation of N-acetylaspartic acid on H-MRS. Urine organic acid analysis shows N-acetylaspartic aciduria, and there is aspartoacylase deficiency on fibroblast enzyme analysis.

An enlarging head with or without spasticity, seizures and regression or developmental arrest may be seen in Alexander disease, in which there is a diffuse white matter signal change predominating anteriorly. A mutation in one allele of the gene for glial fibrillary acidic protein will be found.

Mutations in the *PTEN* gene may be associated with marked macrocephaly and mild developmental delay. Testing for these mutations will usually be guided by the geneticist.

It is often a necessary prerequisite to brain imaging that the physician recognizes the possibility of a disorder which may need prompt treatment. It is worth emphasizing that in chronic increased intracranial pressure in the younger child, an enlarging head and (once the anterior fontanelle has closed) a cracked-pot percussion note over the coronal sutures are more reliable signs than the appearance of the optic discs.

### Further reading

Almgren M, Schalling M, Lavebratt C. (2008) Idiopathic megalencephaly—possible cause and treatment opportunities: from patient to lab. *Eur J Paediatr Neurol* 12: 438–445.

Buxbaum JD, Cai G, Chaste P, et al. (2007) Mutation screening of the PTEN gene in patients with autism spectrum disorders and macrocephaly. *Am J Med Genet* 144: 484–491.

Lachlan KL, Lucassen AM, Bunyan D, et al. (2007) Cowden syndrome and Bannayan Riley Ruvalcaba syndrome represent one condition with variable expression and age-related penetrance: results of a clinical study of PTEN mutation carriers. *J Med Genet* **44**: 579–585.

Tolmie JL, McNay M, Stephenson JB, et al. (1987) Microcephaly: genetic counselling and antenatal diagnosis after the birth of an affected child. *Am J Med Genet* **27**: 583–594.

# Chapter 3.6
# Wobbly-eyed Baby

The baby who seems not to see well or has apparent nystagmus or whose eyes wobble for reasons as yet unexplained will commonly be referred by the paediatrician to the ophthalmologist or the paediatric neurologist, but it is helpful to have some kind of plan of investigation. It is convenient to go through the additional clinical pictures that may suggest further tests. The current recommendation is that the term 'infantile nystagmus syndrome' includes both those with visual system disorders and those with motor control problems. This proposal justifies combining both mechanisms of infantile nystagmus in the same chapter but it is worth making an attempt to distinguish input and output disorders when possible.

## Wobbly eyes as an isolated finding

The younger the baby the more difficult it is to be sure that this is so. However, if the neurological examination suggests *congenital brainstem nystagmus*, as with an otherwise normal infant who has optokinetic nystagmus in the vertical plane while *optokinetic nystagmus is absent in the horizontal plane*, no further investigations are indicated.

## Wobbly eyes and visual defect

Additional clinical features may clarify the situation.

### Photophobia

All such infants deserve referral to a paediatric ophthalmologist to exclude primary ocular disorders (albinism, etc.).

### Optic nerve hypoplasia

In neurologically normal babies optic nerve hypoplasia may occur as an isolated finding or be associated with hypothalamic hypopituitarism. Even when there is septal agenesis as in septo-optic dysplasia, no other neurological abnormality need be present.

However, optic nerve hypoplasia may be a marker for several prenatal disorders (see Chapter 2.11) and may be associated with cerebral malformations, so that brain MRI is indicated even if the baby is otherwise clinically normal.

*Optic atrophy*
As an isolated or apparently isolated finding optic atrophy often represents neurofibromatosis type 1. Brain MRI is indicated. Mitochondrial aetiology would be considered if there were other neurological or systemic features.

Osteopetrosis will be recognized on bone radiograph.

*Eyes may appear normal*

CONGENITAL RETINAL BLINDNESS
In Leber congenital amaurosis and in some cases of Joubert syndrome there will be extinction of the flash ERG. Retinal changes may or may not be seen.

OSTEOPETROSIS
Radiography of skull or any bone will indicate this diagnosis.

CORTICAL BLINDNESS
Brain MRI, EEG and VEP should contribute to diagnosis.

## Wobbly eyes, neurological defects and preserved vision
A number of unrelated disorders have motor rather than sensory defects of eye movement, with additional neurological abnormalities. There may be some impairment of visual acuity but this is not the predominant finding.

*Joubert syndrome*
Neonatal onset of tachypnoea may signify Joubert syndrome in which MRI will show hypoplasia of the cerebellar vermis and the molar tooth sign (manifest because of the deep interpeduncular fossa and thick elongated superior cerebellar peduncles). Some infants with Joubert syndrome also have retinal defect and therefore low vision.

*Pelizaeus–Merzbacher disease*
Early stridor, in an appearance resembling dystonic cerebral palsy with rapid oscillatory eye movements, may indicate X-linked Pelizaeus–Merzbacher disease (PMD), or Pelizaeus–Merzbacher-like disorder (PMLD). Rotatory nystagmus may also be seen. The MRI appearance of the cerebral white matter on T2 is characteristic. Confirmation of the diagnosis of PMD is through finding a mutation in a gene for proteolipid protein (*PLP*).

Autosomal recessive PMLD has been caused by mutations in *GJA12*, which encodes connexin 47, but X-linked PMLD from *MCT8* mutations is more common. What is termed hypomyelination in *MCT8*-related PMLD slowly improves and so is really delayed myelination and not hypomyelination. More genes have yet to be discovered.

*Leigh disease*
The explanation for the wobbly eyes in this mitochondrial disorder, commonly due to *SURF1* mutations, may be in part visual but seems predominantly motor.

*'Dancing eyes' (opsoclonus–myoclonus syndrome)*
We will discuss this further in Chapter 3.20.

## Wobbly eyes, neurological defect, low vision
The associated clinical findings and brain MRI will clarify the cause in most situations, such as in Joubert syndrome and Joubert-like disorders with retinal dysplasia, all of which show the molar tooth sign on brain MRI.

## Further reading
Leigh RJ, Zee DS. (2006) *The Neurology of Eye Movements. 4th edn.* Oxford: Oxford University Press.

# Chapter 3.7
## 'Cerebral Palsy'

We call this chapter 'Cerebral Palsy' because it is not uncommon for infants and children to be labelled with 'cerebral palsy' when they have no such thing. Because such cerebral palsy mimics tend to be genetic disorders, this chapter emphasizes investigations that are of value for genetic purposes, but also draws attention to those disorders that are treatable if the correct diagnosis is made (see also Chapter 3.23).

### Static versus progressive disorders

As in many areas of diagnosis the primary question is whether the disorder is static or represents a progressive or paroxysmal disorder. It is well known that cerebral palsy (CP) evolves from the neonatal period through infancy and childhood. Thus hemiplegic CP may not be apparent until purposeful hand use at the age of 6 months and spastic diplegia might not become obvious until the age of 12–18 months. Those with severe CP are never normal at any age.

The widespread use of *home video recordings* allows retrospective review of the developmental trajectory and clarification of whether a disorder is congenital or acquired. Even the early emergence of strong right or left handedness (as a sign of hemiparesis) may be obvious on video in infancy.

### Importance of a congenital brain lesion

In the absence of a clear-cut aetiology, the appearance of a defined lesion on brain MRI is comforting with respect to correctness of diagnosis. Ideally, destructive lesions or malformations should be visible in *all* cases of true CP.

Bear in mind, however, that true CP from a genuine destructive brain lesion may reflect a genetic defect, such as a mutation in *COL4A1* which is associated with porencephaly.

We will now outline some conditions that may be mistaken for CP.

### Spinal cord tumours

It is important to consider spinal cord tumours in two situations: first, when there is a *'congenital hemiplegia' with normal brain MRI*; and second, when there is *pure paraplegia*. Careful neurological examination and spinal cord MRI should clarify. The same applies to other congenital cord lesions.

### Hyperekplexia

Hyperekplexia may masquerade as tetraplegia in the first months of life because the babies (at any rate those with *GLRA1* dominant mutations) are very stiff and irritable, with thumbs in palms. A positive head retraction response to a tap on the tip of the nose together with prominent auditory startle supports the diagnosis sufficiently to proceed directly to seeking mutations in the glycine receptor gene *GLRA1* and the glycine transporter gene *GlyT2*.

### Hereditary myokymia

This is another ion channelopathy that may convincingly masquerade as 'cerebral palsy'. Brain MRI (if it is undertaken, and it is not necessary) is normal. The presentation is with congenital stiffness and flexion posturing. A confusing aspect is that apparently unequivocal extensor plantar responses have been elicited in affected individuals. The generalized myokymia may be subtle but is obvious on surface EMG.

A similar presentation is seen in others with mutations in potassium channel, *KCNA1* and episodic ataxia type 1 and/or simple partial epilepsy.

### Prader–Willi syndrome

Prader–Willi syndrome may initially give rise to confusion because of the axial hypotonia/atonia and dystonic posture of the limbs. If possible one should make a positive clinical diagnosis of Prader–Willi syndrome before establishing the genetic diagnosis.

### Sandifer syndrome

The neck contortions that are secondary to gastro-oesophageal reflux sometimes mislead. Barium swallow and oesophageal pH studies should clarify.

### Duchenne muscular dystrophy

Early manifesting Duchenne muscular dystrophy is commonly misdiagnosed as diplegia when neurological examination is insufficiently detailed.

Creatine kinase will be grossly elevated, and if genetic studies [dystrophin-targeted multiplex ligation-dependent protein amplification (MLPA) for deletions/duplications – and, if negative, full dystrophin gene sequencing] are unrevealing, then muscle biopsy will show defective dystrophin on specific staining.

## Angelman syndrome, Angelman-like syndrome and Rett syndrome
These conditions are hardly likely to be called 'cerebral palsy' but should be thought of. EEG may aid diagnosis.

## *MECP2* duplication
In boys this condition leads to prominent hypotonia that may evolve into spasticity, usually with absent speech, severe learning disability and often recurrent lower respiratory infections. Boys may very easily be misdiagnosed with CP, particularly if the brain MRI shows white matter signal change that is misinterpreted as prenatal periventricular leukomalacia. Diagnosis is by MLPA and, if negative, *MECP2* gene sequencing.

## Congenital dopa-responsive disorders
Segawa-type dopa-sensitive dystonia is fairly easy to diagnosis when it presents at a toddler age with tip-toe walking, diagnosis being by levodopa therapeutic trial (Chapter 2.16). If CSF monoamine neurotransmitters are not estimated before the levodopa trial it is important to discuss with the parents in advance that this may be necessary later (at least a week after stopping levodopa). Confirmation of reduced levels of the enzyme GTP cyclohydrolase-1 (GCH1) in peripheral blood mononuclear cells is a valuable aid to diagnosis.

Although Segawa disease is the usual expression of autosomal dominant GCH1 deficiency, autosomal dominant GCH1 deficiency may be much more difficult to diagnose in infancy when dopa-responsiveness is less complete. Abnormalities of CSF biogenic amines and pterins and *GCH1* gene mutations need to be sought.

## Autosomal recessive GTP cyclohydrolase (GTP-CH) deficiency
In autosomal recessive GTP-CH deficiency without hyperphenylalaninaemia there is a combination of truncal hypotonia and limb spasticity, with – if untreated (see Chapter 3.23) – drooling, oculogyric crises and some degree of parkinsonism. CSF monoamine neurotransmitter studies may not be grossly abnormal, but pterins are *low*. This example emphasizes the need to estimate pterins in all such cases.

## Sepiapterin reductase deficiency
Sepiapterin reductase deficiency is an uncommon but important cause of 'cerebral palsy' (unexplained central motor disorder, primary motor delay), accompanied by a degree of speech and cognitive disorder and often by oculogyric crises.

Improvement with a trial of levodopa will support the clinical diagnosis of this group of dopa-sensitive disorders, but has the danger of CSF neurotransmitter studies confusing the physician unless one waits at least one week till the lumbar puncture is done. Raised blood prolactin will be a nonspecific finding, but paradoxically *increased* urine homovanillic acid, 5-hydroxyindole acetic acid and vanillylmandelic acid favour this particular diagnosis. CSF analysis of monoamine neurotransmitter metabolites and pterins will show reduced metabolites and biopterin with increased sepiapterin (Chapter 3.23).

### Genetic spastic paraplegia

Recognitition of hereditary spastic paraplegia without a family history may be difficult. The combined clinical and imaging picture is necessary to point towards which gene is analysed. Mutations in the autosomal dominant gene *SPAST* (the disease being called *SPAST*-associated hereditary spastic paraplegia) are most common, while a thin corpus callosum is a pointer to looking for autosomal recessive *SPG11* mutation or X-linked *LICAM* (as in the mental retardation, aphasia, shuffling gait and adducted thumbs or MASA syndrome). In boys, also consider MCT8 disorder (see below). *Biotinidase deficiency* is rarely a cause of spastic paraparesis.

### Glucose transporter 1 (GLUT1) deficiency (syndrome)

The phenotypic spectrum of GLUT1 deficiency is still extending and it may no longer be so useful to talk about GLUT1 deficiency 'syndrome'. One of the more common phenotypes includes spasticity, dystonia and ataxia, almost always with early epilepsy of a myoclonic or atypical absence type (Chapter 3.23). Diagnosis begins through fasting blood glucose taken immediately before lumbar puncture for CSF glucose.

### 'Ataxic cerebral palsy'

This is not a diagnosis, and all such labeled children deserve reinvestigation for one of the conditions in this chapter, or something new.

### Lesch–Nyhan disease

Practitioners imagine that boys affected by Lesch–Nyhan disease must have gross self-mutilation requiring total dental clearance and later gout from hyperuricaemia. Rarely the picture may be almost purely one of athetoid or mixed 'cerebral palsy' without self-mutilation and with only marginal increase in serum urate. However, 24-hour urine urate seems always to be increased, the urine being orange and gritty, and mutations should be detected in the *HPRT1* gene.

### Monocarboxylate transporter 8 (MCT8): mutations in the *SLC16A2* gene

MCT8 mutations in boys usually present as dyskinetic 'cerebral palsy' in what is also called Allan–Herndon–Dudley syndrome. Myopathic face and thin quadriceps may be found, and paroxysmal dyskinesia in early childhood. MRI may show delayed myelination or putaminal signal changes. Abnormal thyroid transporter function is reflected in elevated free triiodothyronine and lowered free thyroxine levels in the blood.

## Purine nucleoside phosphorylase (PNP) deficiency

PNP deficiency presents with what we have called disequilibrium–diplegia. There is a static congenital motor disorder with a combination of truncal unsteadiness and pyramidal signs, there being extensor plantar responses. Serum uric acid is low and PNP deficiency may be demonstrated in red blood cells. The T-lymphocyte deficiency that leads to overwhelming infections appears later.

## Ataxia–telangiectasia

Superficially similar to PNP deficiency, but with mixed movement disorder and flexor plantar responses, ataxia–telangiectasia often manifests with early infections and oculomotor apraxia. The tonsils are flat like tiddlywinks and immune deficiencies are usually present, with increased serum alpha-fetoprotein. The story of the ataxia–telangiectasia mutated gene (*ATM*) is complex, but genetic diagnosis is not difficult.

## Arginase deficiency

This rare urea cyle defect presents as spastic diplegia, abnormal hair, hyperargininaemia and increased blood ammonia.

## Succinic semialdehyde dehydrogenase (SSADH) deficiency (4-hydroxybutyric aciduria)

SSADH deficiency is not a particularly specific neurodevelopmental syndrome but may include learning, language and coordination difficulties, oculomotor apraxia, nonprogressive ataxia, epileptic seizures, chorea, hypotonia and difficult to elicit (but present) tendon reflexes. Brain MRI often shows increased signal in globi pallidi on T2. Urine organic acid analysis will reveal the 4-hydroxybutyric acid (gamma-hydroxybutyric acid or GHB). Confirmation is by mutation analysis of the *ALD5A1* gene.

## Glutaric acidura type 1 (GA1)

The choreoathetoid or dystonic state gradually develops over time or becomes acutely exacerbated after febrile decompensation. Accelerated head circumference growth not simply due to increase in brain size is a clue. Brain imaging (CT/MRI) may show subdural fluid collections, failure of opercularization, and basal ganglia or white matter changes. Urine organic acid analysis will reveal traces of glutaric acid (and 3-hydroxyglutaric acid). Urine organic acid abnormalities are more prominent during an acute episode of encephalopathy and may be difficult to detect otherwise. If GA1 is strongly suspected on clinical grounds then the urine acylcarnitine profile should be obtained looking for glutarylcarnitine. For definitive diagnosis demonstration of deficient glutaryl-coenzyme A dehydrogenase in leukocytes or fibroblasts followed by mutation analysis is indicated. A mutation in the glutaryl-coenzyme A dehydrogenase gene on chromosome 19p13–2 may be found.

### Pelizaeus–Merzbacher disease (PMD)

Pelizaeus–Merzbacher disease in its classic X-linked form may masquerade as severe CP due to perinatal asphyxia. Dystonic features may be prominent with early rotating nystagmus, optic atrophy and often laryngeal stridor. Visual evoked potentials and brainstem auditory evoked responses are markedly diminished. MRI shows a variable white matter abnormality on T2-weighted sequences, sometimes including a tigroid appearance. Confirmation of the diagnosis is by finding mutations in the proteolipid protein (*PLP*) gene.

Female carriers of this X-linked condition may show an evolving paraparesis.

### Pelizaeus–Merzbacher like disease

A very similar presentation with hypomyelination may be seen in both girls and boys with mutations in *GJA12*.

### Canavan disease of mild type

Unlike Canavan disease of classic type (Chapter 3.22), mild Canavan disease may present as a static disorder with mild developmental delay, no megalencephaly, and only subtle changes on MRI. In these children, organic acid analysis showed only a comparatively slight increase (compared with classic Canavan disease) of N-acetylaspartate (NAA), and no gross increase of NAA on H-MRS. However, aspartoacylase activity was deficient in cultured fibroblasts, and mutations were found in the aspartoacylase gene (*ASPA*).

### Hexosaminidase A and B deficiency

Hexosaminidase A and B deficiency as a late-infantile Sandhoff disease (variant GM2 gangliosidosis) may present in this way in one of its many guises. Ataxia predominates and progression may be minimal. Clinical clues include sensorimotor and autonomic neuropathy. The earlier onset, the more rapid is the likely regression and the less likely that CP will be long diagnosed. Lysosomal enzyme studies will demonstrate lack of hexosaminidase A and B, and mutations may be found in the *HEXB* gene.

### Congenital HIV infection

This is an important non-genetic cause of CP worldwide with therapeutic implications, so HIV testing in a child of an affected mother is indicated when appropriate.

### Aicardi–Goutières syndrome

The clinical and neuroimaging features of Aicardi–Goutières syndrome are very similar to congenital infection and to human immunodeficiency virus infection in particular, with calcification of the basal ganglia being almost universal in families. CSF lymphocytes are usually raised, while CSF interferon-alpha is always increased in the first year of life. Gene testing is readily available (*TREX1, RNASEH2, SAMHD1*).

## Congenital defects of glycosylation
Although dysmorphisms are expected, listing these conditions is a reminder to check sialotransferrins.

## Mitochondrial disorders
Last but not least we discuss mitochondrial disorders. The initial presentation may be nonspecific with features such as failure to thrive, but an initial diagnosis of CP or '?CP' would not be unexpected. The progression (regression) may be so slow that this confusion is easy. Hypotonia, dystonia or unexplained ataxia may be features. If the CSF protein is examined, it is usually found to be increased for age (Chapter 2.7), and MRI will often show altered signal in basal ganglia. The most likely genetic defect will be a mutation in *POLG1*.

### Leigh disease
In this common presentation, clinical clues are peculiar eye movements and unusual breathing pattern, and it soon beomes obvious that there is a regressive disorder. Initial investigations will be plasma and CSF lactate (Chapters 2.14, 3.22) and brain MRI for symmetrically altered signal in basal ganglia and brainstem, and the most likely mutation will be in the *SURF1* gene.

### Pyruvate dehydrogenase deficiency
Mitochondrial disorders are ubiquitous imitators of CP of varying severity, and with slow progression may have various specific aetiologies, in particular pyruvate dehydrogenase deficiency. Altered signal in the basal ganglia on MRI will prompt blood and CSF lactate estimations in the first instance. However, some children with PDH deficiency causing dystonia will have normal blood and CSF lactate and even no lactate peak on H-MRS. Further, a normal lactate/pyruvate ratio is expected. In the clinical context of 'dystonic CP' with basal ganglia lesions and normal lactates, enzyme analysis on skin fibroblasts may be indicated.

## Summary
Most cases of 'cerebral palsy' will have CP but it is important not to let this label prevent reconsideration of the diagnosis and appropriate investigations when the course is atypical, whatever the age of the child. The single most important neurological investigation pointing to the CP diagnosis being wrong is a normal brain MRI. It follows that brain MRI (with H-MRS if nothing structural is seen) is indicated in all children said to have CP unless the diagnosis is otherwise absolutely secure.

## Further reading
Bax M, Tydeman C, Flodmark O. (2006) Clinical and MRI correlates of cerebral palsy: the European Cerebral

Palsy Study. *JAMA* **296**: 1602–1608.

Chen H, von Hehn C, Kaczmarek LK, et al. (2007) Functional analysis of a novel potassium channel (KCNA1) mutation in hereditary myokymia. *Neurogenetics* **8**: 131–135.

Depienne C, Stevanin G, Brice A, et al. (2007) Hereditary spastic paraplegias: an update. *Curr Opin Neurol* **20**: 674–680.

Hayakawa F, Okumura A, Kato T, et al. (2007) Interpretation scheme for non-expert pediatricians evaluating magnetic resonance images of children with cerebral palsy. *Pediatr Neurol* **37**: 331–337.

Hendriksz CJ, Corry PC, Wraith JE, et al. (2004) Juvenile Sandhoff disease—nine new cases and a review of the literature. *J Inherit Metab Dis* **27**: 241–249.

Kersnik Levart T. (2007) Rare variant of Lesch–Nyhan syndrome without self-mutilation or nephrolithiasis. *Pediatr Nephrol* **22**: 1975–1978.

Lissens W, Vreken P, Barth PG, et al. (1999) Cerebral palsy and pyruvate dehydrogenase deficiency: identification of two new mutations in the E1alpha gene. *Eur J Pediatr* **158**: 853–857.

Neville, B. (2007) Congential DOPA-responsive disorders: a diagnostic and therapeutic challenge to the cerebral palsies? *Dev Med Child Neurol* **49**: 85.

Neville BGR, Parascandalo R, Farrugia R, et al. (2005) Sepiapterin reductase deficiency: a congenital dopa-responsive motor and cognitive disorder. *Brain* **128**: 2291–2296.

Salinas S, Proukakis C, Crosby A, Warner TT. (2008) Hereditary spastic paraplegia: clinical features and pathogenetic mechanisms. *Lancet Neurol* **7**: 1127–1138.

Sedel F, Fontaine B, Saudubray JM, Lyon-Caen O. (2007) Hereditary spastic paraparesis in adults associated with inborn errors of metabolism: a diagnostic approach. *J Inherit Metab Dis* **30**: 855–864.

# Chapter 3.8
## Peculiar Gait

The first question is whether the peculiar gait seems to have a neurological basis. In many cases there are orthopaedic explanations, or benign variants of gait of no serious significance. The normal neurological examination, including running, walking backwards, getting off the floor and standing on one leg with eyes closed, together with intact tendon reflexes and flexor plantar responses, will be reassuring in this regard. It is extremely valuable to be able to tell from the elicited spoken history or from serial home videos that the gait disorder is either static or progressive, but unfortunately it is quite often not possible to be certain. In this situation one can either wait and follow up, or undertake tests on the presumption that a progressive disorder may be present. Particular attention should be paid to the question: is there *dystonia*? (see below).

A more limited range of possibilities exists when there are clearly marked fluctuations or intervals of complete normality. Diurnal fluctuation occurs in Segawa disease (discussed below), and intermittent ataxia may be a feature of inborn errors of metabolism (notably variants of maple syrup urine disease, isovaleric acidaemia, biotinidase deficiency and urea cycle defects). Blood ammonia, lactate and pyruvate, plasma and urinary amino acids, and urinary organic acids may be measured during attacks.

The various paroxysmal gait disorders that may be seen, including episodic ataxias, will be outlined in Chapter 3.14.

*Toe-walking* is one of the presentations of several of the disorders to be discussed. Most commonly it will be a benign normal variant or a reflection of tight tendo Achillis. Other aetiologies are

- autism spectrum disorder
- Rett syndrome
- diplegia
- neuromuscular, especially Duchenne muscular dystrophy

- spinal dysraphism (asymmetrical)
- dopa-responsive dystonia of Segawa type
- rarely, a progressive disorder such as late infantile metachromatic leukodystrophy.

It is helpful to attempt to clarify whether the disorder is one of weakness or spasticity or ataxia or dystonia. Difficulties arise with this oversimplified classification because more than one pattern of neurological abnormality may occur in the same disorder, and the type of abnormality may also vary within one disorder. For example, children with neuropathy may be weak on the one hand, and on the other may present with predominant sensory ataxia.

## Weakness

### Duchenne muscular dystrophy
Children with Duchenne muscular dystrophy who have not already presented with language delay will have a history of difficulty with running and climbing. Toe-walking and the pattern of weakness should indicate the diagnosis. Early on, very brisk ankle jerks may suggest diplegia. EMG shows myopathic changes but is usually not necessary. Diagnosis is confirmed by creatine kinase (CK) of several thousand units per litre and by genetic studies (dystrophin-targeted multiplex ligation-dependent probe amplification for deletions/duplications – and, if negative, full dystrophin gene sequencing). If genetic studies are unrevealing then muscle biopsy will show defective dystrophin on specific staining.

### Inflammatory myopathy
Juvenile dermatomyositis, when of insidious onset, may present in this way and is an important diagnosis, being eminently treatable. The diagnosis is essentially clinical, based on the triad of misery, violaceous rash (which may be subtle) and proximal weakness. CK and/or muscle histology may be normal in up to one-third of cases, but EMG is invariably abnormal, showing features of myopathy and denervation. CK is of no value in monitoring response to steroid treatment.

### Becker muscular dystrophy
It may be difficult to distinguish more severe cases of Becker muscular dystrophy from milder cases of Duchenne muscular dystrophy early on. In Becker muscular dystrophy, deletions will be detected in the dystrophin gene, and biopsy will show patchy dystrophin immunolabelling.

### Other forms of muscular dystrophy
The pattern of weakness, localization of contractures, degree of elevation of CK, muscle histology and immunolabelling will usually guide targeted molecular genetic testing.

### Congenital myasthenia syndromes
Some of the more recently recognized forms of congenital myasthenia syndromes (such

as that due to *DOK7* mutations – DOK = downstream of kinase) may present like a limb–girdle muscular dystrophy.

*The congenital myopathies*
These are usually recognized long before a question of disturbance of gait arises and are distinguished by electronmicroscopy of biopsied muscle.

*Spinal muscular atrophies*
Type 3 spinal muscular atrophy may be confused with Duchenne muscular dystrophy, early on, because of waddling gait, but is usually clinically distinguished. The CK may be mildly elevated but never to a range of several thousands. Electrophysiological testing may show baseline tremor on ECG, reduction of muscle action potential and features of denervation on EMG and muscle histology. Molecular genetic testing of *SMN* should clarify.

*Distal spinal muscular atrophy*
This closely resembles axonal hereditary motor and sensory neuropathy, below.

*Hereditary motor and sensory neuropathies*
There has been an explosion of neurogenetic knowledge and refinement of the clinical analysis of the hereditary motor and sensory neuropathies, also called Charcot–Marie–Tooth disease (CMT) – see http://neuromuscular.wustl.edu/time/hmsn.html. The website just referenced is so comprehensive that little is to be gained by repeating the information, except to say that in the most common childhood forms, dominantly inherited CMT1A and CMT1B, there is slow nerve conduction typical of myelin disorder, whereas in dominantly inherited CMT2A the nerve conduction velocity is mildly slow and, in keeping with axonal involvement, there is evidence of denervation on EMG.

*Chronic relapsing polyneuropathy*
This disorder may fluctuate little and have insidious onset. Findings on nerve conduction (Chapter 2.3), together with the increased CSF immunoglobulin G and total protein will usually indicate the diagnosis without need for nerve biopsy.

*Spinal dysraphism*
Difference in the size and shape of the feet and/or superficial changes over the lumbar–sacral region will indicate this type of malformation. Spine radiography will usually but not always be abnormal. Spinal MRI will clarify.

**Ataxia** (see Chapter 3.20)

*Minor epileptic status*
Drooling and alterations of behaviour and mentation should give a clue to this situation, which is confirmed by standard EEG showing continuous high-voltage, usually irregular, generalized spike and slow wave activity.

*Chronic phenytoin or other drug intoxications*
Disabling ataxia is still unfortunately seen in children with epilepsy on phenytoin therapy. Blood or saliva phenytoin level will be diagnostic (Chapter 2.15). Occasionally when drug combinations are being used, a high free phenytoin level is sufficient to cause ataxia without the total level being increased, but saliva estimation should clarify this. Otherwise formal free phenytoin estimation may be assayed in plasma.

*Cerebellar hypoplasia*
Cerebellar hypoplasia is likely to be genetic or secondary to a metabolic problem such as a mitochondrial disorder or congenital defect of glycosylation. As in the case of the floppy baby, jerky ocular pursuit suggests this pathology, which brain MRI will clarify.

*Obstructive hydrocephalus*
For this to present as a gait problem in the absence of a cerebral tumour, the duration of the block is likely to have been long and the head size will be increased, with a cracked-pot percussion note. Lateral skull radiography will confirm split sutures, and MRI will confirm the hydrocephalus.

*Posterior fossa tumour*
Symptoms of additional difficulties above the neck (vomiting, head tilt, etc.) will prompt immediate MRI or CT with contrast enhancement, whichever is more rapidly available.

*Basilar impression*
Basilar impression or platybasia is an important treatable cause of ataxic gait. Clues may be neck pain and extensor plantar responses. Lateral skull radiography with specific attention to the odontoid will allow the diagnosis, which may be missed if only brain MRI is done.

*Friedreich ataxia*
The willowy appearance of these children and the combination of neurological features makes the diagnosis virtually certain. It should be noted that they do not usually have pes cavus at presentation. The diagnosis is suggested by (1) absent sural sensory evoked potentials, and (2) thickened septum on echocardiogram, and is confirmed by finding a typical trinucleotide expansion in the *frataxin* gene.

*Ataxia with isolated vitamin E deficiency*
Isolated vitamin E malabsorption may simulate Friedreich ataxia closely, with similar investigation results except there is no cardiomyopathy, the serum vitamin E level is low (<2.5mg/L, normal 6–15) and there are mutations in the alpha-tocopherol transfer protein gene (*TTPA*).

*Ataxia–telangiectasia*
The peculiar head turning due to saccadic eye movement control defect ('oculomotor apraxia') suggests this disorder before conjunctival or ear-lobe telangiectasia appear in later childhood. Alphafetoprotein increase confirms the diagnosis in most cases.

Chromosomal aberrations and abnormal cellular responses to ionizing radiation are found in cultured fibroblasts; these tests are not necessary for diagnosis. Diagnosis will be confirmed by mutations in the *ATM* gene.

### Ataxia with oculomotor apraxia 1 (AOA1)

AOA1 is characterized by early onset and apparently static gait ataxia, eye movements that resemble those in ataxia–telangiectasia, and subtle evidence of motor and sensory neuropathy (such as a combination of cerebellar and sensory ataxia). Choreoathetosis develops later. Investigation abnormalities include low serum albumin, increased cholesterol, neurophysiologicial evidence of motor and sensory axonal neuropathy, and cerebellar and brainstem atrophy on MRI. Confirmation is by finding a mutation in the *APTX* gene that encodes ataxin.

### Ataxia with oculomotor apraxia 2 (AOA2)

This spinocerebellar ataxia presents in late childhood with dystonic posturing when walking occasionally accompanied by oculomotor apraxia. As in ataxia–telangiectasia, alphafetoprotein is increased but radiosensitivity is not seen. Mutations are found in the gene for senataxin (*SETX*).

DNA repair aberrations with various degrees of subtlety are found in the last three disorders – ataxia–telangiectasia, AOA1 and AOA2 – but while these biological phenomena are of scientific interest, identifying them is not necessary for the clinical diagnosis.

### Metachromatic leukodystrophy

Presentation with neuropathy may simulate ataxia, including Friedreich ataxia (see Clinical Vignette 2.9.4), or earlier with toe-walking. T1-weighted MRI with gadolinium may show enhancement of cranial nerves.

### eIF2B-related disorder (vanishing white matter disease)

Ataxic gait in early school age is often the presentation of mutations in the eukaryotic translation initiating factor 2B (eIF2B). All have central white matter signal change on T1 and T2 on brain MRI and low CSF asialotransferrin will then prompt gene studies.

### Other neurometabolic disorders

Juvenile Sandhoff disease and juvenile GM1 gangliosidosis may present with ataxia. Hexosaminidase A and B and beta-galactosidase determinations will clarify these diagnoses.

### Hypothyroidism

This may present with various gait disturbances associated with spastic paraparesis: thyroid function studies confirm the diagnosis.

### Mitochondrial disorders

Affected children may have prominent disturbance of gait, but other clinical signs often suggest the diagnosis (Chapters 2.14, 3.7 and 3.22).

## Spasticity

### Spastic diplegia

Spastic diplegia is a common outcome in survivors of low-birthweight preterm birth but periventricular leukomalacia may occur prenatally in infants born at term. Brain imaging, usually MRI, is indicated and may also reveal a specific malformation such as lobar holoprosencephaly or a structural clue to a metabolic disorder.

### Basilar impression (platybasia)

Platybasia, discussed above, usually presents with predominant ataxia.

### Spinal cord tumour

Cervical cord tumours may simulate diparesis or even hemiparesis. Progression, pain, fixed neck position, and upper-limb signs will suggest the need for spinal cord MRI. Tumours at lower levels may be associated with scoliosis or back stiffness and may be particularly difficult to diagnose in a child with learning disability for another reason.

### Segawa disease (dopa-sensitive dystonia)

This may masquerade as spastic diplegia – see below.

### Down syndrome; Hunter syndrome

Deterioration in gait which includes spastic paraparesis may occur in children with these disorders, due to lesions at the foramen magnum. Careful cervical spine radiography may clarify the situation in Down syndrome; in Hunter syndrome MRI may be helpful.

### Cobalamin disorders

All physicians are familiar with the subacute combined degeneration of the cord that is a sequel to vitamin $B_{12}$ (cyanocobalamin) malabsorption in the older individual with pernicious anaemia. More difficult are the genetic disorders of cobalamin metabolism that may lead to similar spinal cord dysfunction (and to other neurological deficits besides).

One difficulty is that the blood $B_{12}$ (and folic acid) level is normal, with no history indicating a predisposition to $B_{12}$ deficiency. T2-weighted spinal cord MRI will show a bright signal in the posterior columns.

Biochemical studies will almost always show

- excess methylmalonic acid on urine organic acid analysis
- excess homocystine in urine
- hyperhomocysteinaemia.

## Dystonia

### Dystonia with diurnal fluctuations (Segawa disease)

This disorder may present so early that it masquerades as congenital diplegia. The characteristic history of normality in the morning (after sleep) and progression as the day goes on may be absent. It has to be suspected in a young child who variably walks on the toes in a rather diplegic manner without unequivocal extensor plantar responses.

A trial of levodopa is indicated in unexplained gait disorder of this type. While our recommendation is that in *atypical* cases CSF neurotransmitter and pterin studies should be undertaken *before* the levodopa trial, there is an argument for doing the therapeutic trial first, *provided that* the family know that should the levodopa trial be positive the drug will be withdrawn and CSF studies done before gene analysis and lifelong treatment recommendations.

### Sepiapterin reductase deficiency
In contrast to those with Segawa disease patients usually have cognitive difficulties and dysarthria. Motor difficulties may respond to small doses of levoopa, although cognitive impairment is not improved. However, full diagnostic CSF studies (monoamines and pterins) are advisable *before* levodopa trial (Chapters 2.16 and 3.7). Molecular genetic studies will show a mutation in the sepiapterin reductase (*SPR*) gene.

### Idiopathic torsion dystonia
This disorder, commonly due to a mutation in the *torsin A* gene and known as DYT1, often presents in the first decade with abnormal gait due to foot dystonia. A specific mutation in the gene is found in a high percentage of cases with the classic phenotype, but genetic counselling is desirable.

### Myoclonus–dystonia
This is an important cause of gait disorder that manifests usually soon after walking and before the age of 18 months. The gait at this stage has been described as a 'swaggering gait' and might be recognized in retrospect on family home videos. Myoclonus does not manifest until later, but tremulousness is a feature at this age. The diagnosis is much easier when there is a clear family history, but information – such as familial alcohol abuse – may be withheld (Chapter 1.1). Mutations are found in the sarcoglycan epsilon gene (*SGCE*).

### Conversion disorder
When a conversion disorder presents as a gait disturbance the diagnosis should as far as possible be entirely clinical, insofar as neurological investigations may tend to strengthen the idea of 'organicity' of the symptoms. Some clues are sudden onset, incongruity with other features, alteration with distraction, lurching and/or very elaborate gait.

### Paroxysmal gait disorders
Conditions such as benign paroxysmal vertigo, and paroxysmal torticollis, the episodic ataxias and the paroxysmal dyskinesias will all be discussed in Chapter 3.14.

## Summary
Home and hospital videos are important investigational tools in childhood gait

disorders. In part this is because changes over the passage of time become more obvious, and partly because such movies allow sharing between practitioners of varied experience.

## Further reading

Baik JS, Lang AE. (2007) Gait abnormalities in psychogenic movement disorders. *Mov Disord* 22: 395–399.

Carmel R, Green R, Rosenblatt DS, et al. (2003) Update on cobalamin, folate, and homocysteine. *Hematology Am Soc Hematol Educ Program* 62–81.

Cheyette BN, Cheyette SN, Cusmano-Ozog K, et al. (2008) Dopa-responsive dystonia presenting as delayed and awkward gait. *Pediatr Neurol* 38: 273–275.

Criscuolo C, Chessa L, Di Giandomenico S, et al. (2006) Ataxia with oculomotor apraxia type 2: a clinical, pathologic, and genetic study. *Neurology* 66: 1207–1210.

Nicholson GA. (2006) The dominantly inherited motor and sensory neuropathies: clinical and molecular advances. *Muscle Nerve* 33: 589–597.

Ouvrier R, Geevasingha N, Ryan MM. (2007) Autosomal-recessive and X-linked forms of hereditary motor and sensory neuropathy in childhood. *Muscle Nerve* 36: 131–143.

Lo HP, Cooper ST, Evesson FJ, et al. (2008) Limb–girdle muscular dystrophy: diagnostic evaluation, frequency and clues to pathogenesis. *Neuromuscul Disord* 18: 34–44.

Said G. (2006) Chronic inflammatory demyelinating polyneuropathy. *Neuromuscul Disord* 16: 293–303.

Salinas S, Proukakis C, Crosby A, Warner TT. (2008) Hereditary spastic paraplegia: clinical features and pathogenetic mechanisms. *Lancet Neurol* 7: 1127–1138.

Shahwan A, Byrd PJ, Taylor AM, et al. (2006) Atypical presentation of ataxia–oculomotor apraxia type 1. *Dev Med Child Neurol* 48: 529–532.

Soltanzadeh A, Soltanzadeh P, Nafissi S, et al. (2007) Wilson's disease: a great masquerader. *Eur Neurol* 57: 80–85.

# Chapter 3.9

# Learning Disability/ Mental Retardation

The diagnosis of the cause of learning disability is within the province of paediatric neurology, but it is beyond the scope of this book to discuss all known possibilities. It is important that when possible prenatal infection is diagnosed in the neonatal period. When this has not been done, the stored neonatal Guthrie card may be used for retrospective diagnosis, in particular of cytomegalovirus. Static disorders with dysmorphic features may be recognized with the help of the geneticist and dymorphology databases, and through the neurological database SimulConsult (www.simulconsult.com).

In this chapter we try to give some help with a choice of investigations for investigating learning disability when the diagnosis is not obvious. Abnormal head size has been discussed in Chapter 3.5 and profound unresponsiveness in Chapter 3.3. If from the clinical data one is able to obtain a clue to the most probable disorder then one can move quickly to the appropriate test. We have listed in Table 3.9.1 a number of investigations that *might* be helpful, in approximate order of invasiveness, together with thumbnails of the conditions that may be diagnosed. We have included some investigations for progressive, that is to say regressive, disorders where deterioration may be very slow and difficult to notice. The topic of regression is covered more fully in Chapter 3.22.

It is important to remember that the family history, the patient history and the clinical examination will give strong clues as to whether any investigations are likely to prove positive. The following features, particularly in combination, increase the chances of discovering a recognizable aetiology:

- consanguinity
- family history of a similar disorder (Chapter 1.1)
- lack of progress, or regression (see Chapter 3.22)
- head circumference large or small for the family (Chapter 3.5)

- dysmorphism including cutaneous manifestations (Chapter 1.2)
- high myopia (Chapter 3.6)
- certain behavioural phenotypes (Chapter 3.11)
- motor deficits including ataxia (Chapters 3.7 and 3.20)
- epileptic seizures (Chapters 3.12 and 3.15)
- organomegaly (Chapter 1.2).

## Further reading

Archer HL, Evans J, Edwards S, et al. (2006) CDKL5 mutations cause infantile spasms, early onset seizures, and severe mental retardation in female patients. *J Med Genet* **43**: 729–734.

Cruysberg JR, Boers GH, Trijbels JM, et al. (1996) Delay in diagnosis of homocystinuria: retrospective study of consecutive patients. *BMJ* **313**: 1037–1040.

Engbers HM, Berger R, van Hasselt P, et al. (2008) Yield of additional metabolic studies in neurodevelopmental disorders. *Ann Neurol* **64**: 212–217.

Fong CY, Baird G, Wraige E. (2008) Do children with autism and developmental regression need EEG investigation in the absence of clinical seizures? *Arch Dis Child* **93**: 998–999.

Froyen G, Van Esch H, Bauters M, et al. (2007) Detection of genomic copy number changes in patients with idiopathic mental retardation by high-resolution X-array-CGH: important role for increased gene dosage of XLMR genes. *Hum Mutat* **28**: 1034–1042.

Gibson WT, Harvard C, Qiao Y, et al. (2008) Phenotype–genotype characterization of alpha-thalassemia mental retardation syndrome due to isolated monosomy of 16p13.3. *Am J Med Genet* **146**: 225–232.

Gropman AL, Summar M, Leonard JV. (2007) Neurological implications of urea cycle disorders. *J Inherit Metab Dis* **30**: 865–879.

Gyato K, Wray J, Huang ZJ, et al. (2004) Metabolic and neuropsychological phenotype in women heterozygous for ornithine transcarbamylase deficiency. *Ann Neurol* **55**: 80–86.

Jurecka A, Zikanova M, Tylki-Szymanska A, et al. (2008) Clinical, biochemical and molecular findings in seven Polish patients with adenylosuccinate lyase deficiency. *Mol Genet Metab* **94**: 435–442.

Mueller S, Sherr EH. (2008) The importance of metabolic testing in the evaluation of intellectual disability. *Ann Neurol* **64**: 113–114.

Peppink D, Douma-Kloppenburg DD, de Rooij-Askes ES, et al. (2008) Feasibility and outcomes of multiplex ligation-dependent probe amplification on buccal smears as a screening method for microdeletions and duplications among 300 adults with an intellectual disability of unknown aetiology. *J Intellect Disabil Res* **52**: 59–67.

Stockler S, Schutz PW, Salomons GS. (2007) Cerebral creatine deficiency syndromes: clinical aspects, treatment and pathophysiology. *Subcell Biochem* **46**: 149–166.

Troester MM, Trachtenberg T, Narayanan V. (2007) A novel mutation of the ARX gene in a male with nonsyndromic mental retardation. *J Child Neurol* **22**: 744–748.

Table 3.9.1 Investigations in learning disabilities (mental retardation)

| Investigation | Disorder (phenotype) | Comments |
|---|---|---|
| **Urine test** | | |
| Amino acids | Homocystinuria (myopia) | Red colour of urine with sodium nitroprusside is a simpler test. Plasma amino acids may be normal |
| Organic acids | 4-hydroxybutyric aciduria (ataxia) | 4-hydroxybutyric aciduria |
| | Mild Canavan disease (delay) | ↑ NAA is much less than in classic Canavan disease. NAA not ↑ on H-MRS |
| Heparan sulphate | Sanfilippo disease (hyperactive, aggressive) | May masquerade as static disorder. Take 24 hour collection if in doubt |
| Bratton–Marshall test | Adenylosuccinate lyase deficiency* (autism, self-injury) | Purple colour = succinylpurines |
| Sulphite test | Variant molybdenum cofactor deficiency* (usually very severe) | Fresh urine needed. Stix turns pink to orange. May be false negative. |
| Guanidinoacetate | GAMT deficiency* (intellectual disability, speech delay) | ↑ In GAMT deficiency but brain H-MRS desirable. |
| | AGAT deficiency* (less severe than GAMT) | ↓ But also brain H-MRS desirable |
| Urate | Lesch–Nyhan (dyskinesia) | ↑ Even if plasma urate normal |
| **Blood biochemistry (usually plasma)** | | |
| Amino acids in *mother* | Maternal PKU (small head in child) | ↑ Phenylalanine |
| Calcium | Pseudohypoparathyroidism (moon face) | Phenotype subtle Ca ↓ |

Table 3.9.1 continued

| Investigation | Disorder (phenotype) | Comments |
|---|---|---|
| **Blood biochemistry (usually plasma)** | | |
| Calcium | Williams syndrome (friendly) | Ca ↑ |
| Creatinine | GAMT deficiency* (as above) | Creatinine may be low |
| Urate | Atypical molybdenum cofactor deficiency* | Urate ↓ |
| | Atypical Lesch–Nyhan (dyskinesia) | Urate ↑ (but not always) |
| Creatine kinase | Duchenne muscular dystrophy (speech delay) | Weakness may be overlooked |
| Lead | Chronic lead intoxication (might have 'lead lines' at bone ends or abdominal radio opacities) | Depends on environment |
| Amino acids | PKU (low-functioning autistic) | Phenylalanine ↑ in case missed by neonatal screening |
| | Homocystinuria (as above, in urine) | Homocysteine ↑ and methionine ↑: blood should be deproteinized promptly |
| | Serine synthesis disorder* (congenital microcephaly, altered tone) | Serine and glycine may be ↓ but CSF study necessary |
| **Endocrine** | | |
| Thyroid function test | Hypothyroidism (delayed fontanelle closure) | TSH ↑ T3 ↓ T4 ↓ |
| | *MCT8* mutation in boys (dysarthria or no speech, ± reduced muscle mass) | TSH normal or ↑ Free T3 ↑ Free T4 ↓ |

Table 3.9.1 continued

| Investigation | Disorder (phenotype) | Comments |
|---|---|---|
| **Haematology** | | |
| Full blood count | Anaemia (may not be pale) | Iron deficiency is usually correctable |
| Ferritin | Iron deficiency (may not be obvious) | Low ferritin indicates iron deficiency |
| Blood film | Lead intoxication (hyperactivity) | Basophilic stippling |
| | ATRX syndrome (dysmorphism) | HbH bodies on cresyl blue staining indicate need for α-thalassaemia gene studies |
| **Genetic blood tests** | | |
| Chromosome karyotype | Various disorders (need not be dysmorphic) | Geneticist may suggest other tests such as MLPA, telomeric studies, CGH |
| Microdeletion testing | 22q (speech and language) 17p (Smith–Magenis* self-hugging, etc.) | MLPA is superseding FISH |
| Fragile X testing | Fragile X syndrome* (big ears) | Surprisingly uncommon in paediatric neurology clinics |
| *UBE3A* (15q11.3–13) | Angelman syndrome* (jerky) | EEG first with passive eye closure if clinical suspicion |
| *MECP2* mutations | * (handwashing, including Angelman-like) | Rett disorder |
| *MECP2* duplication | *MECP2* duplication syndrome* (boys, severe learning disability, no speech, ± MRI white matter signal change, ± lower respiratory infections) | MLPA usually necessary but if negative, gene sequencing |
| *ARX* | Nonspecific* (may be dystonia) | Occasionally not syndromic |

Table 3.9.1 continued

| Investigation | Disorder (phenotype) | Comments |
|---|---|---|
| **Genetic blood tests** | | |
| *CDKL5* | Epilepsy, spasms* (may be Rett-like) | Phenotype widening |
| *TCF4* mutation | Pitt–Hopkins syndrome* (mid-childhood-onset hyperventilation) | The respiration is the clue |
| **Neurophysiology** | | |
| EEG | Angelman syndrome* (early seizures with fever, jerky movements) | Passive eye closure to induce occipital spike and sharp runs |
| **Structural brain imaging** | | |
| Brain MRI | Learning disability unexplained by above investigations* (especially if dysmorphism including skin signs, abnormal head size, motor deficits or epileptic seizures) | Appearances may point towards more detailed specific biochemistry, but beware irrelevant 'abnormalities' |
| **Functional imaging** | | |
| Brain H-MRS | Creatine synthesis and transport disorders especially GAMT and AGAT (as above in urine biochemistry) | Absent creatine peak in all creatine synthesis disorders |

* Epileptic seizures may be a prominent feature.

Abbreviations: AGAT = L-arginine:glycine amidinotransferase; ATRX = alpha–thalassaemia–mental retardation syndrome, X-linked; CGH = comparative genomic hybridization; FISH = fluorescent in situ hybridization; GAMT = guanidinoacetate methyltransferase; HbH = haemoglobin H; MLPA = multiplex ligation-dependent probe amplification; NAA = N-acetyl aspartate; PKU = phenylketonuria; TSH = thyroid-stimulating hormone.

# Chapter 3.10
# Speech and Language Disorders

Speech may not develop or may be slow to develop or may develop and then be lost. The same applies to language, both as output and as input.

### Speech that has not developed adequately

The solution to this problem usually depends on clinical evaluation including specialist help from the speech and language therapist and the psychologist, but deafness, sensorineural or otherwise, is of prime importance. Once deafness has been diagnosed that is not the end of the evaluation, as cognitive defects may coexist, as in congenital rubella and cytomegalovirus infection. For a sound retrospective diagnosis of congenital infections (especially cytomegalovirus) DNA may be extracted from dried blood on the stored neonatal Guthrie card.

In the absence of deafness if there is a defect of both language comprehension and symbolic understanding then investigations are in order as discussed in Chapter 3.9. When there is isolated speech and language disorder then only a few neurological investigations are likely to prove diagnostic.

#### Duchenne muscular dystrophy

Measuring the creatine kinase has been suggested as an investigation to do when a boy has speech and language impairment, but we would not recommend this unless some weakness is also evident, as with difficulty getting off the floor.

#### Creatine synthesis and transport disorders

Severe speech and language delay may be one of the features of creatine synthesis disorders, especially GAMT (guanidinoacetate methyltransferase) and AGAT (arginine:glycine amidinotransferase) deficiency, but only rarely is it an isolated finding. In this clinical situation urine for guanidinoacetic acid (GAA) is one approach: GAA is increased in GAMT deficiency and decreased in AGAT deficiency. A reduced creatine peak on brain or CSF H-MRS will detect most creatine deficiency disorders.

*Angelman syndrome and Angelman-like syndrome*
Though not an isolated feature, lack of expressive speech is a major feature of both Angelman syndrome and the X-linked Angelman-like syndrome due to mutations in *SLC9A6*.

*MECP2 duplication*
This is another condition in which absence of speech is one of the features, often with respiratory infections, but these boys also have severe learning disability and usually epilepsy. Targeted multiplex ligation-dependent probe amplification (MLPA) or if need be *MECP2* gene sequencing will confirm.

*Sepiapterin reductase deficiency*
Sepiapterin reductase deficiency is an uncommon but important cause of primary motor delay accompanied by speech and cognitive disorder and often by oculogyric crises. L-dopa trial will likely improve, but CSF monogenic amines and pterins – with specific request for sepiapterin analysis – should confirm.

*Anterior opercular syndrome*
Selective speech output disorder with dysarthria or anarthria is found in the anterior opecular syndrome (also known as the Worster-Drought or Foix–Chavany–Marie syndrome). This condition is manifest also by oromotor dysfunction with drooling and swallowing difficulty and may be a consequence of prenatal perisylvian polymicrogyria (which may be either genetic or secondary to some insult such as congenital rubella or cytomegalovirus) or secondary to postnatal herpes simplex encephalitis. It may also be a manifestation of an epilepsy, as in perisylvian epileptic encephalopathy. The investigations of choice are Guthrie card testing for viral DNA, brain MRI and EEG.

## Acquired loss of speech
Once again deafness is a common cause, in this case being acquired as with pyogenic meningitis. This should not present diagnostic difficulties unless the ataxia from the labyrinthine damage is regarded as cerebellar rather than vestibular ataxia.

Initial slow speech development followed by gradual speech and language deterioration is typical of Sanfilippo disease in which there is a behaviour disorder that may include aggression, and very gradual intellectual decline. Suspicion of this disorder warrants urine examination for glycosaminoglycans to look for heparan sulphate, and if that test is negative and suspicion is strong a 24-hour urine for heparan sulphate excretion.

*Mutism*
Elective mutism is well known to child psychiatrists, but not all mutism is elective.

POSTERIOR FOSSA SURGERY

Mutism is common after surgery involving the cerebellum and no further investigations are indicated.

MISCELLANEOUS NEUROLOGICAL DISORDERS

We have seen what is apparently mutism or has been called mutism in disparate conditions such as Aicardi syndrome, double cortex (subcortical heterotopia), after corticosteroid treatment of perisylvian epileptic encephalopathy and particularly in the Landau–Kleffner syndrome to be discussed in the next section.

*Landau–Kleffner syndrome*

Otherwise called epileptic aphasia or epileptic auditory agnosia, this disorder need not be associated with any overt epileptic seizures, and if it is they may be few and trivial such as the isolated hemifacial–salivatory seizures seen in benign focal epilepsy of childhood or absence seizures. The helpful investigation is an EEG, which should not only be 'routine' – often showing frequent bilateral spike complexes – but also a sleep recording and if necessary a 24-hour recording. Spikes are commonly bilateral although on the whole not symmetrical and they may be more frequent on one side particularly the left. Their site is in the mid-head region near or posterior to the rolandic strip. The frequency of these spikes is usually such that there is no difficulty in seeing many of them during a standard recording session, but nonetheless 24-hour recording allows the effect of sleep on spike frequency to be demonstrated, commonly as CSWS (continuous spike and wave in sleep).

## Miscellaneous conditions in which speech and language disorders may be prominent

- *22q– deletion* will be detected either by karyotype or fluorescent in situ hybridization (or MLPA).

- *Monocarboxylate transporter 8 (MCT8) mutations* in boys usually include dyskinetic 'cerebral palsy' and learning disability. Thyroid function tests are abnormal.

## Regressive disorders

Several of the conditions discussed in Chapter 3.22 (Progressive Loss of Skills and Dementia) may present with acquired loss of speech but this is not an isolated phenomenon. Dysarthria (and other oromotor problems) are common in Niemann–Pick disease type C, 'mumbling' in juvenile neuronal ceroid lipofuscinosis, interrupted flow of speech output in subacute sclerosing panencephalitis and dysphasia in adrenoleukodystrophy, mentioned next.

*Adrenoleukodystrophy*

What appears at first sight to be isolated loss of speech and language may be the presenting feature of adrenoleukodystrophy, although careful neurological examination should discover other evidence of neurological deficits. When this disorder is suspected the initial investigations are brain MRI and plasma very long chain fatty acids.

## Summary

Until recently the yield from neurological investigations in speech and language disorders has been very low, but rare treatable disorders are emerging (Chapter 3.23).

## Further reading

Manning MA, Cassidy SB, Clericuzio C, et al. (2004) Terminal 22q deletion syndrome: a newly recognized cause of speech and language disability in the autism spectrum. *Pediatrics* **114**: 451–457.

Roll P, Rudolf G, Pereira S, et al. (2006) SRPX2 mutations in disorders of language cortex and cognition. *Hum Mol Genet* **15**: 1195–1207.

Soltanzadeh A, Soltanzadeh P, Nafissi S, et al. (2007) Wilson's disease: a great masquerader. *Eur Neurol* **57**: 80–85.

Stockler S, Schutz PW, Salomons GS. (2007) Cerebral creatine deficiency syndromes: clinical aspects, treatment and pathophysiology. *Subcell Biochem* **46**: 149–166.

Venkateswaran S, Shevell M. (2008) The case against routine electroencephalography in specific language impairment. *Pediatrics* **122**: e911–e916.

Vodopiutz J, Item CB, Häusler M, et al. (2007) Severe speech delay as the presenting symptom of guanidinoacetate methyltransferase deficiency. *J Child Neurol* **22**: 773–774.

# Chapter 3.11

## 'Psychiatric' Disorders

Most behaviour disorders in childhood and most of the disorders that might be seen by the child psychiatrist do not have a neurological basis, at any rate in the sense that neurological investigations might be helpful.

In this chapter we aim to give guidance on what if any neurological investigations to consider in the various 'psychiatric presentations'.

### Psychiatric presentations

In general it will be *atypical* presentations that lead to consideration of neurological investigations. The common symptom of anxiety is too prevalent to be of any diagnostic value or point to the need for any particular investigation.

The situations in which further studies *might* be helpful are listed now (investigations in parentheses).

### Autism spectrum disorders

Autism without additional features has a *low* yield of useful findings on neurological investigation. (We say useful because while it might be possible to show by 3-dimensional MRI that the volume of the cerebellar components is different to the normal population, this is of no value to the psychiatrist, parents or child.) Additional features which are indications for additional investigations include these:

- Severe learning disability (Chapter 3.9)

- Unequivocal epilepsy of early onset (EEG, urine succinylpurines, guanidinoacetate)

- Sudden acute onset of autism (sleep EEG, brain MRI)

- Onset of autism outside the usual age: either too early or later than usual (sleep EEG)

- Marked fluctuation in autistic symptoms (EEG)
- Hands together stereotypy (EEG, MECP2 – Rett; ERG, EEG, protein palmitoyl thioesterase, leukocyte granular osmiophilic deposits – infantile neuronal ceroid lipofuscinosis)
- Associated movement disorders (urine guanidinoacetate, brain H-MRS)
- Regression (see Chapter 3.22).

*Elective mutism*
- When acquired mutism is at first thought to be elective it is important to consider the alternative diagnosis of Landau–Kleffner syndrome (EEG, sleep EEG).

*Conduct disorder/aggression*
- Urine glycosaminoglycans (Sanfilippo disease).

*Rage*
- EEG (frontotemporal epilepsy)
- MRI (hypothalamic hamartoma)
- Ammonia (urea cycle disorder)
- Plasma amino acids including homocysteine [5,10-methylenetetrahydrofolate reductase (MTHFR) deficiency]
- Folate (MTHFR deficiency).

*Tourette, tics, obsessive–compulsive disorder*
- No neurological investigations are generally indicated, but if there are abnormal neurological signs or evidence of regression do brain MRI (pantothenate kinase-associated neurodegeneration) and blood film for acanthocytes (neuroacanthocytosis).

*Attention-deficit–hyperactivity disorder*
- No neurological investigations are generally indicated, but check serum ferritin.

*Learning disability*
- See Chapter 3.9.

*Self-injurious behaviour*
- Dysmorphism may suggest a cause (e.g. Prader–Willi or Cornelia de Lange syndrome)
- Karyotype/fluorescent in situ hybridization (Smith–Magenis syndrome)
- Nerve conductions (sensory and autonomic neuropathy)

- Urinary uric acid (Lesch–Nyhan) – plasma uric acid is *not* adequate
- Urinary succinylpurines (adenylosuccinate lyase deficiency).

*Psychosis*

- EEG (lesional epilepsy)
- Brain MRI/CSF asialotransferrin (eukaryotic translation initiation factor 2B-related disorders)
- $B_{12}$, amino acids and organic acids (cobalamin disorder)
- Ammonia (urea cycle disorders)
- Very long chain fatty acids (adrenoleukodystrophy)
- Porphyrins (porphyria)
- Thyroid function and anti-thyroperoxidase (anti-TPO) antibody (Hashimoto encephalopathy)
- Fibroblast culture cholesterol esterification + filipin staining (Niemann–Pick C).

*'Hysterical' blindness*

- ERG [juvenile neuronal ceroid lipofuscinosis (NCL) – CLN3 or CLN1 – Batten disease].

*'Psychogenic paralysis'*

- ECG, exercise EMG (hypokalaemic periodic paralysis)

*Hallucinations*

- EEG (ring chromosome 20; subacute sclerosing panencephalitis: SSPE)
- MRI for pulvinar (variant Creuztfeld–Jakob disease)
- Karyotype, including 200 metaphases (ring chromosome 20)
- Ammonia (urea cycle disorder)
- Amino acids (MTHFR deficiency; cobalamin disorders)
- Organic acids (cobalamin disorders)
- Toxins (urine gas chromatography mass spectroscopy, etc.)
- Measles titres in blood and CSF (SSPE)
- Anti-NMDA receptor antibodies (anti-NMDA encephalitis).

*Panic attacks*

- Video-EEG and brain MRI (epileptic seizures, e.g. from cortical dysplasia).

*Depression*

- Neurological investigations not indicated when this is an isolated finding

- MRI for pulvinar (variant Creutzfeld–Jacob disease)
- Borrelia titres (neuroborreliosis – but usually diagnosed first)
- Autoantibodies (systemic lupus erythematosus)
- Axillary biopsy (Lafora disease – but usually epileptic seizures and myoclonus first)
- Lysosomal enzymes (Fabry – but pain bouts precede).

*Acute confusion/agitation/delirium*
Diagnostic yield is higher when attacks are recurrent. By far the most common cause will be drug intoxication of some kind: this may require toxicological analyses.

- Ammonia (urea cycle disorder)
- Amino acids including homocysteine (MTHFR deficiency)
- Urine porphyrins (porphyria).

*'Psychiatric' presentation of encephalitis*
Anti-NMDA receptor encephalitis (hallucinations, anxiety, agitation, bizarre behaviour, delusions, paranoia and the resisting of attempted passive eye opening may accompany orofacial and limb dyskinesia alternating with akinesia together with autonomic instability); anti-NMDA receptor antibodies present.

## Range of investigations in 'psychiatric disorders'
Although as we have emphasized *neurological investigations are rarely indicated*, atypical features may prompt the following to be undertaken on occasions (listed in order of Handbook chapters):

- Video–audio (compulsive Valsalva and most disorders)
- EEG and sleep EEG (Landau–Kleffner and other epilepsies, ring 20, SSPE, Lafora)
- ERG ('Batten disease', especially infantile and juvenile NCL)
- Exercise EMG (hypokalaemic periodic paralysis)
- Nerve conduction velocity (sensory and autonomic neuropathy)
- Brain MRI (hypothalamic hamartoma, tumour, cortical dysplasia, pantothenate kinase-associated neurodegeneration eye-of-the-tiger, pulvinar signal in variant Creutzfeld–Jacob disease)
- Brain H-MRS (creatine disorders, mitochondrial)
- Spinal cord MRI (cobalamin disorders)
- CSF protein, immunoglobulin G, measles titres, oligoclonal bands, lactate, 5-methyltetrahydrofolate (SSPE, cerebral folate deficiency)
- Buffy coat electronmicroscopy (NCL – including atypical variants)
- Axillary skin biopsy (Lafora disease)

- Measles titres, blood and CSF (SSPE)

- Borrelia titres (neuroborreliosis)

- Ferritin (attention-deficit–hyperactivity disorder)

- Autoantibodies (systemic lupus erythematosus, Hashimoto encephalopathy, anti-NMDA receptor encephalitis)

- Genetic investigations (see Chapters 2.13 and 3.9 for details) including karyotype and count sufficient mitoses

- Urine glycosaminoglycans (Sanfilippo syndrome)

- Urine porphyrins (porphyria)

- Urine amino acids (as with plasma amino acids, cobalamin disorders)

- Urine organic acids (cobalamin disorders, succinic semialdehyde deficiency)

- Urine uric acid (Lesch–Nyhan disease)

- Urine guanidinoacetate (guanidinoacetate methyltransferase and L-arginine:glycine amidinotransferase deficiency)

- Urinary copper (Wilson disease)

- Urine toxicology (various)

- Thyroid function (hyper- or hypothyroidism, Hashimoto encephalopathy)

- Ammonia (urea cycle disorders)

- Plasma amino acids (phenylketonuria, homocystinuria, atypical glycine encephalopathy)

- Plasma total homocysteine (cobalamin disorders, MTHFR deficiency)

- Copper and copper oxidase (Wilson disease)

- Cholestanol (cerebrotendinous xanthomatosis)

- Glucose (hypoglycaemia)

- Lactate (mitochondrial disorders)

- Plasma very long chain fatty acids (adrenoleukodystrophy)

- Lysosomal enzymes (Fabry)

- Fibroblast cholesterol esterification studies (Niemann–Pick C).

## Concern that something treatable or genetic is being missed
All child psychiatrists will have worries of this nature from time to time. If practicable, consultation with a paediatric neurologist should *precede* further neurological investigations.

## Further reading

Arnulf I, Lin L, Gadoth N, et al. (2008) Kleine–Levin syndrome: a systematic study of 108 patients. *Ann Neurol* **63**: 482–493.

Carmel R, Green R, Rosenblatt DS, et al. (2003) Update on cobalamin, folate, and homocysteine. *Hematology Am Soc Hematol Educ Program* 62–81.

Dinopoulos A, Kure S, Chuck G, et al. (2005) Glycine decarboxylase mutations: a distinctive phenotype of nonketotic hyperglycinemia in adults. *Neurology* **64**: 1255–1257.

Edelman EA, Girirajan S, Finucane B, et al. (2007) Gender, genotype, and phenotype differences in Smith–Magenis syndrome: a meta-analysis of 105 cases. *Clin Genet* **71**: 540–550.

Feinstein C, Singh S. (2007) Social phenotypes in neurogenetic syndromes. *Child Adolesc Psychiatr Clin N Am* **16**: 631–647.

Görker I, Tüzün U. (2005) Autistic-like findings associated with a urea cycle disorder in a 4-year-old girl. *J Psychiatry Neurosci* **30**: 133–135.

Hallett M. (2006) Psychogenic movement disorders: a crisis for neurology. *Curr Neurol Neurosci Rep* **6**: 269–271.

Jansen AC, Cao H, Kaplan P, et al. (2007) Sanfilippo syndrome type D: natural history and identification of 3 novel mutations in the GNS Gene. *Arch Neurol* **64**: 1629–1634.

Largillière C. (1995) Psychiatric manifestations in girl with ornithine transcarbamylase deficiency. *Lancet* **345**: 1113.

Moog U, van Mierlo I, van Schrojenstein Lantman-de Valk HM, et al. (2007) Is Sanfilippo type B in your mind when you see adults with mental retardation and behavioral problems? *Am J Med Genet C Semin Med Genet* **145C**: 293–301.

Sedel F, Baumann N, Turpin JC, et al. (2007) Psychiatric manifestations revealing inborn errors of metabolism in adolescents and adults. *J Inherit Metab Dis* **30**: 631–641.

Soltanzadeh A, Soltanzadeh P, Nafissi S, et al. (2007) Wilson's disease: a great masquerader. *Eur Neurol* **57**: 80–85.

Thandani H, Deacon A, Peters T. (2000) Diagnosis and management of porphyria. *BMJ* **320**: 1647–1651.

Walker RH, Jung HH, Dobson-Stone C, et al. (2007) Neurologic phenotypes associated with acanthocytosis. *Neurology* **68**: 92–98.

# Chapter 3.12
## Epileptic Seizures and Epilepsy

Because it is not as simple as it seems, the definition of an epileptic seizure is often assumed or skated over. To simplify, an epileptic seizure is the outward manifestation of an abnormal excessive discharge of neurons in the brain. The outward manifestations of such an epileptic seizure would normally be clinical phenomena but if recording electrodes happen to be in place close to the seizure origin then repetitive electrical discharges would be recorded. Again in simple terms, epilepsy implies recurrent unprovoked epileptic seizures or at any rate epileptic seizures provoked only by everyday stimuli (such as television).

The recognition of epileptic seizures is by the appearance or semiology, and the first necessity is to distinguish them from non-epileptic paroxysmal events, a task made easier by seeing the episode or a video – such as a home movie – of the event which has happened. Elsewhere in this book we discuss neonatal seizures (Chapter 3.1), febrile seizures (Chapter 3.13), paroxysmal disorders which are not epilepsy (Chapter 3.14) and – of special interest – epileptic and non-epileptic disorders together (Chapter 3.15). While the detailed clinical description that is possible by videocamera or even mobile phone capture is paramount in diagnosis, other investigation or methods may often be helpful.

The EEG (see Chapter 2.2) is of particular value. It is of conclusive help in diagnosis when an epileptic seizure is actually recorded (ictal recording) but once the diagnosis of epilepsy is established the EEG pattern between seizures (interictal) is one of the components of an epileptic syndrome, the others being age of onset, seizure types and interictal condition of the child.

Before we proceed it is important to emphasize that not all seizures are epileptic seizures. In particular they may be anoxic seizures (non-epileptic convulsive syncope) or psychological (psychogenic non-epileptic seizures otherwise called non-epileptic attack disorder). Although this differential diagnosis seems at first sight complex, in practice the situation is often simple. For example, if a normal child standing in school assembly falls down and has a short tonic seizure with immediate recovery (albeit with pallor) then the diagnosis is non-epileptic convulsive syncope without need for further investigations. It was a fainting fit and not an epileptic seizure. But if the child standing next to him complained of feeling sick and looked pale and five minutes later vomited while still standing and gradually became disorientated before his eyes deviated to the right as he became unresponsive, then neurological investigation *would* be indicated, in this case a standard EEG to look for the spike complexes to be expected in Panayiotopoulos syndrome.

Leaving further aspects of the differential diagnosis to other chapters (3.13–3.15) we will now tabulate some investigational aspects of epileptic seizures and epileptic syndromes and situations.

We will assume that an EEG, preferably with natural sleep, will ordinarily be requested for a child who has had an epileptic seizure and is thought likely to have epilepsy. We will also assume that when the described nature of the epileptic seizure (the semiology) suggests a *lesional* origin, brain MRI will be arranged, bearing in mind that very rarely focal twitching will have a *spinal* origin (see Clinical Vignette 2.1.8).

Now follow two tables.

Table 3.12.1 presents a simple guide to epileptic seizure patterns with clinical and EEG information.

Then the longer Table 3.12.2 lists by approximate age at presentation a number of epileptic syndromes and situations from the very common to the very rare – though unfortunately the median age of onset is often not reported in the published literature. We concentrate on the EEG both as is usual between episodes (interictal) and during seizures (ictal) as is occasionally achieved. We also summarize the ictal EMG findings (predominantly from deltoid recordings) where these are available. In the final column we list additional investigations that sometimes clarify the position further. Not every child will have a seizure history that fits neatly into this table, but we think the attempt is a worthwhile exercise.

We could have made this table longer or shorter: longer because many more syndromes have been postulated, shorter because those who are not epileptologists like it simple and might even wish for the old days when it was either grand mal or petit mal. Our objective has been to shed some light on the place of neurological investigations in epileptic situations.

We realize that for several reasons many children's seizures cannot be pigeon-holed into any particular epilepsy syndrome but making some attempt increases the chance of determining the prognosis and the optimum treatment together with the underlying genetic structural or metabolic basis. Discussion of some specifics follows.

Table 3.12.1 EEG investigation in common epileptic seizures

| Seizure type | Semiology | Ictal EEG | Ictal EMG (both deltoids) | Comments |
|---|---|---|---|---|
| Generalized tonic–clonic | Stiffening → vibration → rapid face and limb twitching → slowing in jerk rate → stupor after 1–1½ minutes | Massive generalized EMG obscures very fast spikes → decelerating generalized spike and wave (S/W) | Generalized high-voltage continuous | Mature seizure type of older children and adolescents. 'Generalized tonic–clonic' is much misused for any infantile convulsion |
| Clonic | Rhythmic or semi-rhythmic or syncopated jerks | Generalized rhythmic or semi-rhythmic S/W | Semi-rhythmic accentuations | Many infantile convulsions including anoxic epileptic seizures (AES) – Chapter 3.15 |
| Hemiclonic | Unilateral semi-rhythmic | Contralateral semi-rhythmic S/W | Contralateral semi-rhythmic accentuations | Many infantile convulsions including anoxic epileptic seizures (AES) – Chapter 3.15 |
| Absence (sudden-onset blank 10s or more duration) | Maybe rhythmic small jerks eyelids or neck | 3/s generalized S/W | None | Inducible by hyperventilation |
| Myoclonic–absence | Upper limbs slowly elevate with rhythmic jerks of shoulders | Generalized 3/s S/W | Incremental tonic activity, superimposed 3/s high-voltage transients | Surface EMG (as bilateral deltoid) is a necessary part of EEG examination |

Table 3.12.1 continued

| Seizure type | Semiology | Ictal EEG | Ictal EMG (both deltoids) | Comments |
|---|---|---|---|---|
| Myoclonic | Isolated clustered or rhythmic jerks | Polyspike–wave or irregular spike/polyspike–wave | Spike-like 10–100ms bursts singly or in groups | Seen in many epileptic syndromes and situations |
| Negative myoclonic (atonic/astatic) | Jerk/drop, singly or clustered | Polyspike followed by a high-amplitude slow wave | Ongoing EMG disappears during drop | Video may add |
| Spasm | Longer than myoclonus, usually in runs | Serial biphasic slow complexes with superimposed fast (beta) often central and time-locked with spasms | Diamond or rhomboidal bursts of 0.5–2s duration | Hypsarrhythmia but not always; also seen in older children |
| Tonic | Several seconds stiffening, agonists and antagonists | Flattening or attenuation of background with superimposed low-voltage fast activity and loss of previously seen interictal discharges | High-voltage continuous ('fuzz') | Seen in severe epilepsies as Lennox–Gastaut syndrome |
| Partial/focal/localization-related | Any site, any semiology | Localized/lateralized morphology varies with age, ± secondarily generalized | Depends on site of origin | Seen in genetic ('idiopathic') and structural epilepies |

Table 3.12.2 Epileptic syndromes

| Epileptic syndrome | Age of onset | Age of offset | Clinical | Interictal EEG | Ictal EEG | Additional investigation |
|---|---|---|---|---|---|---|
| Epileptic encephalopathy with suppression bursts | Prenatal, day 1, first weeks | Not unless abolished by pyridoxine or pyridoxal phosphate | Spasms, jerks; profound delay if untreated | Suppression-burst | Bursts | Pyridoxal phosphate trial or pyridoxine trial if pyridoxal phosphate not available, urine α-AASA, CSF amino acids, copper, copper oxidase, catecholamines, brain MRI, *ARX*, *STXBP1* |
| Hemifacial spasms | Day 1 (but may be later) | Only if surgery | Exceedingly frequent facial contractions with winking, eye movement, autonomic disturbance | Normal | Normal except for eyelid movement artefact | Brain MRI, ictal SPECT (hamartoma of floor of fourth ventricle with neuronal elements on surgery) |
| Gelastic/dacrystic seizures | Day 1 (more often later) | Only if surgery | Exceedingly frequent brief bouts of laughter → crying, autonomic. Behavioural arrest if untreated | Often normal | May be normal | Audio with video, MRI including sagittal T2, ictal SPECT (hypothalamic hamartoma on surgery) |
| Neonatal tonic–clonic seizures | First week | Uncertain | Tonic–clonic or tonic–myoclonic seizures with posturing → focal or multifocal clonic | 'Abnormal' | Flattening → focal or bilateral discharges | Pyridoxal phosphate or pyridoxine trial, urine α-AASA, *KCNQ2* mutations |
| Benign neonatal–infantile seizures | Neonate–3mo | <1y | Convulsive, often clusters ± head and eye deviation | Normal or maybe spikes in sleep | Lateralized then generalization | Mutations in *SCN2A* (diagnosis at 3mo avoids bad prognosis) |
| *CDKL5*-related epilepsy | 4w (1–10w) | ?? Not usually | Stares, flush, tonic ± → clonic; → frequent spasms; ± Rett-like | ± Normal | Flattening | Mutations in *CDKL5* |
| DEND (delay, epilepsy, neonatal diabetes mellitus) | 3mo | ? | Neonatal diabetes mellitus, West syndrome with spasms | Independent spikes | ? | Sulphonylurea-responsive mutations in *Kir6.2* (potassium ATP channel) |

Table 3.12.2 continued

| Epileptic syndrome | Age of onset | Age of offset | Clinical | Interictal EEG | Ictal EEG | Additional investigation |
|---|---|---|---|---|---|---|
| Malignant migrating partial seizures | 40d (neonate –3mo) | ? Never | Partial, autonomic, vary from seizure to seizure, appear with increasing frequency over time | Normal to slow, multifocal sharp | Independent R + L sharp runs in theta or alpha frequency | Candidate for novel investigations |
| GLUT1 deficiency (glucose transporter deficiency without full DeVivo syndrome) | ~3–6mo (more data needed) | If given ketogenic diet | Early absences, myoclonic episodes before feeds | Often focal spikes in infancy, generalized S/W in older children (like idiopathic generalized epilepsy) | S/W runs | Fasting blood and CSF glucose + lactate. *SLCA1* mutation |
| West syndrome (serial epileptic spasms, regression) | 5mo (4–7mo) | Various | Spasm runs with loss of contact and regression – many possible associations, e.g. Down syndrome | Hypsarrhythmia usually | Runs of spasms as in Table 3.12.1 | MRI, karyotype, 1p36 *ARX, CDKL5, SCN1A*, rarely metabolic, incl. D-bifunctional protein defect |
| Benign familial infantile seizures (BFIS)/benign partial epilepsy of infancy | 5–6mo (3–18mo) | <2y | Clusters of brief seizures with loss of contact, motor arrest ± head and eye deviation, some automatisms ± secondary generalization; normal development; ± → paroxysmal kinesigenic dyskinesia | Normal | Fast spikes in various locations ± → generalized S/W | No additional investigations required |
| Benign myoclonic epilepsy of infancy | 6mo | Usually 6mo–5y after | Jerks without falls singly or in clusters; may have later generalized tonic–clonic seizures in adolescence | Normal | Generalized polyspike and wave | None (but not known if might be GLUT1D manifestation) |

Table 3.12.2 continued

| Epileptic syndrome | Age of onset | Age of onset | Clinical | Interictal EEG | Ictal EEG | Additional investigation |
|---|---|---|---|---|---|---|
| Reflex myoclonic epilepsy of infancy | 6–21mo | Within 4–14mo | Run of a few myoclonic jerks if startled as with a tap on the head | Normal | Generalized S/W | None |
| Angelman syndrome | 9mo | ~Never | Seizure onset before Angelman features obvious (median age at diagnosis 60mo); absences, myoclonic | Spike on sharp wave on passive eye closure, frontal slow runs, theta | Various S/W runs | Emphasizes importance of passive eye closure during EEG and at least brief video in all EEG recordings |
| Dravet syndrome [including severe myoclonic epilepsy in infancy (SMEI) and SMEI-borderline] | 3–12mo (<18mo) | No | Long especially hemiclonic febrile seizures, clonic, tonic-clonic later ± myoclonic | Normal early ± photo-sensitivity, background slows with age | Polyspike-wave, generalized S/W, focal discharges | Mutations in SCN1A and less often in PCDH19 |
| Febrile seizures (FS) | 3mo – <6y | <6y | Not rigor febrile syncope, 'breath-holding spell', reflex asystolic syncope; temperature >38°C (101°F) probably clonic or tonic | Normal, later ± hypnagogic S/W, age 3–4y | Very rarely captured | Investigations for infections, etc. (see Chapter 3.13). Brain MRI not required |
| Febrile seizures plus (FS+) | FS <3mo or >6y | ? | ± Afebrile epileptic seizures. NB genetic epilepsy with FS+ (GEFS+) is not a patient diagnosis but is a family one | Usually normal | Not known | Not MRI. SCN1A or other mutation possible |
| Febrile status epilepticus (FSE) | Median 1.3y (interquartile range 0.99–2.2y) | ? | Median duration 68min. Semiology disputed but includes clonic | Probably normal | Prolonged discharges | Brain MRI normally not required unless suspect encephalitis |

Table 3.12.2 continued

| Epileptic syndrome | Age of onset | Age of offset | Clinical | Interictal EEG | Ictal EEG | Additional investigation |
|---|---|---|---|---|---|---|
| Benign convulsions with mild gastroenteritis | Median 23mo with rotavirus | After illness | Asian, especially Japanese clusters within 5d of gastroenteritis | Not known | Not known | Viral studies especially rotavirus |
| Benign focal epilepsy in infancy with midline S/W during sleep | 17mo (4–30mo) | 26mo | Cyanosis (especially perioral), stare, behavioural arrest, not secondary generalization postictal sleep (most don't need therapy) | In sleep vertex (midline) spike and bell-shaped wave | Vertex theta runs | None |
| Late-onset 'juvenile spasms' | >12mo | ? Never | Cryptogenic or structural, e.g. double cortex/subcortical band heterotopia | Varied | Runs of serial complexes: slow + fast superimposed | Brain MRI |
| Myoclonic–astatic epilepsy | 18–50mo | ? 36–100mo | Tonic–clonic, myoclonic–astatic, myoclonic, ± myoclonic status, no tonic seizures, may remit | S/W on falling asleep | Generalized S/W bursts with special EMG features: EMG burst → EMG loss | Brain MRI commonly normal (in severe learning disability consider MECP2 duplication by MLPA) |
| Lennox-Gastaut syndrome | 3–5y | ? Never | Axial tonic in sleep, atypical absences; learning disability; cryptogenic and symptomatic; nonconvulsive status epilepticus common | Slow background, slow S/W awake, high-voltage 10–12Hz in sleep | Flattening with tonic EMG | Brain MRI and possibly other aetiological investigations as not a single-cause diagnosis |

Table 3.12.2 continued

| Epileptic syndrome | Age of onset | Age of offset | Clinical | Interictal EEG | Ictal EEG | Additional investigation |
|---|---|---|---|---|---|---|
| Panayiotopoulos syndrome | 3–6y (1–10y) | Usually within 2y | ± From sleep: ictus emeticus (epileptic seizure with nausea and vomiting at onset) pallor and other autonomic features, eye deviation, flaccidity, ± >30min duration then called autonomic status epilepticus | Spikes may be occipital but other sites, such as rolandic, more likely to be seen in sleep. ± Fixation-off sensitivity with occipital discharges | Spike runs occipital but from other sites; may be cardio-respiratory arrest | Panayiotopoulos syndrome diagnosis prevents many other investigations. Brain MRI only if not certain about neurodevelopmental normality at time of first episode |
| Landau–Kleffner syndrome. Continuous spike–wave in sleep (CSWS) also called ESES (epileptic status epilepticus in sleep) | 2–8y | Varied | Auditory agnosia, cognitive decline; learning difficulties may overshadow subtle epileptic seizures if present. Decline in abilities of a child with shunted hydrocephalus may be due to unrecognized CSWS | Perisylvian spike complexes slow spike–wave in non-REM sleep = CSWS | Various | Brain MRI often done; place of functional imaging uncertain |
| Ring chromosome 20 | 4–8y (day 1–17y) | ? | Most have normal development before seizure onset, typical episodes of terror and hallucination may not begin till after age 4y. Neurobehavioural decline with seizures, potentially reversible | Prominent rhythmic frontal slow (delta, but also theta) ± spikes – may not be seen in early years | Frontal onset discharges | Chromosome karyotype with request to count 200 mitoses |

Table 3.12.2 continued

| Epileptic syndrome | Age of onset | Age of offset | Clinical | Interictal EEG | Ictal EEG | Additional investigation |
|---|---|---|---|---|---|---|
| Childhood absence epilepsy (CAE) | Peak 5–6y (4–10y) | 2–6y after onset | Pure sudden on and sudden off blanks, usually hyperventilation-induced | Normal, not photo-sensitive ± occipital intermittent rhythmic delta activity | Symptomatic bursts of 3/s S/W with one spike per wave, often 10s or more absences | Video during hyperventilation in clinic may suffice, but ictal EEG with video best in case pseudo-epileptic absences. If atypical and food (meal) related consider GLUT1 deficiency |
| Childhood absence epilepsy with photoparoxysmal response | 4–10y | ? As CAE | As for CAE except photoparoxysmal response on EEG | Normal but generalized spike/ polyspike and wave on stroboscopic activation | Symptomatic bursts of 3/s S/W with one spike per wave | Video during hyperventialtion in clinic may suffice, but ictal EEG with video best in case pseudo-epileptic absences. If atypical and food (meal) related consider GLUT1 deficiency |
| Epilepsy with myoclonic absences | 7y (1–12y) | May not | Upper limbs slowly elevate with 3/s jerks | Normal background ± generalized S/W bursts | 3/s S/W with incremental tonic EMG and superimposed 3/s EMG bursts | Video. Consider GLUT1 deficiency and chromosomes (e.g. trisomy 12p) |
| Benign rolandic epilepsy (BRE)/ benign epilepsy with centro-temporal spikes (BECTS) | 7–8y (4–14y) | Within 2–4y of onset (<16y) | Hemifacial-salivatory often from sleep, family holiday in back of car; secondary generalization common | Rolandic or centro-temporal spike complexes | Focal discharge during episodes | No need for brain MRI if history typical and neurologically normal. Rolandic spikes more common in those without epilepsy |

Table 3.12.2 continued

| Epileptic Syndrome | Age of onset | Age of offset | Clinical | Interictal EEG | Ictal EEG | Additional investigation |
|---|---|---|---|---|---|---|
| Childhood occipital epilepsy of Gastaut | 8y (3–15y) | 50% within 2–3y | Seizures ~frequent and diurnal, elementary visual hallucinations: multicoloured circular patterns may be the sole manifestation. Migraine-like | ± Fixation-off sensitivity with occipital discharges | Sudden onset of fast rhythms, fast spikes or both in occipital regions | Brain MRI desirable in case symptomatic. Consider *POLG1* if suggestion of mitochondrial disorder |
| Autosomal dominant nocturnal frontal lobe epilepsy | Mainly 8–14y | May not | From sleep, with several throughout the night (contrast night terrors, 1 or 2 at beginning of sleep) | Normal | Often normal with only ictal EMG and motion artefacts | Nocturnal video preferably with infrared recording; helpful to get night-time video of close or distant family members who may be affected; gene analysis by arrangement |
| Juvenile myoclonic epilepsy | 9–13y (5–20y) | May not | Morning myoclonus, clumsiness, generalized tonic–clonic and clonic–tonic–clonic seizures especially when sleep deprived. In childhood, short absences may precede onset of myoclonus and tonic–clonic seizures | Irregular spike and polyspike wave bursts | 4–6/s polyspike and wave. Absences may have multiple spikes per wave, often <10s, shorter than in CAE | Investigations generally unhelpful (if regression, consider progressive myoclonus epilepsies – Chapter 3.22) |
| Mesial temporal lobe epilepsy with hippocampal sclerosis | 4–16y | Mostly only if surgical resection | Ascending epigastric aura may be fear or panic, déjà vu, dreamy state, oro-elementary automatisms, etc. | Spike and slow complexes in ipsilateral anterior temporal region | Subtle onset with focal crescendo theta | High quality brain MRI targeted to show hippocampi |

*Some common and important syndromes*
It is particularly important to be familiar with some syndromes which are common but not always well understood or easily recognized.

FEBRILE SEIZURES
The following chapter (3.13) deals entirely with febrile seizures but because of their great importance and relationship to epilepsy or epilepsies we have paid special attention to these throughout Table 3.12.2. It cannot be repeated too often that if an episode has occurred with a fever it is necessary to determine both what the temperature was and precisely what the nature was of the paroxysmal episode.

For convenience, Table 3.12.3 lists epilepsies that are associated with febrile seizures.

Table 3.12.3 Epilepsies associated with febrile seizures

| Epilepsy situation | Febrile seizures (rounded percentages) |
| --- | --- |
| Benign familal neonatal seizures | 5%[a] |
| Benign myoclonic epilepsy of infancy | 20% |
| Angelman syndrome | 50%[b] |
| Dravet syndrome | 70–100% |
| GEFS+ (families) | 100% |
| Panayiotopoulos syndrome | 20% |
| Childhood absence epilepsy with or without photoparoxysmal response | 20% |
| Benign rolandic epilepsy/benign epilepsy with centrotemporal spikes | 10–20% |
| Mesial temporal lobe epilepsy with hippocampal sclerosis | 60% |

a Not clear, but different from normal rate

b Fever-associated

Some simple investigations have been outlined in Table 3.12.2 and two of the most important conditions listed – GEFS+ and Panayiotopoulos syndrome – will now be detailed further.

GEFS+

It is always nice when an acronym lends itself to helpful changes in the meaning of the component letters. GEFS+ has for over a decade meant 'generalized epilepsy with febrile seizures plus'. However, since in some families focal seizures may also occur Professors Ingrid Scheffer and Samuel Berkovic have suggested altering the nomenclature to *genetic* epilepsy with febrile seizures plus. GEFS+ has been a most important concept in elucidating the relationship between febrile seizures and epilepsy. The concept led directly to the discovery of mutations in sodium channels and GABA receptors in epilepsy, but discovery of a pathogenic mutation is not necessary for the diagnosis of GEFS+ (*SCN1A* mutations are found in <10%). GEFS+ (a family diagnosis) led to the discovery of *SCN1A* being pathogenic in Dravet syndrome, but although most children with Dravet syndrome have *SCN1A* mutations the detection of such mutations is not necessary for that diagnosis to be established [the diagnosis of Dravet syndrome in infancy is possible with some combination of onset of (1) febrile seizures aged 7 months or earlier; (2) five or more seizures with hemiconvulsions; and/or (3) seizures lasting more than 30 minutes]. Recently mutations in *PCDH19* have been found in *SCN1A*-negative patients, mainly female, with a Dravet-like syndrome.

PANAYIOTOPOULOS SYNDROME

Although, as with GEFS+, Panayiotopoulos syndrome is now recognized worldwide to be a common disorder, practitioners still have difficulty with its recognition. It was originally thought to be a benign occipital epilepsy but although it is benign (in the sense that it remits) it is not necessarily occipital at all. Its importance (for general paediatricians or paediatric neurologists and emergency physicians and those in intensive care units) is that it presents as if it were the onset of a severe or even life-threatening encephalopathy with vomiting at onset, pallor, eye deviation and impairment of consciousness. The most useful neurological investigation is a prompt EEG (with sleep activation if need be), which usually shows multifocal high-amplitude sharp and slow wave complexes on a normal background. *SCN1A* mutations may be sought.

ROLANDIC EPILEPSY

Rolandic epilepsy, also called benign rolandic epilepsy (BRE) and benign epilepsy of childhood with centrotemporal spikes (BECTS), is even more common than Panayiotopoulos syndrome. It is supposedly well known but misconceptions are common and much has still to be learned.

The epileptic seizures of early school-age onset are most typically hemifacial with unilateral tonic contraction of the lower lip and numbness of the lip and perhaps tingling inside the mouth. Inability to speak (anarthria) is accompanied by a gurgly sound and excess saliva that dribbles down the chin. These hemifacial salivatory seizures may wake the child from sleep or typically manifest in the back of a car after a family holiday. They are perhaps best described as sylvian seizures, and the EEG spike complexes that are seen interictally are more sylvian than temporal. Whatever one calls them, these rolandic spikes are much more common in children *without* epilepsy, so that it is essential to have the clinical diagnosis before making inferences from the EEG investigation. Having made the diagnosis clinically and with EEG confirmation, then – unlike the situation in focal epilepsies in general – brain MRI is not indicated. Eventually the seizures remit spontaneously and this is why the epilepsy is called benign. Benign does not mean that no neurodevelopmental problems ever arise. Indeed, language and behavioural difficulties are quite common, and sometimes CSWS may develop, such that all-night EEG is indicated if there is a suggestion of regression.

BRE/BECTS has been reported in fragile X syndrome but testing for *FMR1* is indicated only when other clinical features of the fragile X syndrome are present.

*Metabolic and genetic associations*
There are many other situations in which epileptic seizures or epilepsy are associated with genetic factors including chromosomal aberrations, metabolic disorders and structural lesions. Some of these associations with key neurological investigations are tabulated in Tables 3.12.4 and 3.12.5. Mutations in *neuroserpin* have now been found in a case with epilepsy, regression and CSWS, and the epilepsy phenotype of *neuroserpinopathies* is likely to broaden.

CHROMOSOMES
Other chromosomal abnormalities are associated with epilepsies, in particular infantile spasms but also Lennox–Gastaut syndrome (inv-dup chromosome 15). Either an unusual epilepsy or an unusual EEG appearance should prompt at least standard chromosome karyotype examination.

Table 3.12.4 Some genetic and structural epilepsy associations

| Condition | Clinical | Investigations |
| --- | --- | --- |
| Down syndrome | Infantile spasms common (2%) and easily overlooked | Interictal EEG slow general spike wave or hypsarrhythmia (chromosomes of course) |
| 1p36 deletion | Dysmorphism with straight eyebrows and deep-set eyes, the most common seizure type is infantile spasms | Karyotype, fluorescent in situ hybridization, multiplex ligation-dependent probe amplification |
| Ring chromosome 14 | Very mild dysmorphism, early infantile serial tonic | Count sufficient metaphases |
| Lesional epilepsy | Vast range of lesions especially focal cortical dysplasia; partial epilepsies of any kind with onset at any age | Brain MRI but may need ictal SPECT, PET and high-resolution MRI especially if surgical intervention likely |

Table 3.12.4 continued

| Condition | Clinical | Investigations |
|---|---|---|
| Epilepsia partialis continua | Unilateral with atrophy may suggest Rasmussen encephalitis | Anti-brain antibodies not helpful in diagnosing Rasmussen |
| | Unilateral onset in infancy | High-resolution brain MRI for cortical dysplasia |
| | Variable sites may suggest mitochondrial, especially Alpers, with RHADS (rhythmic high-amplitude delta with superimposed spikes) on EEG | *POLG1* and other mitochondrial investigations |
| Video game epileptic seizures | Situational photic or pattern-sensitive epileptic seizures | EEG/ECG with photic and pattern stimulation including monocular |
| Progressive myoclonus epilepsies | Various – see Chapter 3.22 | See Chapter 3.22 |

Table 3.12.5 Some metabolic epilepsy associations

| Condition | Clinical | Metabolic investigations |
|---|---|---|
| Common metabolic problems (sodium, calcium, glucose, etc.) | Convulsive seizures most likely clonic, perhaps tonic–clonic, depends on age | 'Routine' electrolytes, calcium, phosphorus, glucose |
| Pyridoxine dependency | Neonatal especially with suppression–burst, neonatal tonic–clonic epilepsy with status until age 3y, might be Dravet-like | Pyridoxine trial, plasma and urine alpha-aminoadipic semialdehyde ($\alpha$-AASA), pipecolic acid |
| Pyridoxal phosphate-responsive seizures | Neonatal encephalopathy with suppression–burst, not known if occurs later in infancy | Pyridoxal phosphate trial. CSF amino acids. *PNPO* gene analysis |

Table 3.12.5 continued

| Condition | Clinical | Metabolic investigations |
|---|---|---|
| Folinic acid-responsive seizures | As for pyridoxine dependency | Folinic acid trial but also pyridoxine |
| Adenylosuccinate lyase (ADSL) deficiency | Delay with hypotonia usually precedes epilepsy, autism, self-mutilation, postconvulsive hemiplegia reported, various seizures may be intractable with EEG S/W; MRI may show 'hypomyelination' | Urine succinylpurines, possible *ADSL* mutation |
| Serine synthesis deficiency | Early (first month) intractable seizures ('cyanotic episode') jerking, tonic posturing. Microcephaly. MRI ± hypomyelination | CSF serine and glycine, gene analysis especially *PSAT1* |
| Menkes disease, mild forms possible | Kinky hair detectable on microscopy, bone changes and subdural haemorrhage may simulate child abuse, various seizures including spasms | Copper, copper oxidase |
| Untreated phenylketonuria (PKU) missed | Missed PKU may be seen in countries without neonatal screening tests; autism, stereotypies, developmental delay, infantile spasms | Plasma and urine amino acids |
| Mitochondrial disorder | Seizures especially epilepsia partialis continua; may have basal ganglia signal change or cerebellar atrophy or lesions in cortical grey matter especially in occipital regions; multiorgan involvement | Lactates: see Chapter 2.14. Genes: especially *POLG1* |
| Guanidinoacetate methyltransferase deficiency | Developmental delay; epileptic seizures ± early absences and myoclonus; brain H-MRS: absent creatine peak | ↑ urine guanidinoacetate, ↓ creatine on brain H-MRS |

Table 3.12.5 continued

| Condition | Clinical | Metabolic investigations |
|---|---|---|
| Glucose transporter 1 deficiency | Acquired microcephaly, spasticity and delayed development may be absent; early absences and myoclonic seizures *may* be feed- or meal-related, worse when hungry; epileptic seizures are ketogenic diet-responsive, as may be paroxysmal movements and ataxia | Fasting blood and CSF glucose |

## Metabolic epilepsies

There are numerous metabolic disorders in which epileptic seizures may be a feature. The diagnosis of a metabolic error may often be guided by features other than the epilepsy whereas, in some associations, the epilepsy may be a coincidence. In Table 3.12.5 we have listed some metabolic disorders complicated by epilepsy in which the appropriate investigation is important for a child or family.

## Sudden unexplained death in epilepsy (SUDEP)

Investigations after apparent SUDEP relate to the possibility that the death may actually have been due not to epilepsy but to an undiagnosed cardiac conduction defect. In this situation the ECG channel may be reviewed and the neonatal Guthrie card tested for mutations in the ion channel genes responsible for long-QT and related syndromes.

## Conclusion

While a precise, detailed, consecutive, all-embracing history is paramount in the diagnosis of paroxysmal disorders, neurological investigations from the simplest home video recording through various types of EEG to gene mutation analysis may significantly help in the management of affected children and their families.

## Further reading

Bahi-Buisson N, Guttierrez-Delicado E, Soufflet C, et al. (2008) Spectrum of epilepsy in terminal 1p36 deletion syndrome. *Epilepsia* **49**: 509–515.

Bahi-Buisson N, Nectoux J, Rosas-Vargas H, et al. (2008) Key clinical features to identify girls with CDKL5 mutations. *Brain* **131**: 2647–2661.

Battaglia A, Hoyme HE, Dallapiccola B, et al. (2008) Further delineation of deletion 1p36 syndrome in 60 patients: a recognizable phenotype and common cause of developmental delay and mental retardation. *Pediatrics* **121**: 404–410.

Baxter P, Clarke A, Cross H, et al. (2003) Idiopathic catastrophic epileptic encephalopathy presenting with acute onset intractable status. *Seizure* 12: 379–87.

Capovilla G, Beccaria F, Montagnini A. (2006) 'Benign focal epilepsy in infancy with vertex spikes and waves during sleep'. Delineation of the syndrome and recalling as 'benign infantile focal epilepsy with midline spikes and waves during sleep' (BIMSE). *Brain Dev* 28: 85–91.

Caraballo RH, Cersosimo RO, Fejerman N. (2007) Panayiotopoulos syndrome: a prospective study of 192 patients. *Epilepsia* 48: 1054–1061.

Caraballo RH, Bongiorni L, Cersosimo R, et al. (2008) Epileptic encephalopathy with continuous spikes and waves during sleep in children with shunted hydrocephalus: a study of nine cases. *Epilepsia* 49: 1520–1527.

Caraballo RH, Cersosimo RO, Fejerman N. (2008) Childhood occipital epilepsy of Gastaut: a study of 33 patients. *Epilepsia* 49: 288–297.

Coutelier M, Andries S, Ghariani S, et al. (2008) Neuroserpin mutation causes electrical status epilepticus of slow-wave sleep. *Neurology* 71: 64–66.

Depienne C, Bouteiller D, Keren B, et al. (2009) Sporadic infantile epileptic encephalopathy caused by mutations in PCDH19 resembles Dravet syndrome but mainly affects females. *PLoS Genet* 5: e1000381.

Eisermann MM, Ville D, Soufflet C, et al. (2006) Cryptogenic late-onset epileptic spasms: an overlooked syndrome of early childhood? *Epilepsia* 47: 1035–1042.

Ferrie CD, Caraballo R, Covanis A, et al. (2007) Autonomic status epilepticus in Panayiotopoulos syndrome and other childhood and adult epilepsies: a consensus view. *Epilepsia* 48: 1165–1172.

Gallagher RC, Van Hove JL, Scharer G, et al. (2009) Folinic acid-responsive seizures are identical to pyridoxine-dependent epilepsy. *Ann Neurol* 65: 550–556.

Harkin LA, McMahon JM, Iona X, et al. (2007) The spectrum of SCN1A-related infantile epileptic encephalopathies. *Brain* 130: 843–852.

Hattori J, Ouchida M, Ono J, et al. (2008) A screening test for the prediction of Dravet syndrome before one year of age. *Epilepsia* 49: 626–633.

Kassai B, Chiron C, Augier S, et al. (2008) Severe myoclonic epilepsy in infancy: a systematic review and a meta-analysis of individual patient data. *Epilepsia* 49: 343–348.

Marsh E, Melamed SE, Barron T, Clancy RR. (2005) Migrating partial seizures in infancy: expanding the phenotype of a rare seizure syndrome. *Epilepsia* 46: 568–572.

Mikaeloff Y, Jambaque I, Hertz-Pannier L, et al. (2006) Devastating epileptic encephalopathy in school-aged children (DESC): a pseudo encephalitis. *Epilepsy Res* 69: 67–79.

Minkin K, Tzekov C, Naydenov E, et al. (2008) Cerebellar gangliocytoma presenting with hemifacial spasms: clinical report, literature review and possible mechanisms. *Acta Neurochir* 150: 719–724; discussion 724.

Molinari F, Raas-Rothschild A, Rio M, et al. (2005) Impaired mitochondrial glutamate transport in autosomal recessive neonatal myoclonic epilepsy. *Am J Hum Genet* 76: 334–339.

Nabbout R, Dulac O. (2008) Epileptic syndromes in infancy and childhood. *Curr Opin Neurol* 21: 161–166.

Okanishi T, Mori Y, Kibe T, et al. (2007) Refractory epilepsy accompanying acute encephalitis with multifocal cortical lesions: possible autoimmune etiology. *Brain Dev* 29: 590–594.

Panayiotopoulos CP, Michael M, Sanders S, et al. (2008) Benign childhood focal epilepsies: assessment of established and newly recognized syndromes. *Brain* 131: 2264–2286.

Pintaudi M, Baglietto MG, Gaggero R, et al. (2008) Clinical and electroencephalographic features in patients with CDKL5 mutations: two new Italian cases and review of the literature. *Epilepsy Behav* 12: 326–331.

Roulet-Perez E, Ballhausen D, Bonafé L, et al. (2008) Glut-1 deficiency syndrome masquerading as idiopathic generalized epilepsy. *Epilepsia* 49: 1955–1958.

Sadleir LG, Scheffer IE, Smith S, et al. (2008) Factors influencing clinical features of absence seizures. *Epilepsia* 49: 2100–2107.

Schmitt B, Wohlrab G, Sander T, et al. (2005) Neonatal seizures with tonic clonic sequences and poor developmental outcome. *Epilepsy Res* 65: 161–168.

Stephani U. (2006) The natural history of myoclonic astatic epilepsy (Doose syndrome) and Lennox–Gastaut syndrome. *Epilepsia* 47 Suppl 2: 53–55.

Valentin A, Hindocha N, Osei-Lah A, et al. (2007) Idiopathic generalized epilepsy with absences: syndrome classification. *Epilepsia* 48: 2187–2190.

Ville D, Kaminska A, Bahi-Buisson N. (2006) Early pattern of epilepsy in the ring chromosome 20 syndrome. *Epilepsia* 47: 543–549.

Weber YG, Lerche H. (2008) Genetic mechanisms in idiopathic epilepsies. *Dev Med Child Neurol* 50: 648–654.

Wolf NI, Bast T, Surtees R. (2005) Epilepsy in inborn errors of metabolism. *Epileptic Disord* 7: 67–81.

# Chapter 3.13
## Febrile Seizures

### What is a febrile seizure?

Febrile seizures are so common that they will come into the ambit of almost all doctors dealing with children. There has been prolonged controversy around the question of which tests are appropriate and in what circumstances when a child has a seizure with fever. The subject is more complex than it might seem. It is important neither to make blanket recommendations such that all children with a first febrile seizure should have a lumbar puncture, nor to deprive a child with pyogenic meningitis or herpes encephalitis a lumbar puncture just because the potentially lethal infection happens to present as that child's second or third febrile seizure.

### The nature of the seizure

Most febrile seizures are convulsions. In some studies they are called tonic–clonic, but although they may have tonic components they look more clonic to the observer. However, tonic seizures with fever associated with persisting impairment of consciousness may indicate brainstem herniation and signify inflammatory intracranial disease of grave importance.

### Differential diagnosis of seizures with fever

The following diagnostic possibilities exist, these not being mutually exclusive.

1. The convulsion is not an epileptic seizure nor an anoxic seizure (see Chapter 3.14) but is a rigor or an hallucination or febrile myoclonus or febrile ataxia.

2. The seizure is a febrile syncope similar to a syncope suffered by adults with influenza and fever.

3. The seizure is a syncope due to ventricular tachyarrhythmia precipitated by fever in

Brugada syndrome (a sodium channelopathy with several ECG patterns).

4. The seizure represents the presence of a gene for one or other type of epilepsy, albeit genetic analysis may not be practicable.

5. The febrile seizure, especially if prolonged and lateralized (hemiclonic) may be the start of Dravet syndrome otherwise called severe myoclonic epilepsy of infancy (SMEI), with a mutation in *SCN1A*.

6. The febrile seizure may be a manifestation of an *SCN1A* mutation in a family with GEFS+ (genetic epilepsy with febrile seizures plus).

7. The seizures may reflect static focal pathology even if the infant or child has had no previously known neurological signs.

8. Febrile seizures may represent the onset of a chronic progressive pathology such as Alpers disease due to a mutation in the nuclear mitochondrial gene *POLG1*.

9. The febrile seizures may be a manifestation of an acute encephalopathy due to a central nervous system infection such as pyogenic or tuberculous meningitis, herpes simplex encephalitis or human herpes virus 6 or 7 infection.

10. The febrile seizure may be a manifestation of a metabolic encephalopathy, the encephalopathy having been precipitated by the catabolism of the febrile illness. In this case the febrile seizure may be a tonic non-epileptic one with loss of ability to localize pain due to brain herniation.

As an overview it is likely that the vast majority of febrile seizures are related to viral infections and have a benign outcome. Hence, it follows that for most patients no investigations of any kind are indicated. However, in a few children investigations are helpful or essential.

Investigations relate to the question being asked:

*1. Is there a treatable disorder?*

Irrespective of the age of the child and whether it be the first, second, third or fourth febrile seizure, it is incumbent upon the paediatrician to think whether there could be an underlying pyogenic, tuberculous, herpesvirus or other intracranial infection.

The primary investigation is lumbar puncture with pressure measurement and CSF examination, unless failure to localize pain or other signs suggest that brain herniation is likely.

*2. Is there evidence of acute encephalopathy?*

Blood and CSF studies may indicate viral infections such as human herpes virus 6 but this will not influence management.

*3. Is there evidence of a preexisting static lesion?*

Answering this question is not usually helpful and brain MRI is not indicated.

*4. Is there evidence of an underlying progressive disorder?*

Atypical features, such as unexpectedly high CSF protein, may be a clue to an underlying mitochondrial disorder, in particular mutations in *POLG1*.

*5. Will the febrile seizures recur?*

An EEG examination will not answer this question.

*6. Can one predict later epilepsy?*

EEG examination will not answer this question.

A structural lesion on brain MRI might be predictive but such an investigation is not normally justified.

A pathogenic mutation in *SCN1A* indicates the beginning of Dravet syndrome and may be helpful for guiding antiepileptic therapy later.

*7. Was this vaccine encephalopathy or vaccine damage?*

No investigation can support an allegation of 'vaccine damage', but finding a pathogenic mutation in *SCN1A* is a convincing alternative explanation. The best known explanations for deterioration after DTP vaccine are as follows: (1) the start of Dravet syndrome; (2) a mitochondrial disorder, such as due to a mutation in *POLG1*; (3) metabolic decompensation as in (undiagnosed) glutaric aciduria type 1.

### Febrile regression

The onset of *eIF2B*-related disorders may be with fever-related acute regression but not febrile seizures. MRI and CSF asialotransferrin should clarify. Acute necrotizing encephalopathy and bilateral striatal necrosis – probably related nuclear pore disorders – are discussed in Chapter 3.17.

### Further reading

Hesdorffer DC, Chan, S, Tian H, et al. (2008) Are MRI-detected brain abnormalities associated with febrile seizure type? *Epilepsia* **49**: 765–771.

Shinnar S, Hesdorffer DC, Nordli DR Jr, et al. (2008) Phenomenology of prolonged febrile seizures: results of the FEBSTAT study. *Neurology* **71**: 170–176.

Subramony SH, Schott K, Raike RS, et al. (2003) Novel CACNA1A mutation causes febrile episodic ataxia with interictal cerebellar deficits. *Ann Neurol* **54**: 725–731.

# Chapter 3.14
## Paroxysmal Non-epileptic Disorders

In Chapter 3.12 we emphasized the importance of making a distinction between epileptic seizures and paroxysmal non-epileptic events. Time spent on detailed clinical history is the most important aid to making this distinction.

It is as important to recognize the numerous types of non-epileptic paroxysmal event as it is to distinguish epileptic seizures and syndromes. In Table 3.14.1 we have listed the best known conditions with their appropriate investigations. In the majority the most useful investigation is video, including home video and video with audio (see Chapter 2.1). From this it is obvious that it behoves the practitioner to have seen video recordings of as many of these conditions as possible.

Several of these non-epileptic paroxysmal disorders may coexist with epileptic seizures in the same patient or in the same family; this problem is discussed further in Chapter 3.15.

Table 3.14.1 Paroxysmal non–epileptic events

| Category | Condition | Clinical features | Investigations |
|---|---|---|---|
| Sleep phenomena | Benign neonatal sleep myoclonus (BNSM) | Flurries of limb myoclonia while asleep | Home video, show parents video of another child with BNSM |
| | Repetitive sleep starts | Neurodevelopmentally abnormal children; runs of brief tonic episodes (spasms) (may also have epilepsy) | Video/EEG/EMG in sleep to confirm non–epileptic nature |
| Behaviours | Tonic reflex seizures of early infancy (in otherwise normal infants) | Stiffenings when held upright especially after feeds (some resemblance to awake apnoea of Spitzer – a manifestation of gastro–oesophageal reflux) | Evoke episodes on video |
| | Shuddering | Transient shudders and tremors in infants or toddlers | Home video |
| | Benign non–epileptic infantile spasms (benign myoclonus of early infancy) | Runs of spasms mainly affecting upper limbs – interrupted on distraction | Video, video EEG/EMG to show lack of EEG complexes |
| | Infantile masturbation/gratification | Rhythmic repetitive thigh adduction, 'distant' or absorbed appearance often in car seat, cease with distraction | Home video |
| | Stereotypies | Often in learning disabled or autistic children, excited flapping | Home video |

Table 3.14.1 continued

| Category | Condition | Clinical features | Investigations |
|---|---|---|---|
| 'Psychological' | Daydreams and non-epileptic absences | Often in school | May need EEG with hyperventilation and video, ictal EEG slowing (delta) but no spikes |
| | Pseudoepileptic convulsions | Episodes when others present | Video-EEG |
| 'Benign syncopes' | Prolonged expiratory apnoea (blue breath-holding) | Unpleasant stimuli, rapid cyanosis and opisthotonus | Home video |
| | Reflex asystolic syncope | Head bump or other pain stimulus; tonic episode with spasms, often pallor but not always | If not typical, 12-lead ECG for QTc (cardiac monitoring if very severe) |
| | Vasovagal syncope | Common faint, often 'convulsive' | Head-up tilt not usually required |
| | Vagovagal syncope | Swallowing or vomiting are triggers | ECG/EEG while eating or provoked by vomiting |
| | Convulsive Valsalva | Autistic or asymbolic child; true breath-hold often follows hyperventilation | Video/audio (to hear respiratory noise then silence) |
| 'Malignant' syncopes | Hyperekplexia | Stiff apnoeas in neonate preceded by staccato cry; nose-tap positive, startle | Video–audio; EEG/ECG/EMG (rhythmic 8–30Hz compound muscle action potentials); GLRA1 and GlyT2 gene analysis |

Table 3.14.1 continued

| Category | Condition | Clinical features | Investigations |
|---|---|---|---|
| 'Malignant' syncopes | Paroxysmal extreme pain disorder | Tonic episodes with flushing; often Harlequin in neonate | Video; *SCN9A* mutation need not be detected |
| | Long-QT syndromes | Loss of consciousness, stiffness, anoxic seizure – exercise, fright, sudden sound, sleep, swimming | 12 lead ECG ± implantable ECG monitor ± ion channel gene mutation analysis |
| | Imposed upper airways obstruction | 'Seizure' or syncope in infant in presence of carer alone but shown to others (family or hospital staff) do not occur when carer not with infant | Video (covert) EEG/ECG/EMG recording of episode (covert video *surveillance* requires legal sanction) |
| 'Dizzy' spells | Paroxysmal vertigo | 'Drunk' with nystagmus during episodes | Home video (ask parents to focus videocamera on child's eyes) |
| | Paroxysmal torticollis | Lateral head tilt | Home video. (*CACNA1A* studies not required) |
| | | More prolonged in Sandifer syndrome and in cervical dystonia | If episodes prolonged, gastrointestinal studies |
| | Craniocervical junction disorder | Falls, brief stiffness, headache | MRI especially sagittal for Chiari I and upper cord |

Table 3.14.1 continued

| Category | Condition | Clinical features | Investigations |
|---|---|---|---|
| Alternating hemiplegia | Alternating hemiplegia of childhood | Tonic episodes, nystagmus often monocular/eye deviations onset first 3 months, then alternating hemiplegia (limp or dystonic), may be precipitated by bathing always relieved by sleep, later fixed choreoathetosis | Home video. No more extensive investigations if history not difficult |
| | Benign familial alternating hemiplegia | Autosomal dominant family history: hemiplegia arises from sleep in otherwise normal children | Home video |
| | Moyamoya | Transient hemipareses, migrainous headaches, paroxysmal dyskinesia or torticollis | 'Re-build-up' on EEG after hyperventilation (but avoid hyperventilation if moyamoya known). Brain MRI/MRA |
| Cataplexies | Narcolepsy–cataplexy | Joke-induced; collapses, face and neck muscles first to go. No loss of consciousness (children also have excessive daytime sleepiness) | Video. Sleep latency test ± human leukocyte antigen ± CSF hypocretin |
| | Niemann–Pick type C | Usually but not always defect in vertical gaze | Video, abdominal ultrasound for subtle splenomegaly, plasma chitotriosidase, bone marrow for sea-blue histiocytes, fibroblast culture for cholesterol studies |

Table 3.14.1 continued

| Category | Condition | Clinical Features | Investigations |
|---|---|---|---|
| Cataplexies | Paraneoplastic hypothalamic syndrome | May also have narcolepsy and other neurological features | Body imaging for occult neural crest tumour |
| | Syndromes with dominant cataplexy: Prader–Willi, Coffin–Lowry, etc. | Family history or syndromic phenotype | Home or hospital video |
| Episodic ataxias | Episodic ataxia type 1 (EA1) | Infantile 'cerebral palsy', myokymia, brief staggers | Video, surface EMG for myokymia. *KCN1A* mutations |
| | Episodic ataxia type 2 (EA2) | Vomiting, prolonged unsteadiness, nystagmus + smooth pursuit disruption, acetazolamide-responsive | Video. MRI for vermis atrophy. $^{31}$P-MRS shows increased pH in cerebellum, reversed by acetazolamide. *CACNA1A* mutations possible but time-consuming |
| | Other episodic ataxias | Various neurological accompaniments | Include testing for GLUT1 deficiency (fasting blood and CSF glucose with lactate) and mitochondrial investigations |
| Paroxysmal dyskinesias | Paroxysmal kinesigenic dyskinesia (PKD) | Dyskinesia (choreoathetosis/dystonia) at *onset* of movement | Video |
| | PKD in hypotonic/dystonic young male child ± ocular wobble ± MRI delayed myelination | Dystonia provoked by *passive* movements or lifting the child | Thyroid function: ↑ free T3, ↓ free T4. *MCT8* testing |

302

Table 3.14.1 continued

| Category | Condition | Clinical features | Investigations |
|---|---|---|---|
| Paroxysmal dyskinesias | Paroxysmal non-kinesigenic dyskinesia | Unprovoked episodes of dyskinesia | Video. (Myofibrillogenesis regulator 1 gene involved) |
| | Paroxysmal exertional dyskinesia | Various dyskinesias during strenuous exercise (may also have epileptic seizures; see Chapter 3.15) | Glucose transporter 1 deficiency tests (fasting, blood and CSF glucose); echinocytes may rarely be seen on blood film |
| | Psychogenic dyskinesias | Psychogenic movement disorders cease with distraction if the child does not think he or she is being observed | Share video with movement disorder expert if in doubt |
| Benign tonic upgaze | | Intermittent tonic upgaze in infancy | Video. (No need for neurotransmitter or *CACNA1A* studies) |
| Benign tonic downgaze | Especially in newborn infants | Intermittent tonic downgaze in normal neonate | Video. Head ultrasound would be wise |
| Night terrors | | 1–2 (–3) total in early part of the night | Sleep video (best with infrared) |

## Conclusion

Although a few non-epileptic paroxysmal disorders are serious and even life threatening, requiring prompt diagnosis, many are harmless unless the dangerous misdiagnosis of epilepsy is made. Home video, perhaps shared with others more experienced, is an increasingly useful diagnostic tool.

## Further reading

Bernard G, Shevell MI. (2008) Channelopathies: a review. *Pediatr Neurol* **38**: 73–85.

Bruno MK, Lee HY, Auburger GW, et al. (2007) Genotype–phenotype correlation of paroxysmal nonkinesigenic dyskinesia. *Neurology* **68**: 1782–1789.

Caraballo RH, Capovilla G, Vigevano F, et al. (2009) The spectrum of benign myoclonus of early infancy: Clinical and neurophysiologic features in 102 patients. *Epilepsia* **50**: 1176–1183.

Drenth JP, Waxman SG. (2007) Mutations in sodium-channel gene SCN9A cause a spectrum of human genetic pain disorders. *J Clin Invest* **117**: 3603–3609.

Jen JC, Graves TD, Hess EJ, et al. (2007) Primary episodic ataxias: diagnosis, pathogenesis and treatment. *Brain* **130**: 2484–2493.

Nechay A, Stephenson JBP. (2009) Bath-induced paroxysmal disorders in infancy. *Eur J Paediatr Neurol* **13**: 203–208.

Rees MI, Harvey K, Pearce BR, et al. (2006) Mutations in the gene encoding GlyT2 (SLC6A5) define a presynaptic component of human startle disease. *Nature Genet* **38**: 801–806.

Roubertie A, Echenne B, Leydet J, et al. (2008) Benign paroxysmal tonic upgaze, benign paroxysmal torticollis, episodic ataxia and CACNA1A mutation in a family. *J Neurol* **255**: 1600–1602.

Suls A, Dedeken P, Goffin K, et al. (2008) Paroxysmal exercise-induced dyskinesia and epilepsy is due to mutations in SLC2A1, encoding the glucose transporter GLUT1. *Brain* **131**: 1831–1844.

# Chapter 3.15
# Epileptic and Non-epileptic Disorders Together

In evaluating paroxysmal disorders a first step is deciding whether episodes are epileptic or non-epileptic. In practice, one often finds both epileptic and non-epileptic events in the same child or in the same family. In this chapter we tabulate better known examples and suggested investigations. Once again, video (particularly home) recording plays a prominent part in the early stage in the diagnosis.

In Table 3.15.1 we present examples of common nonspecific combinations of epileptic and non-epileptic paroxysmal phenomena in the same individual. Most of these situations will be seen by the general paediatrician. In Table 3.15.2 we list rarer and more specific combinations of epileptic and non-epileptic events that may require specialized investigation.

A lesson from this chapter is that even with a 'primary' brain disorder and epileptic seizures one may still have non-epileptic events in addition. Further, because video recording, including home recording, is often the most important investigation, clinical acumen remains paramount.

## Further reading

Guerrini R, Moro F, Kato M, et al. (2007) Expansion of the first PolyA tract of ARX causes infantile spasms and status dystonicus. *Neurology* **69**: 427–433.

Horrocks IA, Nechay A, Stephenson JBP, Zuberi SM. (2005) Anoxic–epileptic seizures: observational study of epileptic seizures induced by syncopes. *Arch Dis Child* **90**: 1283–1287.

Ito S, Nakayama T, Ide S, et al. (2008) Aromatic l-amino acid decarboxylase deficiency associated with epilepsy mimicking non-epileptic involuntary movements. *Dev Med Child Neurol* **50**: 876–878.

Poirier K, Eisermann M, Caubel I, et al. (2008) Combination of infantile spasms, non-epileptic seizures and complex movement disorder: A new case of ARX-related epilepsy. *Epilepsy Res* **80**: 224–228.

Santucci M, Ambrosetto G, Scaduto MC, et al. (2001) Ictal and nonictal paroxysmal events in infantile neuroaxonal dystrophy: polygraphic study of a case. *Epilepsia* **42**: 1074–1077.

Table 3.15.1 Nonspecific combinations of epileptic and non-epileptic phenomena

| Condition | Epileptic component | Non-epileptic component | Investigations |
|---|---|---|---|
| Epilepsy in later childhood and adolescence | Any semiology | Pseudoepileptic convulsions (non-epileptic attack disorder) | Video-EEG (video alone may be sufficient) |
| Autism spectrum disorder and asymbolic retardation | History of previous epileptic infantile spasms ± partial | 'Blanks', stereotypies, compulsive Valsalva | Video-audio, may require ictal EEG/ECG/respiration |
| Cerebral palsy and neurodevelopmental impairment | Partial secondarily generalized. Epileptic spasms | Reflex syncopes as found in individuals without cerebral palsy | *Not* EEG (interictal) |
| | | Obstructive sleep apnoea with tonic non-epileptic seizures | Sleep polysomnograph including EEG, ECG, respiration, surface EMG |
| | | Repetitive sleep starts | Video-EEG/ECG/EMG |
| | | Parentally induced apnoeas (imposed upper airways suction) | Perhaps serial imaging |

Table 3.15.1 continued

| Condition | Epileptic component | Non-epileptic component | Investigations |
|---|---|---|---|
| Panayiotopoulos syndrome | Epileptic seizures with vomiting at onset and pallor and lateral eye deviation, often with autonomic status epilepticus | Occasional cardiorespiratory arrest (so-called 'ictal syncope' is not syncope but is an epileptic manifestation) | Interictal EEG shows rolandic or occipital or multifocal spikes. Ictal EEG/ECG rarely required |
| Anoxic–epileptic seizures (AES) | Epileptic component clonic, often with eye deviation, may be absence; status epilepticus not uncommon | Any type of neurally mediated syncope, in particular reflex asystolic; prolonged expiratory apnoea; compulsive Valsalva | Home video, video in EEG dept., prolonged ECG monitoring, opportunistic ictal EEG/ECG recording; imaging or genetic studies if syndromic aetiology suspected |

Table 3.15.2 Special cases of epileptic and non-epileptic events combined

| Condition | Epileptic component | Non-epileptic component | Investigations |
|---|---|---|---|
| Tricyclic poisoning (as in Munchausen by proxy) | 'Generalized tonic–clonic' | Syncope (ventricular tachyarrhythmias) | ECG, toxicology |
| Glucose transporter 1 deficiency | Various, including generalized tonic–clonic, early-onset absences, myoclonic | Episodic ataxia. Paroxysmal exercise-induced dyskinesia and other movement disorders | Fasting, blood and CSF glucose. *SLC2A1* gene analysis |
| Mitochondrial disorders | Epilepsy partialis continua | Non-epileptic tonic seizures | Brain MRI, blood and CSF lactate. *POLG1* analysis |
| Paroxysmal dyskinesia with infantile convulsions | Clonic, in infancy | Paroxysmal kinesigenic dyskinesia | Home video or office video |
| Alternating hemiplegia of childhood | Tonic (but debatable how many true epileptic seizures – very few recorded on EEG) | Non-epileptic tonic attacks, either hemitonic or dystonic episodes or bilateral dystonic attacks. Episodic nystagmus including monocular nystagmus. Limp hemiplegias and double hemiplegias | Video |
| Moyamoya | Various including partial and absence | Transient ischaemic attacks, migrainous headaches, paroxysmal dyskinesia and torticollis | Brain MRI/MRA. Event monitoring with polygraphy to distinguish epileptic from non-epileptic events |

Table 3.15.2 continued

| Condition | Epileptic component | Non-epileptic component | Investigations |
|---|---|---|---|
| Episodic ataxia type 1 (EA1) | Partial | Short-lasting ataxia | Video surface EMG for myokymia (*KCN1A* gene analysis possible) |
| Episodic ataxia type 2 (EA2) | Absence | Prolonged ataxia, vomiting, nystagmus | Video, MRI for midline cerebellum, possible $^{31}$P-MRS (*CACN1A* gene possible but difficult) |
| Hyperekplexia plus | 'Tonic–clonic' | Tonic apnoeas | Video, EEG/ECG/EMG, *GlyT2* gene analysis |
| ARX | Epileptic infantile spasms | Status dystonicus, nocturnal and diurnal dyskinesia | *ARX* trinucleotide repeat analysis |
| Rett syndrome | Various (including anoxic–epileptic) | Complex: includes apnoeas, Valsalvas, tremors, dyskinesia | Ictal video/ECG/respiration (*MECP2* gene analysis, etc.) |
| Angelman syndrome | Atypical absences, etc. | Laughter–asystole with syncope | Ictal EEG, ictal ECG (Angelman syndrome genetics) |
| Coffin–Lowry syndrome | Tonic and generalized tonic–clonic | 'Cataplexy', cataplexy, hyperekplexia, sound-startle falls | Video, video-EEG (gene analysis possible) |

# Chapter 3.16
## Acquired Neurological Deficits

In this chapter we will discuss some of the acquired neurological deficits that deserve consideration as to how they should be investigated. Most acquired deficits may be elucidated by careful clinical neurology with attention to neuroanatomical details. We will not deal with those here, nor with aspects covered in other chapters such as acute encephalopathy (Chapter 3.17) and ataxia (Chapter 3.20).

### Stroke

The term 'stroke' is defined by the World Health Organization as "rapidly developing clinical signs of focal or global disturbance lasting 24 hours or longer or leading to death with no apparent cause other than of vascular origin." While this clinical definition might be useful in the evaluation of acute focal neurological syndromes in adults, at least a third of children presenting in this way will have a non-vascular aetiology. Thus in paediatric practice it is mandatory to undertake brain imaging as a prelude to diagnosis and then to be specific about the vascular stroke syndrome implicated:

- arterial ischaemic stroke

- cerebral venous thrombosis – including cerebral venous sinus thrombosis (CVST) and cortical venous thrombosis ± venous infarction

- non-traumatic intracranial haemorrhage – including extradural, subdural (though this is most commonly traumatic), intraparenchymal and subarachnoid.

Each of these childhood vascular stroke syndromes requires a targeted clinical approach which, moreover, will be influenced by the age of the child. Metabolic 'stroke' (see section on Stroke-like episodes below) has an entirely different aetiology (namely cellular energy failure) and should be considered in the context of a non-vascular distribution of cerebral injury or a history of developmental difficulties or regression. A further point is that children with relatively transient clinical symptoms or signs (who would be considered as having transient ischaemic attacks if adults) might well have radiologically apparent brain injury and should not be dismissed without adequate assessment.

*Vascular stroke syndromes in childhood*
The incidences of ischaemic and haemorrhagic stroke syndromes are virtually equal in children, and differentiation between them, and distinction from other causes of a clinical 'stroke' presentation cannot be made without brain imaging. In the real world this would generally involve acute brain CT, which will, at the very least, identify intracranial haemorrhage requiring neurosurgical intervention and may well identify some of the other aetiologies mentioned. For example, with administration of contrast, CT is around 85% sensitive for a diagnosis of CVST. Negative CT in the context of persistent neurological impairment should prompt further investigation with MRI or, if this proves impossible, repeat CT, as pathologies such as arterial ischaemic stroke become more apparent on CT with time.

*Arterial ischaemic stroke (AIS)*
AIS is defined as an acute focal neurological deficit with radiological evidence of cerebral infarction in an arterial distribution. In neonates the presenting features may be subtle; infarction before or around the time of birth may never present acutely and may only manifest as emergent hemiparesis in the first year of life. The clinical approach to neonatal and 'presumed perinatal' AIS is distinct from that which should be adopted in older children. As well as brain imaging, investigation should include evaluation for thrombophilia (including anticardiolipin antibodies). The history should include enquiry about previous thrombosis or fetal loss, and consideration should be given to referring the mother for haematological evaluation, especially if she intends to have further pregnancies.

Beyond the neonatal period at least 50% of affected children will have another medical condition rendering them at risk of AIS (for example, sickle cell disease or congenital cardiac disease). It is helpful to consider childhood AIS a multifactorial disorder and to comprehensively investigate the child for vascular and non-vascular risk factors. This is best achieved by undertaking MRI (including diffusion-weighted imaging, which will help to improve lesion definition and timing) and MR angiography of the cerebral circulation from the aortic arch to the circle of Willis. The presence and morphology of arterial disease is one of the most important determinants of subsequent treatment (for example, anticoagulation for dissection, aspirin for focal cerebral arteriopathy, revascularization for moyamoya). The other important determinants of acute management are identification of sickle cell disease (though AIS rarely presents in this way) and the presence of cardiac disease (which might lead to anticoagulation).

Other than vascular imaging and echocardiography the following investigations could be considered:

- full blood count and ferritin (to detect anaemia)

- haemoglobin electrophoresis in Black and South Asian children

- thrombophilia evaluation (protein C, S, antithrombin, factor V Leiden, t-MTHFR, PT20210, lupus anticoagulant and anticardiolipin antibodies)

- total plasma homocysteine (significant if >13.5µmol/L)

- random cholesterol and triglycerides

- transferrin isoforms

- serology: mycoplasma, borellia, varicella zoster.

AIS in the distribution of the posterior circulation (mostly seen in boys) requires exclusion of vertebral artery dissection, which may necessitate catheter cerebral angiography (see Clinical Vignette 2.5.3) and screening for Fabry disease (measure plasma alpha-galactosidase A).

Recurrence of AIS should always prompt reviewing the diagnosis, specifically to exclude a non-vascular cause (see Stroke-like episodes below), and evaluation for potentially treatable conditions such as cerebral vasculitis or moyamoya.

*Cerebral venous sinus thrombosis*
CVST should be considered in the child presenting with clinical 'stroke' who also has features of raised intracranial pressure, e.g. headache or seizures, especially in the context of an acute predisposing illness (e.g. head and neck infection or dehydration) and in whom ischaemic brain injury does not conform to an arterial territory. As previously mentioned, CT with contrast is highly sensitive but if there is doubt MRI, including MR venography, should be undertaken. Anticoagulation is advocated even in the presence of microhaemorrhage (though not haematoma exerting mass effect). Thrombophilia is much more prevalent than in children with AIS and should be sought as it may guide duration of therapy and future management.

*Non-traumatic intracranial haemorrhage*
While acute management of acute non-traumatic intracranial haemorrhage will generally comprise neurosurgical intervention, the paediatrician may need to advise on investigation for underlying aetiology. By far the most common of these is a structural malformation of the cerebral vasculature (most commonly arteriovenous malformations). Aneurysms are much less common in children, even those presenting with subarachnoid haemorrhage, but may be familial (if there are more than two affected first-degree relatives), associated with polycystic kidney disease or with infection. Bleeding diatheses should always be excluded, especially in newborn infants, in whom haemorrhagic disease or haemophilia may present in this way. It is always important to consider inflicted head trauma, which is usually associated with subdural haemorrhage.

In the acute stage the priority is to identify any underlying structural malformation; unless urgent haematoma evacuation is clinically indicated (in which case catheter angiography should be undertaken), CT angiography is currently the initial investigation of choice. MRI should be undertaken if CT angiography is negative as, rarely, pathologies not apparent on CT may be identified (for example, brain tumour with secondary haemorrhage). It is generally advisable to defer catheter angiography to a time at which the acute haematoma will have resolved and when the diagnostic examination might be combined with endovascular intervention.

### 'Stroke-like' episodes
Stroke mimics are not rare and 'stroke-like' episodes are important to recognize. Hemiplegic migraine and Sturge–Weber syndrome will have been diagnosed on clinical grounds. We list the best-known conditions which may include stroke-like episodes, with suggested investigations:

- space-occupying lesion (tumour) (brain MRI)
- encephalitis (brain MRI, CSF, microbiology)
- acure disseminated encephalomyelitis (ADEM) (brain MRI)
- mitochondrial myopathy, encephalopathy, lactic acidosis and stroke-like episodes (MELAS) (lactate, mtDNA analysis)
- epilepsia partialis continua (EEG, *POLG1*, etc.)
- ornithine transcarbamylase and such-like (ammonia, urine orotic acid and uracil)
- Hashimoto encephalopathy (thyroid peroxidase antibody)
- hypoglycaemia (blood glucose, and – if not insulin induced – urinary organic acids and acylcarnitines)
- congenital defect of glycosylation (CDG) (serum sialotransferrins, EEG during episode: shows spike and wave)
- eIF2B-related (brain MRI ±CSF asialotransferrin).

NOTE ON EEG EXAMINATION
It is worth emphasizing that stroke-like episodes may be associated with hemispheric non-convulsive status epilepticus only detectable by ictal EEG. This is a feature of the stroke-like episodes in CDG type 1a and is likely to be a feature of mitochondrial disorders such as with *POLG1* mutations.


## Multiple sclerosis and related conditions
The most common acute demyelinating condition in childhood is ADEM, which is discussed in detail in Chapter 3.17. Some comments are in order here on the current working definition of multiple sclerosis, and of so-called clinically isolated syndrome (CIS) and its subtypes neuromyelitis optica and neuromyelitis without optic neuritis.

### Paediatric multiple sclerosis
The new operational definition of paediatric multiple sclerosis (not agreed by everyone) requires multiple episodes of CNS demyelination separated in time and

space as in adults but with no lower age limit. The risk increases at puberty, especially in girls.

The MRI can be used to meet the dissemination in space requirement if the McDonald criteria for a positive MRI are applied. The MRI must show three of the following four features: (1) nine or more white matter lesions or one gadolinium-enhancing lesion, (2) three or more periventricular lesions, (3) a juxtacortical lesion, (4) an infratentorial lesion.

The combination of an abnormal CSF finding and two lesions on the MRI, of which one must be in brain, can also meet the dissemination in space criteria; the CSF must show either oligoclonal bands or an elevated IgG index.

MRI can be used to satisfy criteria for dissemination in time after the initial clinical event, even in the absence of a new clinical demyelinating event; abnormal T2 or gadolinium-enhancing lesions must develop 3 months after the initial clinical event.

An episode consistent with the clinical features of ADEM cannot be considered as a first event of multiple sclerosis in most circumstances.

*Clinically isolated syndrome*
CIS is defined as a first acute clinical episode of CNS symptoms with a presumed inflammatory demyelinating cause for which there is no prior history of a demyelinating event. This clinical event may be either monofocal or multifocal, but usually does not include encephalopathy (except in cases of brainstem syndromes). Examples include, but are not limited to, the following:

- optic neuritis (unilateral or bilateral)

- transverse myelitis (typically partial)

- brainstem, cerebellar and/or hemispheric dysfunction.

In each of these situations testing for increased antibody to NMO (NMO-IgG), that is to say antibodies to aquaporin protein 4 (AQP4), is indicated.

*Aquaporin-4 (AQP4) autoimmunity*
AQP4 is a water channel that is localized, appropriately, at CSF–brain junctions. It is thus expressed throughout the linings of the CSF compartment, notably in periventricular regions, on the pia, in the Virchow–Robin spaces, and of course in relation to the optic nerves and spinal cord. Antibodies to AQP4 are known both as AQP4-IgG and as NMO-IgG, and were originally decribed in adults specifically with neuromyelitis optica. AQP4 autoimmunity in children (mainly non-Caucasian and mainly girls) seems to be more pleomorphic, with brainstem (including ophthalmoparesis, cerebellar ataxia, intractable vomiting and hiccups) and encephalopathic presentations, but so far almost all develop recurrent optic neuritis and/or transverse myelitis.

CNS MRI shows increased T2 signal in areas predicted from the expression of AQP4, especially in periventricular sites (in descending order of frequency the medulla, supratentorial and infratentorial white matter, midbrain, cerebellum, thalamus, and hypothalamus), and as tentacle-like lesions in the central white matter along the course of the Virchow–Robin spaces.

Testing for AQP4-IgG/NMO-IgG is becoming readily available, and should be considered in ADEM, CIS and multiple sclerosis when clinical and MRI features are consistent.

*Cerebellitis*
Acute cerebellitis (to be distinguished from the usually benign and often varicella-related acute cerebellar ataxia) is an uncommon dangerous disorder that we have not included in rare treatable disorders insofar as it is often *surgical decompression* that effects a cure. Cerebellar swelling is apparent on MRI (or CT) and if it is not post-varicella the agent triggering this parainfectious response may not be detected.

# Paraplegia
The priority in evaluating the child with acute paraplegia is to exclude a compressive lesion of the spinal cord, and urgent cord imaging (MRI or helical CT) should be undertaken. It can sometimes be difficult to distinguish between a lesion localizing to the cord and ascending polyneuropathy, so occasionally nerve conduction studies will be needed to clarify.

# Flaccid paralysis
As indicated in the introductory paragraph to this chapter, clinical neurology is paramount in the diagnosis of most acute neurological deficits. However, the distinction between acute myelitis or myelopathy and acute polyneuropathy as in Guillain–Barré syndrome may require neurological investigations.

- Spinal MRI may or may not show acute changes in acute myelopathy/myelitis but will demonstrate acute lesions that may require surgery (bleeding, etc.).

- Nerve conduction studies will show motor nerves that are difficult to stimulate, or small induced muscle action potentials, or conduction block.

- CSF in Guillain–Barré syndrome classically has increased protein without cells, whereas it is the converse in transverse myelitis.

Rarely, mitochondrial disease – such as pyruvate dehydrogenase deficiency – or *biotinidase deficiency* may masquerade as acute flaccid paralysis. Although increased CSF protein is a frequent feature in CNS mitochondrial disorders, sometimes – paradoxically – CSF protein is normal when Guillain–Barré syndrome is a manifestation of a mitochondrial disorder.

## Facial palsy

When a child develops unilateral lower motor neuron facial weakness with no additional neurological signs on careful examination and normal blood pressure then no further neurological investigations are needed.

Borrelia titres are indicated if there is a history of tick bites and/or erythema migrans.

## Further reading

Al-Hassnan ZN, Rashed MS, Al-Dirbashi OY, et al. (2008) Hyperornithinemia–hyperammonemia–homocitrullinuria syndrome with stroke-like imaging presentation: clinical, biochemical and molecular analysis. *J Neurol Sci* 264: 187–194.

Amlie-Lefond C, Sebire G, Fullerton HJ. (2008) Recent developments in childhood arterial ischaemic stroke. *Lancet Neurol* 7: 425–435.

Banwell B, Ghezzi A, Bar-Or A, et al. (2007) Multiple sclerosis in children: clinical diagnosis, therapeutic strategies, and future directions. *Lancet Neurol* 6: 887–902.

Braun KP, Kappelle LJ, Kirkham FJ, Deveber G. (2006) Diagnostic pitfalls in paediatric ischaemic stroke. *Dev Med Child Neurol* 48: 985–990.

Coker SB. (1993) Leigh disease presenting as Guillain–Barré syndrome. *Pediatr Neurol* 9: 61–63.

Cox MG, Wolfs TF, Lo TH, et al. (2005) Neuroborreliosis causing focal cerebral arteriopathy in a child. *Neuropediatrics* 36: 104–107.

Dale RC, Pillai SC. (2007) Early relapse risk after a first CNS inflammatory demyelination episode: examining international consensus definitions. *Dev Med Child Neurol* 49: 887–893.

Fullerton HJ, Wu YW, Sidney S, Johnston SC. (2007) Risk of recurrent childhood arterial ischemic stroke in a population-based cohort: the importance of cerebrovascular imaging. *Pediatrics* 119: 495–501.

Ganesan V, Prengler M, McShane MA, et al. (2003) Investigation of risk factors in children with arterial ischemic stroke. *Ann Neurol* 53: 167–173.

Ganesan V, Prengler M, Wade, A, et al. (2006) Clinical and radiological recurrence after childhood arterial ischemic stroke. *Circulation* 114: 2170–2177.

Haywood S, Liesner R, Pindora S, Ganesan V. (2005) Thrombophilia and first arterial ischaemic stroke: a systematic review. *Arch Dis Child* 90: 402–405.

Klingebiel R, Benndorf G, Schmitt M, et al. (2002) Large cerebral vessel occlusive disease in Lyme neuroborreliosis. *Neuropediatrics* 33: 37–40.

Kelly PJ, Furie KL, Kistler JP, et al. (2003) Stroke in young patients with hyperhomocysteinemia due to cystathionine beta-synthase deficiency. *Neurology* 60: 275–279.

Kenet G, Kirkham F, Niederstadt T, et al. (2007) Risk factors for recurrent venous thromboembolism in the European collaborative paediatric database on cerebral venous thrombosis: a multicentre cohort study. *Lancet Neurol* 6: 595–603.

Krupp LB, Banwell B, Tenembaum S. (2007) Consensus definitions proposed for pediatric multiple sclerosis and related disorders. *Neurology* 68 (Suppl 2): S7–12.

Liu AC, Segaren N, Cox TS, et al. (2006) Is there a role for magnetic resonance imaging in the evaluation of non-traumatic intraparenchymal haemorrhage in children? *Pediatr Radiol* 36: 940–946.

McGlennan C, Ganesan V. (2008) Delays in investigation and management of acute arterial ischaemic stroke in children. *Dev Med Child Neurol* 50: 537–540.

McKeon A, Lennon VA, Lotze T, et al. (2008) CNS aquaporin-4 autoimmunity in children. *Neurology* **71**: 93–100.

Miravet E, Danchaivijitr N, Basu H, et al. (2007) Clinical and radiological features of childhood cerebral infarction following varicella zoster virus infection. *Dev Med Child Neurol* **49**: 417–422.

Riou EM, Amlie-Lefond C, Echenne B, et al. (2008) Cerebrospinal fluid analysis in the diagnosis and treatment of arterial ischemic stroke. *Pediatr Neurol* **38**: 1–9.

Roach ES, Golomb MR, Adams R, et al. (2008) Management of stroke in infants and children: a scientific statement from a Special Writing Group of the American Heart Association Stroke Council and the Council on Cardiovascular Disease in the Young. *Stroke* **39**: 2644–2691.

Shellhaas RA, Smith SE, O'Tool E, et al. (2006) Mimics of childhood stroke: characteristics of a prospective cohort. *Pediatrics* **118**: 704–709.

# Chapter 3.17

## Acute Encephalopathy

In this chapter we discuss children who present with a short history of altered consciousness, often with focal neurological signs with or without seizures. They do not all have a true acute encephalopathy in the sense of a new pathology but at the onset one does not know: hence the range of investigations which need to be applied. Most of these children present a long way from paediatric neurointensive care units and most of them present outside working hours. Clinical observations, investigations and treatment have to be carried out in parallel. Coincident fever is possible in virtually all situations but paradoxically may be absent in encephalopathies of infective origin.

In many situations the cause will be already apparent from the history and examination: for example meningococcal septicaemia in the presence of purpura fulminans, or blocked shunt in hydrocephalus.

In all cases the clinician will have to make some sort of guess about the intracranial pressure knowing that if a child is flexing rather than localizing to pain then the cerebral perfusion pressure is likely to be too low. Since the cerebral perfusion pressure approximates to the difference between the arterial pressure and the intracranial pressure, measurement of the arterial pressure by a reliable method is mandatory.

Conditions which may present as acute encephalopathy are listed with comments on recognition and key investigations. We will not discuss primary cerebrovascular conditions, which have been dealt with in Chapter 3.16.

### Infectious disorders

*Pyogenic meningitis or septicaemia (when the presence or absence of meningitis is not clear)*
The question of importance is whether or not it is essential to obtain CSF and if so is it

safe to get it via the lumbar route? Provided blood culture is done and antibiotic treatment is started immediately such a decision may be deferred.

*Brain abscess*
Brain imaging with contrast enhancement of the abscess rim will be suggestive.

*Tuberculous meningitis*
The CSF will have increased protein and lymphocytes, possibly some neutrophils, a low but not extremely low glucose and often increased pressure. MRI may show ventricular dilatation and meningeal enhancement with contrast. Microbiological confirmation remains difficult, and treatment is begun when the diagnosis seems possible. In countries where such infection is rare, a mitochondrial disorder may be a more common explanation of this presentation.

*Herpes simplex encephalitis*
Aciclovir will have been started as soon as this diagnosis is considered. However, it is important to recognize the significance of the tests which confirm diagnosis as otherwise aciclovir treatment may be abandoned too early with serious consequences. Initial CSF might be normal but usually shows increase in protein, some lymphocytes, some neutrophils and some red cells. Interferon-alpha (INF-α) may be increased but not necessarily so. Herpes simplex virus polymerase chain reaction (PCR) lends a high sensitivity but this does not reach 100%, with false negative results. Serial blood and CSF herpes simplex virus (HSV) titres should increase from those found at presentation and also the ratio of CSF to blood HSV titres will increase.

The EEG may show periodic lateralized epileptiform discharges but these are not specific.

Brain imaging may be normal at onset, but brain MRI signal change with evidence of associated haemorrhage may suggest vascular infarction or the effects of trauma or even a mass lesion. The virus has a predilection for the anterior opercular region.

Relapse in herpes encephalitis may be due to recrudescence of HSV infection or to an autoimmune phenomenon. CSF INF-α is not increased in the autoimmune relapse.

Chronic herpes simplex encephalitis may be confirmed by the finding of herpes simplex DNA by PCR in CSF. It is not yet known how long acyclovir treatment must be continued to prevent this phenomenon.

*Other viral encephalitides*
Worldwide, arthropod-borne (arbo-)viruses are the leading cause of viral encephalitis. PCR tests or viral cultures are available.

When the CSF INF-α is increased in an acute encephalopathy without evidence of systemic lupus erythematosus and with no positive viral PCR culture or serological evidence the diagnosis *might* be anti-NMDA-receptor encephalitis (see Clinical Vignette 2.10.4).

*Toxoplasma*
This cause of encephalitis may be substantiated if the blood serology is repeated serially over several weeks.

*Malaria*
The diagnosis depends on thinking of this cause. Anaemia is usual if the encephalopathy is severe.

## Parainfectious disorders

Meningoencephalitis or encephalomyelitis complicates the well-known infectious fevers of childhood (varicella, etc.) and diagnostic difficulties do not usually arise. In the case of mumps the usual situation is a lymphocytic meningitis (sometimes with a modest lowering of the glucose) and isolation of the mumps virus from the CSF.

*Mycoplasma pneumoniae*
*M. pneumoniae* infection (clues are rash, hepatitis, pneumonia, otitis) causes an encephalomyelitis with very prominent blood neutrophil leukocytosis and lymphocytes in the CSF. Chest radiograph tends to reflect pneumonia.

*Acute disseminated encephalomyelitis (ADEM)*
ADEM used to be considered as an acute inflammatory (but not infectious) neurological disorder with multiple areas of demyelination in the CNS and corticosteroid responsiveness. The realization that multiple sclerosis often begins in childhood has prompted attempts at more precise definitions of ADEM and multiple sclerosis. Insofar as the differential diagnosis is more difficult when there is more than one episode of ADEM, operational definitions have been agreed for monophasic ADEM, recurrent ADEM and multiphasic ADEM. Definitions have also been made for clinically isolated syndrome (CIS) and paediatric multiple sclerosis (see Chapter 3.16).

MONOPHASIC ADEM
This is defined as a first clinical event with presumed demyelinating cause, with acute or subacute onset, affecting multiple areas of the CNS. The clinical presentation must be polysymptomatic (including polyfocal deficits, more than one locus in the CNS affected) and must include encephalopathy, which is defined as one or more of the following:

- behavioural change, e.g. confusion, excessive irritability

- alteration in consciousness, e.g. somnolence, lethargy, coma.

There may also be fever, meningism or seizures (a comment, not part of the definition).

In our opinion (albeit not in the definition), *slowing of the EEG* is a good indicator of *encephalopathy*.

Events should be followed by improvement either clinically or on MRI or both, but there may be residual deficits.

There should be no history of a clinical episode with features of a prior demyelinating event, and no other aetiologies should explain the event.

New fluctuating symptoms/signs or MRI findings occurring within three months of the inciting ADEM event are considered part of the acute event.

Brain MRI, with FLAIR or T2-weighted images, reveals large (1–2cm) lesions that are multifocal, hyperintense and located in the supratentorial or infratentorial white matter regions; grey matter, especially the basal ganglia and thalamus, is frequently involved. There should not be radiological evidence of destructive white matter changes.

In the rarest cases, brain MRI shows a large single lesion (≥2cm) predominantly affecting white matter.

Spinal cord MRI may show intramedullary lesions with variable enhancement in addition to the abnormal brain MRI findings specified.

RECURRENT ADEM
By the new definition, this is a new event of ADEM with a recurrence of the initial symptoms and signs, 3 or more months after the first ADEM event, without involvement of new clinical areas by history, examination or neuroimaging.

The event does not occur while on steroids, and occurs at least 1 month after stopping steroid therapy.

MRI shows no new lesions, but the original lesions may have enlarged.

No better explanation exists.

MULTIPHASIC ADEM
This is defined as ADEM followed by a new clinical event also meeting criteria for ADEM, but involving new anatomical areas of the central nervous system as confirmed by history, neurological examination and neuroimaging.

A subsequent event must occur (1) at least 3 months after the onset of the initial ADEM event, and (2) at least 1 month after stopping steroid therapy.

A subsequent event must include a polyfocal presentation including encephalopathy with neurological symptoms or signs that differ from the initial event (but mental status changes need not differ from the initial event).

Brain MRI must show new areas of involvement but also demonstrate complete or partial resolution of those lesions associated with the first ADEM event.

CLINICALLY ISOLATED SYNDROME AND PAEDIATRIC MULTIPLE SCLEROSIS
See Chapter 3.16 for descriptions and definitions, including the section on aquaporin-4 autoimmunity.

INVESTIGATIONS IN ADEM

- *EEG* – Although the EEG is almost always slow in ADEM, this is not one of the 'official' criteria for there being encephalopathy as proposed in the current definition. EEG slowing is said to have occurred in children with multiple sclerosis, but data are limited.

- *Evoked potentials* – Prolonged VEP does not distinguish between ADEM and multiple sclerosis.

- *Brain MRI* – Large lesions involving the grey and white matter are frequent in ADEM and rare in multiple sclerosis, but contrast enhancement is frequent in both.

- *CSF* – Increased cell count including lymphocytes but also neutrophils is frequent in ADEM but rare in multiple sclerosis. Oligoclonal bands are frequent in multiple sclerosis but may occasionally be found in ADEM.

- *Microbiology* – Microbiological investigations in ADEM are usually negative despite clinical evidence of a previous influenza-like illness. *M. pneumoniae* markers may be detected.

INVESTIGATIONS FOR ADEM-LIKE OR ADEM-RELATED DISORDERS

- Neuroborreliosis may present in a similar manner to ADEM. Erythema migrans and/or a history of tick bite will prompt borrelia titres in blood and CSF.

- Macrophage activation syndrome – A very young age at onset, parental consanguinity or associated hepatosplenomegaly may suggest familial haemophagocytic lymphohistiocytosis. Elevated ferritin and triglycerides may be clues, followed by haematological investigations including bone marrow, and then mutation analysis of the perforin gene.

- Primary angiitis of the central nervous system – This is a rare differential diagnosis. Clinical clues are persistent headache and malaise, and recurrence of symptoms after corticosteroids are tapered. Catheter cerebral angiography may show abnormalities if medium to large vessels are involved, but has low sensitivity, and ultimately meningeal or brain biopsy may be necessary.

- Neuro-Behçet disease will be suggested by additional clinical features, such as ulcers of mouth and genitalia.

ACUTE HAEMORRHAGIC LEUKOENCEPHALITIS

Acute haemorrhagic leukoencephalitis, also called acute necrotizing haemorrhagic leukoencephalitis, is a more rapid form of ADEM in which haemorrhage and oedema may also be seen on MRI with demyelination frequently sparing the basal ganglia.

### Chorea–encephalopathy

Chorea–encephalopathy has been described as an acquired condition that includes oligoclonal bands in the CSF. It is not clear whether this is different from anti-NMDA receptor antibody encephalitis (see Clinical Vignette 2.12.4).

## Bilateral striatal necrosis (BSN)

Often after an infection a young infant presents with acute illness including encephalopathy, hypotonia and dyskinesia.

MRI shows signal changes in the striatum.

CSF may show mild leukocytosis.

Investigations include microbiology especially for viral infections, metabolic studies including blood and CSF lactate and urine organic acids, and genetic studies of *nup62*, a gene for one of the nuclear pore complex proteins Nup62. Possible biotin responsiveness has been reported.

## Acute necrotizing encephalopathy (ANE)

This is another condition in which infants or young children become comatose after the onset of a febrile illness.

MRI signal changes are seen in the *thalami* and brainstem. Infants with autosomal or dominant inheritance have to be distinguished from sporadic cases and from mitochondrial disorders, in particular Leigh syndrome.

The question has been put as to whether ANE and BSN are completely different disorders. Mutations in a gene encoding a nuclear pore protein (RANBP2) have now been known to be responsible for ANE. Since it is already known that the gene for another nuclear pore protein (Nup62) is involved in BSN, there is an argument for lumping rather than splitting here.

## Haemolytic–uraemic syndrome

The diagnosis is made by the biochemical and haematological findings. Brain MRI may show lesions in basal ganglia, thalami, brainstem and cerebellum – especially in those provoked by *Streptococcus pneumoniae* or *Shigella* – but these do not necessarily imply bad prognosis. When there is secondary renal hypertension, MRI may instead show features of posterior reversible leukoencephalopathy syndrome. Rare hereditary forms exist, such as related to deficiency of the von Willebrand factor-cleaving protease, more usually associated with thrombotic thrombocytopenia.

## Hypoxic–ischaemic encephalopathy

In most instances diagnosis will be apparent from the history but when there has been covert intentional suffocation by a parent (usually the mother) then one will be presented with watershed infarcts on imaging without apparent explanation (this appearance is *not* seen in epilepsy).

### Trauma

Once again a history of trauma will be absent when there has been child abuse. Ophthalmoscopy is an essential early examination. Brain imaging will commonly show subdural haemorrhage and brain swelling but those who interpret images should beware of overinterpreting the explanations of the changes seen. We say this in part because diffuse axonal injury is no longer considered a feature of so-called 'shaken baby syndrome'.

It should be borne in mind that mild head trauma may precipitate subdural (and retinal) haemorrhage.

Head trauma may precipitate acute regression in certain leukodystrophies, especially vanishing white matter disorder and L-hydroxyglutaric aciduria, arterial ischaemic stroke and hemiplegic migraine.

### Tumours

Occasionally brain tumours, especially when there is coincident fever may be confused with meningitis. However, neck stiffness from tonsillar herniation tends to be more of a feature than depression of consciousness.

Urgent brain imaging will show the tumour and the hydrocephalus and lumbar CSF examination should be avoided.

### Toxic disorders

Various chemicals may be ingested or inhaled giving the clinical picture of an encephalopathy. The most common causes are poisoning by benzodiazepines, opiates, barbiturates, antiepileptic drugs and tricyclics. Metabolites of these substances may be detected in samples of blood and urine.

Simple investigations sometimes direct one to the class of chemical involved:

- diffuse fast (beta) activity on EEG suggests benzodiazepine poisoning
- prolonged QTc goes along with tricyclic poisoning.

*Carbon monoxide poisoning*
Carbon monoxide-induced encephalopathy sometimes presents without the tell-tale history. Early estimation of carboxyhaemoglobin confirms the diagnosis. Follow-up MRI may show atrophy of the caudate.

*Lead poisoning*
Papilloedema may be present even when the encephalopathy appears to be acute. Reduced haemoglobin and increased density at the end of long bones are usually present. An increased CSF protein is a constant finding but lumbar puncture is not advised. Blood lead estimation confirms the diagnosis.

## Metabolic disorders

When an otherwise unexplained encephalopathy is not due to an infective or inflammatory cause, then a simple range of blood and urine investigations will indicate most types of metabolic disorder:

- blood urea and electrolytes, acid-base balance, anion gap, glucose, liver function tests, creatine kinase, ammonia, lactate, biotinidase, amino acids, carnitine
- urine amino acids, organic acids, acylcarnitines, orotic acid, uracil
- CSF lactate will have been estimated at the initial lumbar puncture.

## Explosive onset of neurological disease

A number of neurological disorders may present in such an acute, dramatic manner that they masquerade completely as acute encephalopathy. These disorders may be truly progressive or completely static in the pathological sense.

### Epilepsy onset

Epilepsy may present de novo, masquerading as an acute encephalopathy. This may be the mode of presentation of Dravet syndrome. In the context of prolonged hemiclonic seizures with fever in infancy, mutation analysis of the gene *SCN1A* supports the diagnosis and may help management.

### 'Vaccine damage'

An apparent encephalopathy shortly after some sort of immunization makes parents think that the vaccine is causal.

- So-called 'pertussis vaccine encephalopathy' is associated with *SCN1A* mutations.
- Neurodevelopmental deterioration after immunization may be a feature of a mitochondrial disorder but the eventual outcome is due to the mutation (such as *POLG1* – see Clinical Vignette 2.14.1) rather than to the vaccine.

### Alpers disease

Whether or not there is a prolonged history of subtle neurodevelopmental impairment, Alpers disease (otherwise known as Alpers–Huttenlocher disease or progressive neuronal degeneration of childhood with liver disease) commonly presents in an explosive manner with repeated epileptic seizures and impaired consciousness. CSF protein is increased, and EEG may show lateralized runs of slow waves with multiple spike notches. Liver function tests and clotting studies are not necessarily abnormal early in the course of the disease.

Most cases are due to mutations in nuclear mitochondrial gene *POLG1* and DNA should be taken in life, as well as fibroblasts for culture.

### Prenatal brain lesions

Prenatal brain lesions may present after the neonatal period with symptoms of acute encephalopathy. For example, hemimegalencephaly or hemipachygyria may present with repeated seizures and an apparently acquired hemisyndrome and decline in consciousness associated with a febrile illness. The EEG in these disorders may show repetitive high-voltage stereotyped lateralized complexes very closely resembling those seen in herpes encephalitis. Brain MRI will clarify promptly.

## Summary
Many of these conditions cause great family worry, but neurological investigations lead to improved understanding and often a happier outlook.

## Further reading

Alink J, de Vries TW. (2008) Unexplained seizures, confusion or hallucinations: think Hashimoto encephalopathy. *Acta Paediatr* **97**: 451–453.

Basel-Vanagaite L, Muncher L, Straussberg R, et al. (2006) Mutated nup62 causes autosomal recessive infantile bilateral striatal necrosis. *Ann Neurol* **60**: 214–222.

Dale RC, de Sousa C, Chong WK, et al. (2000) Acute disseminated encephalomyelitis, multiphasic disseminated encephalomyelitis and multiple sclerosis in children. *Brain* **123**: 2407–2422.

Dale RC. (2008) Acute disseminated encephalomyelitis: where does it start and where does it stop? *Dev Med Child Neurol* **50**: 326–327.

De Tiege X, Rozenberg F, Heron B. (2008) The spectrum of herpes simplex encephalitis in children. *Eur J Paediatr Neurol* **12**: 72–81.

Glaser CA, Honarmand S, Anderson LJ, et al. (2006) Beyond viruses: clinical profiles and etiologies associated with encephalitis. *Clin Infect Dis* **43**: 1565–1577.

Hahn JS, Pohl D, Rensel M, Rao S. (2007) Differential diagnosis and evaluation in pediatric multiple sclerosis. *Neurology* **68** Suppl 2: S13–22.

Hartley LM, Ng SY, Dale RC, et al. (2002) Immune mediated chorea encephalopathy syndrome in childhood. *Dev Med Child Neurol* **44**: 273–277.

Neilson DE, Eiben RM, Waniewski S, et al. (2003) Autosomal dominant acute necrotizing encephalopathy. *Neurology* **61**: 226–230.

Neilson DE, Adams MD, Orr CM, et al. (2009) Infection-triggered familial or recurrent cases of acute necrotizing encephalopathy caused by mutations in a component of the nuclear pore, RANBP2. *Am J Hum Genet* **84**: 44–51.

Oehmichen M, Schleiss D, Pedal I, et al. (2008) Shaken baby syndrome: re-examination of diffuse axonal injury as cause of death. *Acta Neuropathol* **116**: 317–329.

Orcesi S, Pessagno A, Biancheri R, et al. (2008) Aicardi–Goutières syndrome presenting atypically as a sub-acute leukoencephalopathy. *Eur J Paediatr Neurol* **12**: 408–411.

Sébire G, Devictor D, Huault G, et al. (1992) Coma associated with intense bursts of abnormal movements and long-lasting cognitive disturbances: an acute encephalopathy of obscure origin. *J Pediatr* **121**: 845–851; erratum 1993 122: 491.

Straussberg R, Shorer Z, Weitz R. (2002) Familial infantile bilateral striatal necrosis: clinical features and response to biotin treatment. *Neurology* **59**: 983–989.

Tenembaum S, Chitnis T, Ness J, Hahn JS. (2007) Acute disseminated encephalomyelitis. *Neurology* **68** Suppl 2: S23–S36.

# Chapter 3.18
## Headache

Commonly the clinical history and physical examination of the child with headache lead to the diagnosis without neurological investigations.

Brain MRI is often requested in headache, but there are hazards:

- normal features may be misinterpreted as abnormal
- irrelevant findings may be interpreted as causative for the headache.

That being said, brain MRI is indicated when there is:

- a history of headache that is sudden, atypical, unusual or intense
- any additional atypical features in the history
- any hint of increased intracranial pressure
- evidence of disturbance of the visual system (other than in migraine)
- impairment of balance including one-leg stance
- any alteration of linear growth either excessive or diminished.

In summary, brain MRI is indicated when there are atypical features other than headache in the history, or when there are abnormalities on general, visual or neurological examinations.

That having been said, certain clinical scenarios are worth further discussion.

### Brain tumour
An intracranial tumour would not be expected to cause headache as the sole manifestation, but any hint of increased intracranial pressure such as an odd position of the head or a cracked-pot percussion note on coronal percussion or any neurological

signs such as impaired one-leg stance would prompt immediate brain imaging. One would look for obstructive hydrocephalus.

Pituitary tumours commonly have headache at presentation but not as an isolated symptom.

## Systemic arterial hypertension

What high blood pressure does to the brain used to be called hypertensive encephalopathy but is now known as posterior reversible encephalopathy syndrome. MRI will clarify the posterior circulation predominance of the abnormal signal, but normalizing the arterial pressure will take priority.

## Idiopathic intracranial hypertension

This condition, previously known as benign intracranial hypertension (but not benign), is not a rare cause of headache and/or visual impairment. Vomiting, papilloedema and VIth nerve palsies may coexist, often on a background of obesity or ingestion of various medications such as tetracycline or corticosteroid by any route.

*Investigations*
- Brain imaging (MRI) if possible. CT (immediately if MRI is not available) will precede lumbar puncture.

- The diagnosis is made by finding CSF hypertension. Increased pressure is regarded as an opening pressure >25 cm CSF in the relaxed child lying in the lateral decubitus position. Some advocate a cut-off of 30 cm $H_2O$.

- When there are no associated risk factors yet the lumbar CSF pressure is high, then magnetic resonance venography is indicated to exclude the occurrence of cerebral venous thrombosis. (Venous thrombosis may be a presenting sign of neuro-Behçet disease before ocular, oral and skin lesions, but there are no convenient investigations to determine this.)

## Tonsillar ectopia/Chiari I

Whether cough-induced or post-stool-straining headache, or headache with change in posture, the simple clinical investigation of having a child strain for 10 seconds and then relax may induce a headache. However, MRI to determine descent of the cerebellar tonsils is the best way of being precise about this.

## Panayiotopoulos syndrome

Autonomic features, vomiting and headache may be most obvious features of the seizures that occur predominantly at night in Panayiotopoulos syndrome. Awake EEG usually shows spike discharges, often occipital in location but variable – if need be sleep EEG should be performed.

## Migraine mimics

Rarely, certain metabolic disorders may present rather like migraine, before the development of florid encephalopathy. Attacks may be triggered by fever, fasting or stress. Vomiting tends to precede the headache, and coincident mood change is frequent. Headache with vomiting is rarely the sole manifestation of these conditions.

- MELAS syndrome – mitochondrial myopathy, encephalopathy, lactic acidosis and stroke-like episodes (increased lactate → mutation analysis).

- *POLG* mutations may present with migraine-like headaches.

- OTC deficiency (blood ammonia and amino acids, urine orotic acid and uracil).

- L-2-hydroxyglutaric aciduria (whether this is a true association is uncertain but urine organic acids will reveal).

## Primary angiitis of the central nervous system

Primary angiitis of the central nervous system may present with headaches with no other organs overtly involved and no abnormality in any blood tests. It is most common in those of South Asian descent. Additional features such as papilloedema or focal neurological signs are expected with focal signal changes on MRI (sometimes resembling the demyelination seen in acute disseminated encephalomyelitis), but catheter cerebral angiography may be normal. When this disorder is seriously suspected the investigation of choice is brain biopsy, albeit this has a sensitivity of only 40%.

## Other vascular episodes

Moyamoya may rarely present with headache with migrainous features. MRI/MRA would clarify.

## Summary

Evidence is gradually coming to the aid of 'clinical impression' in the decision to investigate or not in the child with headache.

## Further reading

Abu-Arafeh I. (2002) *Childhood Headache*. London: Mac Keith Press.

Graf WD, Kayyali HR, Alexander JJ, et al. (2008) Neuroimaging-use trends in nonacute pediatric headache before and after clinical practice parameters. *Pediatrics* **122**: e1001–e1005.

Hajj-Ali RA, Furlan A, Abou-Chebel A, Calabrese LH. (2002) Benign angiopathy of the central nervous system: cohort of 16 patients with clinical course and long-term followup. *Arthritis Rheum* **47**: 662–669.

Kossoff EH, Keswani SC, Raymond GV. (2001) L-2-hyroxyglutaric aciduria presenting as migraine. *Neurology* **57**: 1731–1732.

Webb C, Prayson RA. (2008) Pediatric pituitary adenomas. *Arch Pathol Lap Med* **132**: 77–80.

Yaari R, Anselm IA, Szer IS, et al. (2004) Childhood primary angiitis of the central nervous system: two biopsy-proven cases. *J Pediatr* **145**: 693–697.

# Chapter 3.19
## Weakness and Fatigue

Here we discuss aspects of a neurological investigation in children with fatigue and weakness that have not been covered in earlier chapters (2.3, 3.2, 3.3, 3.4, 3.7, 3.8).

### Weakness
Depending on the fine clinical detail, combinations of EMG, nerve conduction studies, muscle imaging, muscle (sometimes nerve) biopsy, biochemistry (especially creatine kinase but also on occasion potassium, thyroid hormones and urine myoglobin) coupled with directed genetic studies will facilitate diagnosis.

### Fatigue
The child with any sort of neuromuscular disorder may be described as having fatigue or being fatigued but it is important to separate those with true fatiguability.

#### Myasthenia
The fatiguability in myasthenia gravis or late-onset 'congenital' myasthenic syndrome may be subtle and require thinking about.

INVESTIGATIONS
- Edrophonium (Tensilon test – advisable to video for future reference, and perform the testing at hospital).

- Anti-acetylcholine receptor antibodies.

- If the above investigations are negative and myasthenia gravis seems probable: go to anti-MuSK antibodies.

The various rare congenital myasthenic syndromes may present throughout childhood.

- Critical to the precise diagnosis is evaluation by a specialist in EMG with paediatric expertise. EMG is most safely undertaken with no sedation, and the most useful initial investigation appears to be stimulation single-fibre electromyography (stimSFEMG). stimSFEMG is reported to have a sensitivity of ~90% and specificity of ~80% for a diagnosis of congenital myasthenia.

- Genetic evaluation is best undertaken in collaboration with a myasthenia reference laboratory.

*Chronic fatigue syndrome*
Children with supposed chronic fatigue syndrome (otherwise 'myalgic encephalomyelitis' or ME in the lay literature) may be referred for neurological investigations. Any investigations undertaken will be to determine whether there is an infective, autoimmune, inflammatory, neoplastic, toxic, metabolic, endocrine, neuromuscular or other physical cause for symptoms. There are no neurological investigations to support the diagnosis of chronic fatigue syndrome/ME, and making this diagnosis in childhood has the danger that identifiable and possibly treatable disorders may be overlooked.

## Stiffness
Myotonic dystrophy, myotonia congenita, paramyotonia, myokymia and hyperekplexia are genetic disorders often with autosomal dominant inheritance and with channelopathy as a mechanism.

Family history and clinical evaluation will usually clarify the diagnosis in these conditions and guide towards genetic testing.

*Dystonic stiffness*
In the young child there may be difficulty in distinguishing between muscle stiffness and dystonia. Video recordings at home and in clinic may speed clarification of the diagnosis.

## Cramps
Cramps at rest are usually not neuromuscular.

Cramps on exercise are a feature of some muscular dystrophies and miscellaneous conditions as follows:

- muscular dystrophies, especially dystrophinopathy and limb–girdle (creatine kinase, mutation ± biopsy)

- phosphorylase deficiency/mitochondrial myopathies (ischaemic forearm test, lacate ± biopsy)

- lipid myopathy (creatine kinase, urine organic acids ± muscle biopsy)

- Fabry disease (white blood cells, alpha-galactosidase)

- porphyria (urine porphyrins).

## Episodic weakness

The periodic paralyses may be associated either with increased (hyperkalaemic) or decreased (hypokalaemic) plasma potassium at the time of the weakness.

## Conversion disorder

In 'impossible' weakness or paralysis (i.e. that not explicable on a neuroanatomical basis), the prognosis may be better if neurological investigations are strictly limited, but beware resistance to eye opening in the 'coma' of anti-NMDA encephalitis.

## Further reading

Benatar M. (2006) A systematic review of diagnostic studies in myasthenia gravis. *Neuromuscul Disord* **16**: 459–467.

Kinali M, Beeson D, Pitt MC, et al. (2008) Congenital myasthenic syndromes in childhood: diagnostic and management challenges. *J Neuroimmunol* **201–202**: 6–12.

Mihaylova V, Müller JS, Vilchez JJ, et al. (2008) Clinical and molecular genetic findings in COLQ-mutant congenital myasthenic syndromes. *Brain* **131**: 747–759.

Müller JS, Herczegfalvi A, Vilchez JJ, et al. (2007) Phenotypical spectrum of DOK7 mutations in congenital myasthenic syndromes. *Brain* **130**: 1497–1506.

Newsom-Davis J. (2007) The emerging diversity of neuromuscular junction disorders. *Acta Myol* **26**: 5–10.

Palace J, Lashley D, Newsom-Davis J, et al. (2007) Clinical features of the DOK7 neuromuscular junction synaptopathy. *Brain* **130**: 1507–1515.

Parr JR, Jayawant S. (2007) Childhood myasthenia: clinical subtypes and practical management. Dev Med *Child Neurol* **49**: 629–635.

Sedel F, Barnerias C, Dubourg O, et al. (2007) Peripheral neuropathy and inborn errors of metabolism in adults. *J Inherit Metab Dis* **30**: 642–653.

# Chapter 3.20

# Ataxia

We offer some clinical points about the diagnosis of ataxia before discussing the appropriate neurological investigations.

The motor component of the coordination circuit is not regarded as playing a key part in ataxia, but in young children weakness may be confused with ataxia.

Although some texts confine discussion of ataxia to cerebellar ataxia, there are several types of ataxia that are worth distinguishing, albeit some may be combined:

- *cerebellar ataxia* (incoordination despite adequate visual, vestibular, posterior column function)
- *vestibular ataxia* (vertigo expected, and may have high-tone hearing loss and/or non-fatiguing nystagmus)
- *sensory ataxia* from peripheral nerve or posterior column dysfunction (rombergism and incoordination with the eyes closed)
- *visuomotor ataxia* (rare finding in disconnection syndromes: incoordination in a visual field – might be expected in adrenoleukodystrophy)
- *epileptic ataxia* (EEG will clarify)
- *'functional' or psychogenic ataxia* (sudden onset of astasia–abasia with impossible neurological signs).

Combinations of these subtypes are possible, most commonly as *spinocerebellar ataxia*.

Aspects of the neurological investigation of ataxia – in particular sensory and spinocerebellar – have been discussed in Chapter 3.8. This chapter deals mainly with cerebellar ataxia. Disorders with progressive ataxia are mentioned in Chapter 3.22.

### Acute ataxia

The common scenario is acute onset of unsteadiness in a toddler or preschool child that is termed *acute cerebellar ataxia* and is a frequent consequence of varicella (chickenpox) infection.

Notes on investigations follow.

*Intoxication*

- Urine or other toxicology (e.g. benzodiazepines, barbiturates, carbamazepine, phenytoin, tricyclics, alcohol, solvents, lindane/benzene hexachloride, mercury). At the time of wrting there is not a test for the brevetoxins that may be ingested via shellfish harvested during red-tide algal bloom.

- EEG for beta activity, especially from benzodiazepines.

*Infections*

Acute ataxia may occasionally be the result of infections, especially viral, for which microbiological investigations are available. With the recent decline in MMR (measles, mumps and rubella) immunization rates, the incidence of subacute sclerosing panencephalitis presenting in this way before EEG changes is likely to increase. Nonetheless, parainfectious causes are likely to remain predominant.

*Parainfectious*

This is the usual mechanism, with the *acute cerebellar ataxia* following a clinical viral infection, most often varicella.

- Brain imaging is not mandatory but MRI is usual especially when ataxia is severe, with or without a history of varicella to exclude acute cerebellar swelling.

- Nerve conduction studies looking for conduction block are indicated if Guillain–Barré syndrome might be the diagnosis: ataxia is said to be a presenting feature in 50%.

- Microbiological investigations do not aid management but may be useful for epidemiological purposes.

*Opsoclonus–myoclonus (dancing eye syndrome)*

The clinical picture varies from pure acute cerebellar ataxia to predominant postural and intention myoclonus with marked irritability. Eye movements vary from normal through very subtle saccadic intrusions to ocular flutter to full-blown opsoclonus.

- Brain imaging is not mandatory but MRI usually done.

- Urine catecholamines.

- Full-body MRI or CT to seek neural crest tumour.

- Meta-iodobenzylguanidine scan.

With current methodology very small neural crest tumours will not be detected, and if a previous neural crest tumour has completely regressed then it will be impossible to detect.

*Vertebral artery dissection*
This important condition should be considered when there is acute onset of cerebellar ataxia with no preceding history of an infection (such as varicella), although headache, neck or facial pain may precede or accompany the ataxia.

- Brain MRI (infarction in the posterior circulation distribution).

- Brain MRA (may show the dissection but if normal proceed to next test).

- Catheter cerebral angiography.

*Miller–Fisher syndrome*
Miller–Fisher syndrome includes some degree of external ophthalmoplegia, tendon areflexia and ataxia. The ataxia is sensory rather than cerebellar. The condition may be the same as Bickerstaff encephalitis.

- Soleus H reflexes are absent on neurophysiological testing (Chapter 2.3).

- Anti-GQ1b antibodies are likely to be present.

## Subacute ataxia
A major concern is cerebellar ataxia of fairly short duration and whether this is due to a posterior fossa tumour.

- Brain CT or MRI will be sufficient in the first instance.

## Episodic ataxia
Benign paroxysmal vertigo of childhood may look like ataxia but the diagnosis is by history not by neurological investigations. Although episodic ataxias are increasingly subdivided, the following are best known.

*Episodic ataxia type 1 (EA1)*
The presentation of this potassium channelopathy includes stiff baby, fluctuating myokymia, very brief episodes of ataxia (rarely with dyspnoea) and sometimes partial epilepsy.

- Surface EMG (myokymia will be detected).

- DNA mutation analysis (*KCNA1*).

*Episodic ataxia type 2 (EA2)*
Clinical presentation may be migraine-like, with long periods of episodic ataxia and nystagmus, possibly progressive fixed ataxia and sometimes absence epilepsy. Oculovestibular studies may clarify.

- DNA for mutations in *CACNA1A* but the gene is large and difficult to study.

*Pyruvate dehydrogenase deficiency*
Mitochondrial disorders may show intermittent ataxia, sometimes as an isolated feature.

- Blood and CSF lactate may be normal.
- Pyruvate dehydrogenase activity will be reduced in cultured fibroblasts.

*Intermittent maple syrup urine disease*
Vomiting may be present.

- Plasma and urine amino acids.
- Urine organic acids.

Intermittent ataxia is also seen in *GLUT1 deficiency* and *mitochondrial disorders*.

## Genetic ataxias

There are many predominantly autosomal recessive ataxias, ataxia-plus syndromes and spinocerebellar ataxias for which genetic tests are available (see Chapter 3.8).

One genetic ataxia or ataxia-plus syndrome for which it is impracticable (because there are too many possible mutations) – or too expensive – to investigate genetically is eIF2B-related disorder. When this is suspected after brain MRI then CSF asialotransferrin estimation is the investigation of choice.

## Further reading

Debray FG, Lambert M, Gagne R, et al. (2008) Pyruvate dehydrogenase deficiency presenting as intermittent isolated acute ataxia. *Neuropediatrics* **39**: 20–23.

Gribaa M, Salih M, Anheim M, et al. (2007) A new form of childhood onset, autosomal recessive spinocerebellar ataxia and epilepsy is localized at 16q21–q23. *Brain* **130**: 1921–1928.

Jen JC, Graves TD, Hess EJ, et al. (2007) Primary episodic ataxias: diagnosis, pathogenesis and treatment. *Brain* **130**: 2484–2493.

Kuwabara S, Asahina M, Nakajima M, et al. (1999) Special sensory ataxia in Miller Fisher syndrome detected by postural body sway analysis. *Ann Neurol* **45**: 533–536.

Mitchell WG, Davalos-Gonzalez Y, Brumm VL, et al. (2002) Opsoclonus–ataxia caused by childhood neuroblastoma: developmental and neurologic sequelae. *Pediatrics* **109**: 86–98.

Morrison PJ. (2006) Paediatric and adult ataxias (update 5). *Eur J Paediatr Neurol* **10**: 249–53.

Palace J, Lashley D, Newsom-Davis J, et al. (2007) Clinical features of the DOK7 neuromuscular junction synaptopathy. *Brain* **130**: 1507–1515.

Shook SJ, Mamsa H, Jen JC, et al. (2008) Novel mutation in KCNA1 causes episodic ataxia with paroxysmal dyspnea. *Muscle Nerve* **37**: 399–402.

Tonelli A, D'Angelo MG, Salati R, et al. (2006) Early onset, non- fluctuating spinocerebellar ataxia and a novel missense mutation in CACNA1A gene. *J Neurol Sci* **241**: 13–17.

Vanderver A, Hathout Y, Maletkovic J, et al. (2008) Sensitivity and specificity of decreased CSF asialotransferrin for eIF2B-related disorder. *Neurology* **70**: 2226–2232.

# Chapter 3.21
## Movement Disorders

In this chapter we concentrate on the neurological investigation of disorders in which abnormal movements (or movements perceived to be abnormal) are the predominant feature.

We will deal with infancy (the first two years of life) and later ages separately. We will not discuss congenital movement disorder such as is seen in cerebral palsy (Chapter 3.7).

### Infancy (first 2 years of life)

- Neonatal Prader–Willi syndrome – hypokinesia and limb dystonia – fluorescent in situ hybridization/multiplex ligation-dependent probe amplification for deletion of paternally inherited chromosome 15.

- Neonatal hyperekplexia/startle – *GLRA1* and *GlyT2* mutations.

- Disorders of monoamine metabolism – temperature instability, oculogyric crises, lethargy and parkinsonism – plasma amino acids, CSF neurotransmitters and pterins.

- Although dopa-responsive dystonia usually presents later, this disorder should be considered in any infant with a pure dystonic disorder and oral levodopa trial initiated.

- Glutaric acidura type 1 – usually after acute encephalopathy but not always; dystonia and choreoathetosis – urine organic acids.

- Mitochondrial disorders – dystonias – MRI, lactates, enzyme activities, genes (e.g. pyruvate dehydrogenase, *POLG1*).

- Methaemoglobinaemia type 2 – microcephaly, dystonia, mild cyanosis – red cell methaemoglobin, gene NADH – cytochrome b 5 reductase.

- Post-herpes encephalitis – ballismus – CSF, herpes simplex virus polymerase chain reaction though likely negative.

- Lesch–Nyhan syndrome – choreoathetosis superimposed on gross motor delay (usually followed by self-mutilation) – urine uric acid, hypoxanthine phosphoribosyltransferase 1 assay red cells or cultured fibroblasts.

- Shuddering and benign infantile spasms – tremor-like spasms – video, video-EEG if in doubt.

- Infantile masturbation – repeated dystonic adduction of the thighs – video.

- Transient dystonia of infancy – episodes of dystonic posturing especially of upper limbs distally – home video.

### Older children
Movement disorders may be a component of many progressive disorders which are discussed in Chapter 3.22. Some paroxysmal events have been mentioned in Chapters 3.14 and 3.15.

In Tables 3.21.1–3.21.3 we deal with situations where movement disorders are a prominent feature. Table 3.21.1 lists those with acute onset, Table 3.21.2 lists paroxysmal disorders, and Table 3.21.3 includes movement disorders which may be more or less chronic and in most cases progressive, at any rate without adequate treatment.

Table 3.21.1 Acute-onset movement disorders

| Condition | Movement disorder(s) | Investigations |
|---|---|---|
| Drugs (neuroleptic) | Dystonia, oculogyric crises, torticollis | Video |
| Arterial ischaemic stroke | Chorea, dystonia, etc. | Brain MRI, MRA ± catheter cerebral angiography |
| Sydenham chorea | Chorea | ECG, antistreptolysin O titre, anti-DNAaseB titre |
| Anti-NMDA receptor encephalitis | Orofacial dyskinesia, and alternating violent limb dyskinesia and akinesia | Anti-NMDA receptor antibodies, CSF oligoclonal bands |
| Immune-mediated chorea encephalopathy | Chorea ± oculogyric crises, rigidity (not clear if different from anti-NMDA receptor encephalitis) | CSF oligoclonal bands |

Table 3.21.1 continued

| Condition | Movement disorder(s) | Investigations |
|---|---|---|
| Systemic lupus erythematosus | Chorea | Anti-DNA antibodies, etc. (auto-antibody battery), CSF, INF-$\alpha$ |
| Glutaric aciduria type 1 | Choreoathetosis, dystonia (usually postencephalopathy) | Brain MRI, urine organic acids |
| Mitochondrial | Dystonia | MRI, and see Chapter 2.14 |
| Pyruvate dehydrogenase deficiency | Dystonia (may be paroxysmal) | MRI (globus pallidus signal change), $\pm$ H-MRS, lactates, PDH activity in fibroblasts |
| Rapid-onset dystonia parkinsonism (DYT12) | Upper-limb dystonia, bulbar symptoms (parkinsonism later) | Video. Gene test: *ATP1A3* |
| Psychogenic ('functional') | Any movement disorder, sudden onset, cease when not observed | Minimum |

Table 3.21.2 Paroxysmal movement disorders

| Condition | Movement disorder(s) | Investigations |
|---|---|---|
| Alternating hemiplegia of childhood | Dystonia, ocular deviation and monocular nystagmus, limp attacks, bath-induced in one third | Home video |
| Paroxysmal kinesigenic dyskinesia | Choreoathetosis on sudden voluntary movement, family history | Home video (gene[a]) |
| Paroxysmal non-kinesigenic dyskinesia | Chorea and dystonia, family history, alcohol and caffeine provocation in family members | Home video (gene[a]) |

Table 3.21.2 continued

| Condition | Movement disorder(s) | Investigations |
|---|---|---|
| Paroxysmal exertional dyskinesia | Choreoathetosis during sustained exercise, family history | Family video. Blood film (echinocytes). GLUT1 deficiency (fasting blood and CSF glucose) |
| Infantile convulsions with paroxysmal dyskinesia | Choreoathetosis, kinesigenic or exercise induced, with history of infantile clonic epileptic seizures | Home video (gene[b]) |
| GLUT1 deficiency | Variable, usually with epilepsy also, meal related | Low fasting CSF/blood glucose ratio; red cell GLUT1 assay; *SLC2A1* gene |

a Gene test may be available but not normally indicated.

b Gene localized to centromere of chromosome 16 but not helpful in individual diagnosis.

Table 3.21.3 Chronic or progressive movement disorder

| Type of movement disorder | Condition | Investigations |
|---|---|---|
| Mixed movement disorder | Wilson disease (onset over age 5 years, usually over 7 years) | Serum copper, copper oxidase, 24h urine copper ± liver copper. Gene mutation |
| | Guanidinoacetate methyltransferase deficiency (dystonia, ballismus) | Brain H-MRS ± urine guanidinoacetate |
| | Mitochondrial | Brain MRI, H-MRS. See Chapter 2.14 |
| | Myoclonus–dystonia (DYT11) | Video. *SGCE* gene mutation |
| | Rapid-onset dystonia parkinsonsim (DYT12) | Video. *ATP1A3* gene mutation |
| | Dystonia–parkinsonism (DYT16), *not* rapid onset | *PRKRA* gene mutation |
| | Juvenile parkinsonism | Fluoride-PET. Several genes |

Table 3.21.3 continued

| Type of movement disorder | Condition | Investigations |
|---|---|---|
| Dystonia | Idiopathic torsion dystonia (DYT1) | Gene – *Torsin A* |
| | Dopa-responsive dystonia (DRD=DYT5) | Levodopa trial, *GCH1* gene |
| Chorea | Benign hereditary chorea | *TITF-1* gene mutation |
| | Hypoparathyroidism | Plasma calcium and phosphorus, ECG for QTc, CT/MRI (calcification of basal ganglia and white matter), better seen on CT |
| | Lesch–Nyhan (choreoathetosis) | Urine uric acid, red-cell hypoxanthine phosphoribosyltransferase |
| Tremor | Essential tremor | Frequency analysis possible, gene test available but not required |
| | Hyperthyroidism | Thyroid function tests |
| | $B_{12}$ deficiency (also after treatment) | Blood film, $B_{12}$, urine organic acids, spinal cord MRI |
| Myoclonus | Many metabolic and epileptic conditions | Biochemistry, EEG |
| | Myoclonus–dystonia (DYT11) – begins with dystonic toddler gait (under age 3y) that may be forgotten, later lightning jerks of upper limbs dominate | Home video including archival footage. *SGCE* gene mutation |
| | Restless legs syndrome | Night video; levodopa trial has not been evaluated as a diagnostic test in children; polysomnography might add |
| Tics | Tourette syndrome | No tests (significance of anti-basal ganglia antibodies unclear) |

341

## Movement disorders in individuals with learning disability

Most of the abnormal movements in those with severe learning disability, in particular various kinds of stereotypy, do not help in clinical diagnosis and do not suggest particular neurological investigations. However, sound-startle induced falls that resemble cataplexy or hyperekplexia point to Coffin–Lowry syndrome (investigation: home or clinic video, possible gene analysis see Chapter 3.14), and status dystonicus in a boy with epileptic infantile spasms will prompt *ARX* mutation analysis (see Chapter 3.15).

In another *ARX* phenotype boys have focal dystonia with an X-linked inheritance. A prominent movement disorder in a boy with mild facial dysmorphism will prompt estimation of free T3 (triiodothyroxine) and, if elevated, mutation analysis of *MCT8* (monocarboxylate transporter 8 gene).

## Further reading

Ahmed MA, Martinez A, Yee A, et al. (2008) Psychogenic and organic movement disorders in children. *Dev Med Child Neurol* **50**: 300–304.

Assmann B, Surtees R, Hoffmann GF. (2003) Approach to the diagnosis of neurotransmitter diseases exemplified by the differential diagnosis of childhood-onset dystonia. *Ann Neurol* 54 Suppl 6: S18–S24.

Bhidayasiri R, Pulst SM. (2005) Dystonia (DYT) genetic loci. *Eur J Paediatr Neurol* **9**: 367–370.

Bruno MK, Lee HY, Auburger GW, et al. (2007) Genotype–phenotype correlation of paroxysmal nonkinesigenic dyskinesia. *Neurology* **68**: 1782–1789.

Canavese C, Ciano C, Zorzi G, et al. (2008) Polymyography in the diagnosis of childhood onset movement disorders. *Eur J Paediatr Neurol* **12**: 480–483.

Dalmau J, Gleichman AJ, Hughes EG. (2008) Anti-NMDA-receptor encephalitis: case series and analysis of the effects of antibodies. *Lancet Neurol* **7**: 1091–1098.

Dressler D, Benecke R. (2005) Diagnosis and management of acute movement disorders. *J Neurol* **252**: 1299–1306.

Echenne B, Roubertie A, Assmann B, et al. (2006) Sepiapterin reductase deficiency: clinical presentation and evaluation of long-term therapy. *Pediatr Neurol* **35**: 308–313.

Ewenczyk C, Leroux A, Roubergue A, et al. (2008) Recessive hereditary methaemoglobinaemia, type II: delineation of the clinical spectrum. *Brain* **131**: 760–761.

Friedman J, Hyland K, Blau N, MacCollin M. (2006) Dopa-responsive hypersomnia and mixed movement disorder due to sepiapterin reductase deficiency. *Neurology* **67**: 2032–2035.

Geyer HL, Bressman SB. (2006) The diagnosis of dystonia. *Lancet Neurol* **5**: 780–790.

Guerrini R, Moro F, Kato M, et al. (2007) Expansion of the first PolyA tract of ARX causes infantile spasms and status dystonicus. *Neurology* **69**: 427–433.

Hartley LM, Ng SY, Dale RC, et al. (2002) Immune mediated chorea encephalopathy syndrome in childhood. *Dev Med Child Neurol* **44**: 273–277.

Horvath GA, Stockler-Ipsiroglu SG, Salvarinova-Zivkovic R, et al. (2008) Autosomal recessive GTP cyclohydrolase I deficiency without hyperphenylalaninemia: evidence of a phenotypic continuum between dominant and recessive forms. *Mol Genet Metab* **94**: 127–31.

Kullnat MW, Morse RP. (2008) Choreoathetosis after herpes simplex encephalitis with basal ganglia involvement on MRI. *Pediatrics* **121**: e1003–e1007.

McFarland R, Chinnery PF, Blakely EL, et al. (2007) Homoplasmy, heteroplasmy, and mitochondrial dystonia. *Neurology* 69: 911–916.

Morrison PJ. (2008) Paediatric and adult movement disorders (update 2). *Eur J Paediatr Neurol* 12: 253–256.

Neville BG, Parascandalo R, Farrugia R. (2005) Sepiapterin reductase deficiency: a congenital dopa-responsive motor and cognitive disorder. *Brain* 128: 2291–2296.

Pearl PL, Taylor JL, Trzcinski S, Sokohl A. (2007) The pediatric neurotransmitter disorders. *J Child Neurol* 22: 606–616.

Pfeiffer RF (2007) Wilson's disease. *Semin Neurol* 27: 123–132.

Picchietti MA, Picchietti DL. (2008) Restless legs syndrome and periodic limb movement disorder in children and adolescents. *Semin Pediatr Neurol* 15: 91–99.

Pons R, Ford B, Chiriboga CA, et al. (2004) Aromatic L-amino acid decarboxylase deficiency: clinical features, treatment, and prognosis. *Neurology* 62: 1058–1065.

Roberts EA, Schilsky ML. (2008) Diagnosis and treatment of Wilson disease: an update. *Hepatology* 47: 2089–2111.

Wolf DS, Singer HS. (2008) Pediatric movement disorders: an update. *Curr Opin Neurol* 21: 491–496.

# Chapter 3.22

# Progressive Loss of Skills and Dementia

The process of development is such that it is often difficult to distinguish disorders with true neurological regression from those which are static and non-progressive. The causes of regression are most important to recognize and differentiate because some are treatable (Chapter 3.23) and many more have specific genetic implications. In others, the provision of a diagnostic label is helpful to families, even many years after the death of their child.

Some clinical clues are helpful in reducing the range of investigations necessary for diagnosis.

- *Age:*
  At any given age some disorders are likely, others unlikely, others almost impossible. Thus we deal with the more important disorders in approximate age order.

- *Somatic features:*
  Certain somatic features found on physical examination will narrow the diagnostic possibilities. Computer-based resources such as SimulConsult (www.simulconsult.com) deal with this aspect well. For example, most of the mucopolysaccharidoses have somatic features that allow a rapid route to diagnosis, whereas Sanfilippo syndrome is often purely neurological (or neuropsychiatric) and is given more attention here.

- *With or without epilepsy:*
  The pattern of neurological involvement – whether with or without epilepsy – will distinguish others.

Where precise differentiation is not possible on the basis of these three aspects, the battery of 'screening' tests may still be reduced to manageable proportions.

The more one knows about this subject, the more one may be able to discriminate between individual disorders and thus reduce the number of neurological investigations required. This is an argument for onward referral.

It is also an argument for wide consultation, including if need be at an international level. The experience of the older physician may complement the technological expertise of the younger. What follows includes a discursive element and is not in table form to highlight the philosophy that discussion and reflection are a prelude to focusing on the key diagnostic investigations.

There is an argument also for keeping a record of undiagnosed child patients so that the quest for a diagnosis is never abandoned.

## Outline of diagnostic process
We will concentrate on deteriorating neurological disorders for which the choice of neurological investigations is important. We will pay less attention to disorders with extraneurological features because these are more readily diagnosed through databases such as SimulConsult. We admit to bias towards the frequency of diagnoses made in developed countries and recognize that in parts of the world where measles vaccine does not approach total coverage subacute sclerosing panencephalitis (SSPE) will be common rather than rare as in our experience.

When epilepsy is present, we emphasize that regression (sometimes called pseudoregression) may be a common feature and happily sometimes may be a reversible feature. These situations we will not discuss here (see Chapter 3.12).

Thanks to Dr Chris Verity, lead investigator of the PIND (Progressive Intellectual and Neurological Deterioration) study of the BPSU (British Paediatric Surveillance Unit), we are aware of the first approximately 1000 'confirmed' diagnoses. Of these, the total number of children with neuronal ceroid lipofuscinoses marginally exceeds the total of those with mitochondrial cytopathy to take first place, ahead of combined 'neurological' lysosomal disorders (metachromatic leukodystrophy, Niemann–Pick type C and Krabbe), mucopolysaccharidoses, GM gangliosidoses and peroxisomal disorders. However, we suspect that with the emerging facility for the diagnosis of nuclear encoded mitochondrial diseases (due to mutations in *POLG1* in particular), mitochondrial disorders as a group might take first place in the future.

The prominence of mitochondrial disorders at all ages leads us to be concise in the individual citations and instead refer readers for further details to Chapter 2.14 and to recent cited key references on mitochondrial diagnosis.

## Too early to know whether condition is regressive or static
When the presentation is from the neonatal period or in very early infancy it may be difficult to be sure that there really is a progressive (regressive) disorder. Some of these conditions have been discussed in previous chapters, especially 3.1, 3.2 and 3.7.

*Hypothyroidism*
Untreated or unrecognized hypothyroidism is detected by thyroid function tests.

*Phenylketonuria*
Undetected phenylketonuria and related metabolic disorders are detected by plasma amino acids.

*Vitamin B$_{12}$ disorders*
B$_{12}$ disorders are suggested by plasma amino acids (homocysteine) and/or urine organic acids (methylmalonic).

*Creatine synthesis disorders*
GAMT deficiency may be detected by urine guanidinoacetate, but the fact that some creatine synthesis disorders may be detected only by finding a reduced creatine peak on proton MRS of brain means that this investigation should be considered whenever MRI is done for an unexplained condition with developmental regression.

*Pelizaeus–Merzbacher disease and Pelizaeus–Merzbacher-like disease*
These have been discussed in Chapter 3.7. They are examples of disorders with hypomyelination. Insofar as hypomyelination is defined as no change in lack of myelin over time, one might expect a truly static disorder rather than the clinical progression that may be evident.

*Aicardi–Goutières syndrome*
This was also discussed in Chapter 3.7. It is an example of a disease which may be both progressive on imaging and non-progressive clinically, especially with mutations in *RNASEH2B*.

## Deterioration in infancy – infantile
Several of these conditions have suffiently characteristic features to point to the investigation or investigations of choice.

*GM2 gangliosidosis*
Tay–Sachs disease presents with sound-startle, and the cherry-red spot at the macula prompts hexosaminidase estimation. Infantile Sandhoff disease is similar but with variable hepatosplenomegaly.

*Krabbe disease*
An irritable infant with extended posture is surprisingly found to have absent tendon reflexes. Increased CSF protein suggests demyelinating neuropathy which is confirmed by very slow motor nerve conduction velocity. Confirmation of the diagnosis is by galactocerebrosidase beta-galactosidase estimation using a natural substrate.

*GM1 gangliosidosis*
The dysmorphism is sufficient to prompt white cell enzyme assay looking for deficient beta-galactosidase. If urine glycosaminoglycans are tested for, keratan sulphate will be found to be increased.

*Menkes disease*
Pili torti is usually a sufficient clue but in more subtle cases reduced serum copper and copper oxidase will show the diagnosis. Biochemical evaluation alone is needed when presymptomatic newborn infants are evaluated in known affected families: here abnormal plasma catecholamines reflect the disease.

*Canavan disease*
Visual loss and megalencephaly will be identified by huge amounts of N-acetylaspartate on urine organic acid analysis. If MRI and H-MRS have been done first, the extensive white matter abnormality and N-acetylaspartate peak will be obvious. As mentioned in Chapter 3.7, mild Canavan disease is a static disorder with only developmental delay and a modest N-acetylaspartic aciduria.

*Molybdenum cofactor deficiency*
Milder cases of molybdenum cofactor deficiency may present in infancy not necessarily with dislocated lenses. Sulphite test of fresh urine will often but not always be positive. Plasma uric acid will be low, and total homocysteine should be estimated at the same time in case this is isolated sulphite oxidase deficiency.

*Infantile neuronal ceroid lipofuscinosis*
This condition (most common in Finland) overlaps the first and second year of life in its time of presentation which is mainly around 1 year to 18 months. Normal development ceases before a subtle regression. Clinical clues include impaired visual awareness and repetitive movements of the hands rubbed together – these movements were originally described as knitting movements but closely resemble the so-called hand-washing movements of Rett syndrome. Short bursts of myoclonic activity (myoclonic epileptic seizures) may be subtle as developmental skills are gradually lost. The ERG declines in amplitude before the EEG flattens. MRI shows atrophy and increased signal in the thalami. Electronmicroscopy of white cell pellets will show granular osmiophilic deposits (GRODs). Protein palmitoyl thioesterase (PPT) activity is reduced in plasma and in leukocytes – this will not normally be detected on routine white cell enzyme analyses and needs to be targeted specifically.

As with serious neurodegenerative disorders in general, it is wise not to rely on a single abnormal neurological investigation. In this case, one should have at least the appearance of GRODs and very low PPT activity, and if possible, a *CLN1* mutation.

## Deterioration in infancy – late infantile

*Rett syndrome*
This is not a true regressive disorder but it certainly presents as loss of skills, particularly hand function, usually in the second year of life, with hand-washing movements and often bruxism and salivation, and acquired microcephaly. EEG is nonspecific but may show spikes and sharp waves at first only in sleep. Most affected girls have mutation in *MECP2* but other genetic variants are recognized.

*Late infantile neuronal ceroid lipofuscinosis*
This disorder may start beyond the age of 2 years but we mention it now as it is in many countries one of the most common neurodegenerative disorders at about this age. It presents as epilepsy and may include stimulus-sensitive myoclonus. Ataxia and loss of skills may be attributed to either the epilepsy or the antiepileptic medication. Brain imaging shows cerebellar atrophy but the most important simple investigation is slow stroboscopic activation at 0.5Hz during EEG, so this test should never be omitted. In late infantile neuronal ceroid lipofuscinosis, giant occipital potentials are induced with each slowly repeated flash. Curvilinear inclusions on electronmicroscopy of white cell pellet or other tissues can be found and should be looked for, but it is easier to go direct to gene analysis of *CLN2*.

*Metachromatic leukodystrophy*
The main clinical clue is evidence of peripheral neuropathy (impaired tendon reflexes) especially accompanying subtle dementia, cerebellar ataxia and bulbar signs. Toe-walking may be the presentation. The CSF protein is increased. Nerve conduction velocities will be slow, metachromatic material found in tubular epithelial cells in urine, and aryl sulphatase A (ARSA) will be deficient in leukocytes or fibroblasts (a clinical diagnosis, aided by the demonstration of metachromatic material, will not be negated by normal white-cell ARSA). If brain MRI is done with gadolinium contrast, the cranial nerves may enhance (as they do in Krabbe leukodystrophy).

*Infantile neuroaxonal dystrophy*
Completely normal development is followed by regression in central and peripheral nervous functions at around the end of the second year of life. There is usually a plateau before this regression. Clinical features include subtle ocular wobble, distal weakness with tendon hyporeflexia or areflexia and emerging extensor plantar responses. EEG shows diffuse beta activity but at first this is not obvious when it is still of rather low voltage. Nerve conduction velocities are normal but EMG shows evidence of denervation. Brain imaging reveals a degree of cerebellar atrophy. Biopsies are necessary only if mutations are not found in *PLA2G6*.


# Middle childhood

*Sanfilippo disease*
In this common condition there is subtle dementia with more prominent behaviour difficulties, in particular aggression. Dysmorphisms such as difficulty extending the fingers are subtle. Urine glycosaminoglycans should reveal the diagnosis but 24 hour urine for heparan sulphate should be requested specifically if in doubt. Gene tests are available, but the various genotypes are phenotypically indistinguishable.

*Adrenoleukodystrophy*
By far the most common of the peroxisomopathies, this condition in boys may present with gradual loss of higher functions. Not only may there be 'cortical' visual impairment, but choroiditis or other ocular abnormalities may be detected on

ophthalmological examination. Brain MRI usually shows predominantly posterior white matter change, the margins of which may enhance with contrast (there is an inflammatory reaction). Very long chain fatty acids should be increased in blood.

*Niemann–Pick type C*
This disorder may or may not have manifested in the neonatal period with jaundice and splenomegaly. Clumsiness and mild learning difficulties are common. Decline is associated with some degree of vertical supranuclear ophthalmoplegia and often with true cataplexy, but epilepsy may be the presenting symptom. Dysphagia is also frequently noted. Chitotriosidase is nonspecifically increased.

Sea-blue histiocytes are often but not always seen on bone marrow examination, and storage material may also be found in other tissues such as appendix or rectal biopsy, but if cultured fibroblasts show severely abnormal intracellular cholesterol homeostasis, then biopsy confirmation is not necessary. Genetic confirmation by examination of *NPC1* and *NPC2* is possible, but is unnecessary if the fibroblast cholesterol studies are unequivocal.

When fibroblast cholesterol studies are atypical or equivocal, additional studies – biopsy, gene analysis – may be needed for secure diagnosis.

*Pantothenate kinase-associated neurodegeneration (Hallevorden–Spatz disease)*
In this disease dystonia may become extreme with gross opisthotonus. Brain MRI eventually shows the eye of the tiger sign in the basal ganglia. Genetic diagnosis is through *PANK2* (pantothenate kinase-associated neurodegeneration).

*Cerebellar leukoencephalopathy, presumed histiocytosis-related*
This regressive disorder begins with cerebellar and pyramidal and extrapyramidal features but with later behavioural difficulties and cognitive decline, and shows first on MRI as a striking cerebellar white matter signal change, followed by brainstem and basal ganglia abnormalities. Eventually hypopituitarism may suggest histiocytosis, and sometimes biopsy will confirm this (see also Chapter 2.12).

*Subacute sclerosing panencephalitis (SSPE)*
Regression is usually gradual (but occasionally fulminant), often with behavioural change. School performance declines. Periodic subtle changes of expression may be apparent on close observation. EEG usually shows periodic complexes each associated with EMG change of spasm duration. Measles titres are elevated in blood and CSF, and CSF immunoglobulins are increased also, with oligoclonal bands.

While this disorder appears very rare in countries with excellent infant immunization programs, it is common elsewhere in the world. A report from India evaluated 307 patients with SSPE admitted to a tertiary care hospital over a 10-year period. The initial diagnosis by various health care professionals was other than SSPE in 79%. These misdiagnoses included epilepsy, metachromatic leukodystrophy, Schilder disease, cerebral palsy, hemiparkinsonism, Wilson disease, vasculitis, spinocerebellar ataxia, motor neuron disease, nutritional amblyopia, tapetoretinal degeneration, catatonic schizophrenia, and malingering. The median interval between first reported symptom and precise diagnosis was 3 months.

## Older child and adolescent
Several of the disorders already mentioned may appear in different forms in older childhood and adolescence. Enzyme deficiencies which manifest with dysmorphism and/or visceromegaly in the very young tend to have *only* neurological features at later ages. Dystonia emerges as a prominent neurological sign, without specific disease implications.

### Juvenile neuronal ceroid lipofuscinosis
Visual impairment is almost always the presenting sign and because there is so little to explain the visual difficulty these affected schoolchildren may be falsely labelled with psychiatric diagnoses including 'hysterical blindness' or 'functional visual loss'. However, pigmentary macular changes eventually appear. Carefully performed ERG (Chapter 2.4) will show impaired retinal function from the start and in all classical cases examination of blood film will show large vacuoles (which contain fingerprint bodies on electronmicroscopy). In such children mutations in the gene *CLN3* should be detected. In the much less common Scottish variant with GRODs the same biochemical and genetic tests should be used as in infantile neuronal ceroid lipofuscinosis looking for a modest reduction of protein palmitoyl thioesterase in plasma or leukocytes and mutations in *CLN1*.

### Huntington disease
Juvenile Huntington disease is surprisingly common, presenting with parkinsonism and on examination oculomotor apraxia in horizontal gaze, with caudate atrophy on brain MRI. Testing for repeat in the Huntington gene is easy, albeit tragic.

### Wilson disease
Dysarthria, subtle behavioural change and school problems, choreoathetosis and other movement disorders are some of many presentations of this rare treatable disorder (Chapter 3.23). Slit-lamp microscopy almost always shows Kayser–Fleischer rings. Signal changes are seen in lentiform nuclei, usually with low plasma copper and copper oxidase.

### Variant Creutzfeld–Jacob disease
Although very rare, this has been recognized in older children. 'Psychiatric' symptoms and paraesthesiae are seen with regression, and MRI shows altered signal in the pulvinar. Any CSF or other invasive studies need to be done with very special precautions against disease transmission. Cases in the UK and Ireland are reported to the PIND study.

## Progressive myoclonus epilepsies

### Unverricht–Lundborg disease

Generalized epilepsy with tonic–clonic and clonic seizures is complicated by action myoclonus. EEG commonly includes a photoparoxysmal response and an increased potential in response to sensory stimulation that is different to that seen in Lafora disease (Chapter 2.4). Mutations may be found in *CSTB*.

### Lafora disease

This disorder also presents with adolescent convulsive epilepsy but with even more severe myoclonus, before the emergence of unsteadiness and dementia. Somatosensory evoked potentials are large and different in detail from those in Unverricht–Lundborg disease. Axillary skin biopsy – or standard skin biopsy – usually but not always shows Lafora bodies. Mutations may not be easy to detect in *EPM2A* and *EPM2B*.

## Leukodystrophies and leukoencephalopathies

We have said little about leukodystrophies and leukoencephalopathies, whether often recognizable – as for instance vanishing white matter (VWM) disease or Alexander disease – or one of the many as yet undiagnosable conditions. Pattern recognition is a major strategy for the identification of these white matter disorders. We recommend the article by van der Knaap and Valk (2005) together with numerous articles by the first author to be found on PubMed, including Schiffmann and van der Knaap (2009). In one condition or group of conditions, the eIF2B-related disorders, more than pattern recognition is often necessary.

### eIF2B-related disorders

VWM (vanishing white matter) and CACH (childhood-onset ataxia with CNS hypomyelination) were earlier acronyms for *eIF2B*-related disorders but it has become apparent that these common autosomal recessive leukoencephalopathies have a wide phenotypic spectrum. Even when brain MRI shows 'typical' features of VWM disease (T2 signal intensity of white matter equivalent to CSF, FLAIR images consistent with attenuation of involved white matter, and striae or strands in the white matter on T1), the explanation need not be a mutation in one of the five subunits of *EIF2B*. Estimation of CSF asialotransferrin is a simple way of clarifying this: if the CSF asialotransferrin is below 8% of total transferrin then it is highly likely that an *EIF2B* mutation will be found, if it is over 8% then *EIF2B* genetic testing may not be justified.

## Deteriorating disorders without dementia

### Friedreich ataxia

Friedreich ataxia has been mentioned in earlier chapters. A willowy gait with a combination of cerebellar and sensory ataxia, ocular dysmetria, absent caudal tendon reflexes and extensor plantar reflexes make the diagnosis likely. Nerve conduction studies reveal evidence of a sensory axonal neuropathy. Most have an abnormal echocardiogram with thick septum. A novel MRI technique using tract-based spatial statistics and voxel-based morphometry may have wider diagnostic application. Direct genetic testing for GAA repeats in *FXN* will confirm the Friedreich diagnosis.

*Spinocerebellar ataxias*
A lack of symptom specificity sometimes makes it necessary to use a spinocerebellar ataxia gene test battery, but see Chapter 3.8 for specific suggestions. It should not be forgotten, however, that mitochondrial disease, especially mutations in *POLG1*, may cause spinocerebellar ataxia (see Clinical Vignette Introduction.1).

*eIF2B-related ataxia*
Because *eIF2B*-related disorders may present with motor regression – especially progressive ataxia – without obvious cognitive problems, we mention them again here. Whether or not there are the well-known provocations of fever, head bump or fright, the finding of central white matter signal changes on brain MRI should prompt CSF asialotransferrin estimation as a diagnostic tool.

*Progressive spastic parapareses*
A number of genetic causes of progressive or ascending spastic paraparesis are known. A rare treatable cause is biotinidase deficiency, detectable by direct plasma biotinidase assay. Ascending spastic paraplegia may be due to mutations in the *alcin* gene.

## Deterioration in a child with a 'static' disorder

It is not uncommon for regression to occur from early childhood to adolescence in children with 'static' learning difficulties or apparent cerebral palsy with or without epilepsy. Neurological investigations do not necessarily help in the situation where the cause of the disability is known, such as with deterioration in Down syndrome.

When the cause of the supposedly static disorder is unknown then it is more likely that the cause of regression will emerge through renewed neurological investigations. Some examples follow, with clues and key investigations.

- *MECP2* duplication – recurrent severe respiratory infections, slow EEG, nonspecific MRI white matter changes – multiplex ligation-dependent probe amplification.

- *POLG1* mutation – deterioration is with myoclonus or epilepsy – *POLG1* mutation analysis.

- Pyruvate dehydrogense (PDH) deficiency – often globus pallidus changes – PDH activity in fibroblasts.

- GAMT deficiency – acquired movement disorder – brain or CSF H-MRS.

- Organic aciduria (e.g. L-2-OH-glutaricaciduria) – white matter and dentate changes – urine organic acids.

Beware nutritional deficiencies, especially with enteral assisted feeding.

## Approaches when the diagnosis seems too difficult

If an enzyme thought to be deficient seems to be present, consider tissue examination, even old-fashioned tests like full thickness rectal biopsy. Don't omit electronmicroscopy of buffy coat to exclude atypical neuronal ceroid lipofuscinosis. When an expected mutation should be present but isn't found, consider another mutation. Go back to the history, start again and make a systematic summary. Discuss that with international colleagues and/or place the details on a forum such as the Child-Neuro listserve (https://listserver.itd.umich.edu/cgi-bin/lyris.pl?enter=child-neuro). Never give up!

## Further reading

Canafoglia L, Ciano C, Panzica F, et al. (2004) Sensorimotor cortex excitability in Unverricht–Lundborg disease and Lafora body disease. *Neurology* **63**: 2309–2315.

Carrilho I, Santos M, Guimarães A. (2008) Infantile neuroaxonal dystrophy: What's most important for the diagnosis? *Eur J Paediatr Neurol* **12**: 491–500.

Chedrawi AK, Ali A, Al Hassnan ZN, et al. (2008) Profound biotinidase deficiency in a child with predominantly spinal cord disease. *J Child Neurol* **23**: 1043–1048.

Coutelier M, Andries S, Ghariani S. (2008) Neuroserpin mutation causes electrical status epilepticus of slow-wave sleep. *Neurology* **71**: 64–66.

Della Nave R, Ginestroni A, Tessa C, et al. (2008) Brain white matter tracts degeneration in Friedreich ataxia. An in vivo MRI study using tract-based spatial statistics and voxel-based morphometry. *Neuroimage* **40**: 19–25.

Eymard-Pierre E, Lesca G, Dollet S, et al. (2002) Infantile-onset ascending hereditary spastic paralysis is associated with mutations in the alsin gene. *Am J Hum Genet* **71**: 518–527.

Finsterer J. (2008) Leigh and Leigh-like syndrome in children and adults. *Pediatr Neurol* **39**: 223–235.

Gregory A, Westaway SK, Holm IE. (2008) Neurodegeneration associated with genetic defects in phospholipase A(2). *Neurology* **71**: 1402–1409.

Kälviäinen R, Eriksson K, Losekoot M, et al. (2007) Juvenile-onset neuronal ceroid lipofuscinosis with infantile CLN1 mutation and palmitoyl-protein thioesterase deficiency. *Eur J Neurol* **14**: 367–372.

Kurian MA, Morgan NV, MacPherson L, et al. (2008) Phenotypic spectrum of neurodegeneration associated with mutations in the PLA2G6 gene (PLAN). *Neurology* **70**: 1623–1629.

Maegawa GHB, Stockley T, Tropak M, et al. (2006) The natural history of juvenile or subacute GM2 gangliosidosis: 21 new cases and literature review of 134 previously reported. *Pediatrics* **118**: 1550–1560.

Miller RJ, Roos RP. (2000) What happens when mutant neuroserpins get into bad shape. *Lancet* **355**: 590–591.

Prashanth LK, Taly AB, Sinha S, Ravi V. (2007) Subacute sclerosing panencephalitis (SSPE): an insight into the diagnostic errors from a tertiary care university hospital. *J Child Neurol* **22**: 683–688.

Roberts EA, Schilsky ML. (2008) Diagnosis and treatment of Wilson disease: an update. *Hepatology* **47**: 2089–2111.

Schiffmann R, van der Knaap MS. (2009) Invited article: an MRI-based approach to the diagnosis of white matter disorders. *Neurology* **72**: 750–759.

Shahwan A, Farrell M, Delanty N. (2005) Progressive myoclonic epilepsies: a review of genetic and therapeutic aspects. *Lancet Neurol* **4**: 239–248.

Soltanzadeh A, Soltanzadeh P, Nafissi S, et al. (2007) Wilson's disease: a great masquerader. *Eur Neurol* **57**: 80–85.

van der Knapp MS, Valk J. (2005) *Magnetic Resonance of Myelination and Myelin Disorders, 3rd edn.* Berlin, Heidelberg, New York: Springer.

van der Knaap MS, Arts WF, Garbern JY, et al. (2008) Cerebellar leukoencephalopathy most likely histiocytosis-related. *Neurology* **71**: 1361–1367.

Velinov M, Zellers N, Styles J, et al. (2007) Homozygosity for mutation G212A of the gene for aspartoacylase is associated with atypical form of Canavan's disease. *Clin Genet* **73**: 288–289.

Vanderver A, Hathout Y, Maletkovic J, et al. (2008) Sensitivity and specificity of decreased CSF asialotransferrin for eIF2B-related disorder. *Neurology* **70**: 2226–2232.

Walker RH, Jung HH, Dobson-Stone C, et al. (2007) Neurologic phenotypes associated with acanthocytosis. *Neurology* **68**: 92–98.

# Chapter 3.23
## Rare Treatable Disorders

In this book we have tried to emphasize targeting investigations to specific conditions or disorders. In this chapter we go over in table form some of the rarer treatable conditions previously discussed, arranged in alphabetical order (Table 3.23.1). We have grouped them together because often there are minimal clues on clinical evaluation or on 'routine' investigations and they are thereby easily missed.

We have not included more straightforward treatable disorders nor those in which therapies are mainly symptomatic. Nor have we included those in which bone marrow transplant is reported to be effective only in presymptomatic cases.

Metabolic errors such as phenylketonuria and homocystinuria have been left out because they should always be detected by blood and urine amino acids examination, as will all the other metabolic errors with elevated phenylalanine or homocysteine.

Also excluded are tumours that may have either direct or paraneoplastic effects (Chapter 2.12) and may be treatable and curable by surgery and chemotherapy, such as the hypothalamic syndromes caused by occult ganglioneuroblastoma (see Clinical Vignette 2.12.3).

We have tried to focus on conditions in which it matters whether the clinician thinks of the possibility, where thinking of the disorder and the right neurological investigations might help the child's life and future development.

### Further reading

Biancheri R, Cerone R, Schiaffino MC. (2001) Cobalamin (Cbl) C/D deficiency: clinical, neurophysiological and neuroradiologic findings in 14 cases. *Neuropediatrics* **32**: 14–22.

Biancheri R, Cerone R, Rossi A. (2002) Early-onset cobalamin C/D deficiency: epilepsy and electroencephalographic features. *Epilepsia* **43**: 616–622.

Carmel R, Green R, Rosenblatt DS, et al. (2003) Update on cobalamin, folate, and homocysteine. *Hematology Am Soc Hematol Educ Program,* 62–81.

Cooper EC, Pan Z. (2007) Putting an end to DEND: a severe neonatal-onset epilepsy is treatable if recognized early. *Neurology* **69**: 1310–1311.

Gallagher RC, Van Hove JL, Scharer G, et al. (2009) Folinic acid-responsive seizures are identical to pyridoxine-dependent epilepsy. *Ann Neurol* **65**: 550–556.

Gamstrop I. (1991) Lyme borreliosis from a patient's view-point. *Scand J Infect Dis Suppl* **77**: 15–16.

Olsen RK, Olpin SE, Andresen BS, et al. (2007) ETFDH mutations as a major cause of riboflavin-responsive multiple acyl-CoA dehydrogenation deficiency. *Brain* **130**: 2045–2054.

Ozand PT, Gascon GG, Al Essa M, et al. (1998) Biotin-responsive basal ganglia disease: a novel entity. *Brain* **121**: 1267–1279.

Rötig A, Mollet J, Rio M, et al. (2007) Infantile and pediatric quinone deficiency diseases. *Mitochondrion* **7** Suppl: S112–S121.

Saudubray JM, Sedel F, Walter JH. (2006) Clinical approach to treatable inborn metabolic diseases: an introduction. *J Inherit Metab Dis* **29**: 261–274.

Sedel F, Lyon-Caen O, Saudubray JM. (2007) Therapy insight: inborn errors of metabolism in adult neurology—a clinical approach focused on treatable diseases. *Nat Clin Pract Neurol* **3**: 279–90.

Surtees R, Wolf N. (2007) Treatable neonatal epilepsy. *Arch Dis Child* **92**: 659–661.

Tuchman M, Lee B, Lichter-Konecki U, et al. (2008) Cross-sectional multicenter study of patients with urea cycle disorders in the United States. *Mol Genet Metab* **94**: 397–402.

Zeng WQ, Al-Yamani E, Acierno JS Jr, et al. (2005) Biotin-responsive basal ganglia disease maps to 2q36.3 and is due to mutations in SLC19A3. *Am J Hum Genet* **77**: 16–26.

Table 3.23.1 Neurological investigations in rare treatable disorders

| Condition | Presentation | Key investigations | Treatment |
|---|---|---|---|
| Autosomal-recessive guanosine triphosphate (GTP) cyclohydrolase 1 (AR-GCH1) deficiency without hyperphenylalaninaemia (those with high blood phenylalanine will have been detected by neonatal screening test) | 'Cerebral palsy'; oculogyric crises, tremulousness, bradykinesia | Avoid levodopa trial to prevent diagnostic confusion, phenylalanine loading test is simple to perform (Chapter 2.14): 4 hour blood spot phenylalanine level will be high as will phenylalanine/tyrosine ratio. CSF pterins low, monoamine neurotransmitters may be normal. Definitive diagnosis is by either peripheral blood mononuclear or fibroblast GTP cyclohydrolase enzyme assay or directly through mutation analysis on DNA | BH$_4$ (tetrahydrobiopterin), levodopa; 5-hydroxy-tryptophan and folinic acid will allow normal development if started sufficiently early |
| Adrenocorticotrophic hormone (ACTH) unresponsiveness | Recurrent encephalopathy with hypoglycaemia, secondary epilepsy. Joint hyperpigmentation may be subtle | ↓ glucose, ↓ cortisol, ↑ ACTH | Cortisol |
| Biotinidase deficiency (or biotin deficiency) | Epilepsy, developmental delay, various acquired neurological deficits (cerebrum, brainstem, cord), mimics Leigh syndrome (± alopecia, rash) | Brain and spinal cord MRI, urine organic acids, blood and CSF lactate, biotin trial, plasma biotinidase | Biotin |
| Biotin-responsive basal ganglia disease | Vague illness → rapid loss of motor skills → quadriparesis; seizures, akinetic, no speech | Brain MRI: head of caudate and putamen 'necrosis'. Response to biotin trial 5–10mg/kg/d. Mutations in *SLC19A3* | Biotin |

Table 3.23.1 continued

| Condition | Presentation | Key investigations | Treatment |
|---|---|---|---|
| Cerebrotendinous xanthomatosis | Combined central and peripheral nervous system degeneration. Xanthomata may not be apparent. Juvenile cataracts | Plasma cholestanol ↑ | Chenodeoxycholic acid |
| Cobalamin disorders, especially deficiency of cobalamin complementation groups c and d | Infantile epilepsy, delay, hypotonia, poor head growth, encephalopathy, 'psychiatric', myelopathy (pyramidal and posterior column), neuropathy | Spinal cord MRI, especially T2 posterior columns; plasma homocysteine; urine methylmalonic acid | Hydroxycobalamin |
| DEND (delay, epilepsy, neonatal diabetes mellitus) | Neonatal diabetes mellitus, delay, epileptic spasms | *KCNJ11* mutations | Sulphonylurea (tolbutamide) |
| Dopa-responsive dystonia (Segawa disease) | Dystonia any time from early childhood | Levodopa trial, CSF pterins and monoamine neurotransmitters | Levodopa/carbidopa |
| Familial haemophagocytic lymphohistiocytosis | May not show macrophage activation syndrome. Fever and multiple neurological presentations: acute disseminated encephalomyelitis (ADEM)-like, Aicardi–Goutières-like and peripheral neuropathy. Brain lesions asymmetrical | Complete blood count and film; ↑ ferritin; bone marrow; CSF cells for perforin marker | Allogenic bone marrow transplant |

Table 3.23.1 continued

| Condition | Presentation | Key investigations | Treatment |
|---|---|---|---|
| Folate deficiency (cerebral folate deficiency) | Supposed manifestations include nonspecific neurodevelopmental delays and deviations ± autism | CSF 5 methyl-tetradydrofolate (5-MTHF) low with normal serum folate | Folinic acid |
| Guanidine methyltransferase (GAMT) deficiency | Epilepsy, learning disability, possible acquired movement disorder (may have false aminoaciduria, or glycoamino-glycanuria) | Urine guanidinoacetate ↑ ↓ Creatine peak on brain H-MRS ↓ Creatine peak on in vitro CSF H-MRS | Creatine |
| Glucose transporter 1 (GLUT1) deficiency | Epilepsy not drug-controlled: absences, myoclonus, drops; ± early infancy paroxysmal 'opsoclonus' movement disorder. Ataxia, especially intermittent ataxia. Paroxysmal exertional dyskinesia | Fasting blood glucose immediately before CSF; low CSF glucose, low CSF/blood glucose ratio (0.19–0.49) and normal to low lactate | Ketogenic diet |
| Hashimoto encephalopathy | Older girls, seizures, stroke-like episodes, confusion, hallucinations | Anti-thyroperoxidase (anti-TPO) antibodies | Corticosteroids |
| Hyperekplexia | Neonatal apnoeas, stiffness, startle, nose-tap head retraction | Video surface EMG as part of ictal EEG/ECG; *GLRA1*, GlyT2 (*SLC6A5*) mutations | Clonazepam |
| Long-QT syndromes (LQT) | 'Seizures' especially fright or sound startle induced, including nocturnal in sleep | ECG for QTc but may not always be long; implantable ECG monitoring; LQT mutation analysis | Beta blockers (± implantable defibrillator) |

Table 3.23.1 continued

| Condition | Presentation | Key investigations | Treatment |
|---|---|---|---|
| Myasthenia (congenital myasthenia) | Neonatal and infantile apnoeas, floppy baby | Edrophonium test. Stimulation single-fibre EMG (stimSFEMG) orbicularis oculi. Mutation analysis at specialist myasthenia laboratory | Pyridostigimine, etc. |
| Neuroborreliosis | Facial palsy, headache, meningitis without neck stiffness, ADEM-like, arterial ischaemic stroke, cerebellar ataxia, sensorimotor neuropathy | Borrelia titres, CSF, polymerase chain reaction borrelia | Specific antibiotics (such as ceftriaxone) |
| Neuroleptospirosis | Aseptic meningitis, cerebellar ataxia, neuropathy; hepato-renal dysfunction ± conjunctival injection | Leptospira serology | Specific antibiotics (such as crystalline penicillin) |
| Ornithine transcarbamylase heterozygotes | Stroke-like episodes, headache, vomiting, acute encephalopathy | Blood ammonia, urine orotic acid and uracil | Low protein diet, etc. |
| Paroxysmal extreme pain disorder | Neonatal flushing, apnoea, anoxic seizures, tonic attacks | Home video, SCN9A mutation analysis | Carbamazepine |

Table 3.23.1 continued

| Condition | Presentation | Key investigations | Treatment |
|---|---|---|---|
| Poisoning (exogenous and endogenous): accidental ingestion or exposure, covert poisoning; gut and urinary tract bacterial overgrowth syndromes) | Acute encephalopathy, seizures, syncope, central and peripheral deficits, bizarre history | EEG, ECG, radiography knees, abdominal imaging, urine culture, blood film, ammonia (and toxicology of course for tricyclics, etc.) | Remove source |
| Pyridoxine–dependent epilepsy | Neonatal, infantile or later infantile seizures, polymorphous may be Dravet-like | Pyridoxine trial (or pyridoxal phosphate trial), urine ↑ alpha-aminoadipic semialdehyde ($\alpha$-AASA), ↑ pipecolic acid in all body fluids, antiquitin (*ALDH7A1*) gene mutation (check alkaline phosphatase to exclude untreatable hypophosphatasia) | Pyridoxine |
| Pyridoxal phosphate-responsive seizures | Neonatal seizures, usually suppression–burst EEG (not yet known if infantile, late infantile or childhood presentation possible) | Pyridoxal phosphate trial. If seizures cease investigate as in pyridoxine-dependent epilepsy; if $\alpha$-AASA and pipecolic acid normal go to *PNPO* gene (pyridoxal-5′-phosphate may also be measured in CSF) | Pyridoxal phosphate |

Table 3.23.1 continued

| Condition | Presentation | Key investigations | Treatment |
|---|---|---|---|
| Pyruvate dehydrogenase (PDH) deficiency | 'Mitochondrial' presentations, episodic ataxia, dystonia, flaccid paralysis | MRI altered signal in globus pallidus; CSF lactate may be normal but lactate/pyruvate ratio low; fibroblast PDH | Ketogenic diet |
| Riboflavin-responsive multiple acyl-coenzyme A dehydrogenase deficiency (MADD) | Encephalopathy, muscle weakness or both. Might be multiple sclerosis-like; may be earlier history of cyclical vomiting | Urine acylcarnitines, mutations in one of the electron transfer flavoprotein genes | Riboflavin |
| Sepiapterin reductase deficiency | 'Cerebral palsy' oculogyric crises (might be mistaken for atypical absences), dystonic episodes, learning disability | Although dopa responsive, avoid levodopa trial if possible; CSF monoamine neurotransmitters and biopterins + specific analysis of CSF sepiapterin | Levodopa, carbidopa, 5-hydroxytryptophan $\pm$ BH$_4$ |
| Serine synthesis disorders (phosphoserine aminotransferase deficiency is treatable postnatally) | Early epileptic seizures, microcephaly | CSF amino acids for low serine and glycine | Serine and glycine supplements |

Table 3.23.1 continued

| Condition | Presentation | Key investigations | Treatment |
|---|---|---|---|
| Ubiquinone (CoQ10) deficiency | Clinically and probably genetically heterogeneous. Severe infantile encephalopathy with renal disease, encephalomyopathy, myopathy, ataxia, cerebellar atrophy | White cell CoQ10, muscle electron transport chain studies, muscle CoQ10, fibroblast CoQ10 | Oral CoQ10 (only some variants are treatable: arguably CoQ10 should be used as a therapeutic trial) |
| Vitamin $B_{12}$ deficiency (may not be as obvious as it might seem – see also Cobalamin disorders, above) | Infantile tremor or odd movement disorder, mother vegan | $B_{12}$, organic acids | Hydroxycobalamin |
| | Subacute combined degeneration of the cord – may be difficult because of psychosocial factors | Spinal cord MRI for posterior column signal change, $B_{12}$, organic acids | Hydroxycobalamin |
| Vitamin E deficiency (especially isolated vitamin E malabsorption) | Ataxia, neuropathy, retinopathy, spinocerebellar features, deafness | Blood vitamin E | Vitamin E |
| Wilson disease | Older child and adolescent, almost always Kayser–Fleischer rings, behavioural, extra pyramidal, tremor dysarthria, basal ganglia signal change on MRI | Ceruloplasmin, urine and plasma Cu, 24-h urine Cu, liver Cu if necessary. *ATP7B* gene mutation *once neurological investigations have established diagnosis* (too many mutations to screen) | D-penicillamine, zinc, trientine |

# Appendix 1
# Predictive Value of Investigation Results

In the Introduction and in the body of the book, stress has been put on making the significance of a test result depend on the likelihood of the disease or disorder being present. In this section some simple calculations of likelihood or probability are preceded by definitions of the terms employed. A binary table (Table A.1) helps to clarify the simple algebra used in this section.

Table A.1  Algebraic representation of true and false investigation results

|  |  | Disease | |  |
|---|---|---|---|---|
|  |  | Present | Absent |  |
| Investigation | Positive | True positive  a | False positive  b | a + b |
|  | Negative | False negative  c | True negative  d | c + d |
|  |  | a + c | b + d | a + b + c + d |

## Definitions

*Sensitivity.* The probability that the investigation result will be positive when the disease is present, i.e. the true positive rate [a/(a+c)].

*Specificity.* The probability that the investigation result will be negative when the disease is not present, i.e. the true negative rate [d/(b+d)].

In the definitions listed here an asterisk (*) indicates that *prediction depends on the prevalence* of the disease or disorder, that is, how probable the clinician expects that to be the diagnosis. The major exception is the ROC (receiver operating characteristic) curve (see below), which is ideal for comparing the diagnostic power of two investigations such as CT and ultrasound or CT and MRI. Unfortunately, at the time of writing the literature on neurological investigations in children still contains very few studies backed by ROC evidence. The remainder of this section will thus be confined to some calculated examples of the effect of estimates of prevalence on the interpretation of neurological investigations. Many further calculations are available to the interested reader.

* *False positive rate.* The probability that the investigation will be positive when the disease is not present (1 = minus specificity, i.e. 1 − [d/(b+d)].

* *False negative rate.* The probability that the investigation will be negative when the disease is present (1 = minus sensitivity, i.e. 1 − [a/(a+c)].

*Positive likelihood ratio (LR+).* This is the likelihood ratio for a positive investigation and equals the sensitivity divided by [1 − specificity], i.e. [a/(a+c)]/ [1 − d/(b+d)].

*Negative likelihood ratio (LR−).* This is the likelihood ratio for a negative investigation and equals [1 − sensitivity] divided by specificity, i.e. 1 − [a/(a+c)]/[d/(b+d)].

* *Prevalence.* The proportion of patients in the population investigated who have the disease in question, i.e. (a+c)/(a+b+c+d). Commonly this has to be interpreted as the proportion who are expected to have the disease or disorder in question, thus becoming the *prior probability*.

* *Prior odds.* The odds that a disease or disorder is present as estimated before obtaining the result of the investigation in question. It is the probability of the disease being present divided by the probability of the disease not being present.

* *Posterior odds.* The odds that the disorder is present as estimated after the result of the investigation in question, on the basis of the assumed sensitivity and specificity of the investigation. The posterior odds equals the prior odds multiplied by the likelihood ratio. If the investigation is *positive*, posterior odds = (prior odds × LR+). If the test is *negative*, posterior odds = (prior odds × LR−).

* *Probability.* This is another way, besides odds, of describing the frequency or expected frequency of a disorder. Mathematically, probability = odds/(1 + odds).

* *Positive predictive value (PV+).* The probability that the disease is present if the investigation result is positive, i.e. a/(a+b).

* *Negative predictive value (PV−).* The probability that the disease is not present if the investigation result is negative, i.e. d/(c+d).

*True positive proportion (pTP).* The proportion of true positive results at any particular degree of diagnostic confidence. This is also called the true positive fraction. It is the same as the true positive rate, i.e. sensitivity.

*False positive proportion (pFP).* The proportion of false positive results at any particular degree of diagnostic confidence. This is also called the false negative fraction. It is *not* the same as the false positive rate, the latter being dependent on the prevalence of the disorder.

*True negative proportion (pTN).* The proportion of true negative results at any degree of diagnostic confidence (also called the true negative fraction). It is the same as the true negative rate, i.e. specificity.

*False negative proportion (pFN).* The proportion of false negative results at any degree of diagnostic confidence (also called the false positive fraction). It is *not* the same as the false negative rate, the latter being dependent on the prevalence of the disorder.

*Cut-off point.* An arbitrary value separating positive and negative results in any given investigation.

*Receiver operating characteristic (ROC) curve.* A graphic plot of the true positive proportion (pTP) against the false positive proportion (pFP) at each of a number of cut-off points. This is the same as a plot of the false negative proportion (pFN) against the true negative proportion (pTN). Put another way, the ROC curve is a graph of sensitivity $[a/(a+c)]$ plotted against one minus specificity $(1 - [d/(b+d)])$ at different levels of diagnostic confidence in one's ability to discriminate a and d.

### Example 1. Does a convulsion at age 3 years signify epilepsy?
Let us assume (1) that EEG spikes are seen in 80% of those with epilepsy, (2) that 2% of normal children at this age have EEG spikes, and (3) that there is no positive evidence in the clinical history to support epilepsy of any kind. Nonetheless, the physician obtains an EEG 'for reassurance', only to discover that clear-cut spikes are recorded.

From the first two assumptions, the sensitivity of the EEG is 80% or 0.8, and the specificity is 98% or 0.98. The likelihood ratio for epilepsy given the presence of spikes (LR+) is thus $0.8/(1 - 0.98) = 0.8/0.02 = 40$. However, from the third assumption the expected prevalence has to be regarded as no different from that in the general population, say 5/1000 or 0.005. The prior odds are thus $0.005/0.995 = 0.005$ to 1, and the posterior odds $0.005 \times 40 = 0.2$ to 1. The posterior probability, being odds/(1 + odds), is thus $0.2/1.2 = 0.17$, or 17% in favour of epilepsy and 83% against.

In this example the probability of epilepsy remains low despite the presence of EEG spikes, so that the EEG is not of value as a positive diagnostic tool. Had spikes been absent, the likelihood ratio of epilepsy (LR–) would have been $[1 - 0.8]/0.98 = 0.2/0.98 = 0.2$, and the posterior odds $0.005 \times 0.2 = 0.001$ to 1, or 0.001 probability. This is the result the physician wants, but in the example the prior odds were so low that the EEG result was a luxury.

## Example 2. Does a very preterm neonate have brain damage?

For this example we make use of the data of Hope et al. (1988). These authors compared blind (uninformed) the results of ultrasound brain scanning and the criterion standard of neuropathology in an unselected series of babies with a gestational age of less than 33 weeks. For the diagnosis of any intraparenchymal brain lesion (haemorrhagic or hypoxic–ischaemic) sensitivity was 0.44 (44%), specificity 0.82 (82%), LR+ 2.4 and LR– 0.68. For intraparenchymal haemorrhage separately, sensitivity was 0.82 (82%), specificity 0.97 (97%), LR+ 27.3 and LR– 0.19, whereas for hypoxic–ischaemic damage sensitivity was 0.28 (28%), specificity 0.86 (86%), LR+ 2.0, and LR– 0.83. The low likelihood ratios for hypoxic–ischaemic lesions mean that when the prior odds are low the posterior odds will not change in a useful manner. If such a lesion seems more than probable, a positive scan may be helpful, as follows: prior probability 0.55 (55%) equals odds 1.22 to 1; posterior odds = 1.22 × 2.0 = 2.44 to 1, giving a posterior probability of 0.71 (71%). However, a negative scan would leave the probability at around 0.5 (50%).

## Further reading

Hope PL, Gould SJ, Howard S, et al. (1988) Precision of ultrasound diagnosis of pathologically verified lesions in the brains of very preterm infants. *Dev Med Child Neurol* **30**: 457–471.

# Appendix 2
## Some Normal Values

A selected number of 'normal' value are included in this section. In many instances the available data are based on statistical assumptions of normality, such as coming within two standard deviations (SD) of the mean or between the 2nd and 98th centiles. In practice, the concepts of likelihood ratio related to prior odds or the positive and negative predictive value, as defined in the previous section, are more helpful in deciding whether a particular test result influences a clinical diagnosis.

### Motor nerve conduction velocity (metres per second)
Velocities are fastest in the ulnar, slowest in the posterior tibial, and intermediate in the median and common peroneal nerves. The lower limit is based on 2 SD below the mean, but pathological slowing may require a velocity of 60% of the mean, or less. Values for the ulnar (U) and posterior tibial (T) are listed as −2 SD (mean). Places of decimals are not used since the basis of the measurements does not allow for such accuracy.

| | | | | | |
|---|---|---|---|---|---|
| Neonate | U | 20–22 (28) | 1 year | U | 40 (46) |
| | T | 17 (22) | | T | 31 (38) |
| 3 months | U | 31 (35) | 3 years | U | 45 (55) |
| | T | 22 (26) | | T | 40 (44) |
| 6 months | U | 35–37 (42) | Adult | U | 49 (60) |
| | T | 26 (32) | | T | 40 (45) |

### Sensory nerve conduction velocity
Velocities in sural and median nerves approximate to those in the faster motor nerves.

*Flash VEP (latency in m/s)*

| | |
|---|---|
| Neonate | 190 |
| 3 months onward | 100 |

*BAEP: I–V latency (ms) [mean and (upper limit)]*

| | | | |
|---|---|---|---|
| Neonate | 5.1 (6.0) | 1 year | 4.2 (4.9) |
| 3 months | 4.8 (5.6) | Adult | 4.1 (4.8) |
| 6 months | 4.6 (5.3) | | |

*BAEP: V/I ratio [mean and (lower limit)]*

| | | | |
|---|---|---|---|
| Neonate | 1.2 (0.4) | 6 months | 2.3 (0.5) |
| 3 months | 1.7 (0.5) | 1 year | 2.8 (0.5) |

## Cortical grey matter maximum depth

5mm

## CSF protein (g/L)

Upper limit is based on 2 SD above the mean, 95th centile

| | | | |
|---|---|---|---|
| Neonate | 1.08 | 3–6 months | 0.40 |
| 1–2 months | 0.77 | 6 months – 10 years | 0.32 [range (N=599) 0.10–0.44] |
| 2–3 months | 0.60 | 10–16 years | 0.41 |

To convert g/L to mg/dL multiply by 100, e.g. 0.32g/L = 32mg/dL.

*CSF:serum IgG index ($Q_{IgG}/Q_{alb}$)*

<18 months: up to 1.02; >18 months: up to 0.78

*CSF special biochemistry*

| | |
|---|---|
| 1gG:albumin ratio < 0.27 | Glycine up to 15µmol/L |
| Lactate 0.8–2.4mmol/L | CSF:plasma glycine ratio ≤0.025, i.e. plasma:CSF glycine ratio ≥40. |

## Note on haematology
In USA a blood film is called a smear.

## Further reading

Biou D, Benoist JF, Huong CNX. (2000) Cerebrospinal fluid protein concentrations in children: age-related values in patients without disorders of the central nervous system. *Clin Chem* **46**: 399–403.

Gamstorp I. (1963) Normal conduction velocity of ulnar, median and peoneal nerves in infancy, childhood and adolescence. *Acta Paediatr Suppl* **146**: 68–76.

Gamstorp I, Shelburne SA. (1965) Peripheral sensory conduction in ulnar and median nerves of normal infants, children and adolescents. *Acta Paediatr Scand* **54**: 309–313.

Lenassi E, Likar K, Stirn-Kranjc B, Brecelj J. (2008) VEP maturation and visual acuity in infants and preschool children. *Doc Ophthalmol* **117**: 111–20.

# Appendix 3
## List of Clinical Vignettes

Introduction.1 *POLG1* – finally
         diagnosed!

1.1.1 Neonatal hyperekplexia (glycine
      transporter 2 dominant)

1.1.2 Paroxysmal kinesigenic dyskinesia

1.2.1 Rett syndrome

1.2.2 Opsoclonus–myoclonus

2.1.1 Infantile masturbation/
      gratification

2.1.2 Paroxysmal extreme pain
      disorder

2.1.3 Compulsive Valsalva manoeuvre

2.1.4 Compulsive Valsalva with
      anoxic–epileptic seizures

2.1.5 Shuddering

2.1.6 Benign non-epileptic infantile
      spasms

2.1.7 Myoclonus–dystonia

2.1.8 Cervical cord tumour

2.2.1 Vasovagal syncope

2.2.2 Long-QT type 1

2.2.3 Tuberous sclerosis

2.2.4 Landau–Kleffner syndrome

2.2.5 Ring chromosome 20

2.3.1 Vaccine-associated poliomyelitis

2.3.2 Charcot–Marie–Tooth type 1

2.3.3 Congenital myasthenic syndrome:
      slow channel syndrome

2.3.4 Congenital myasthenic syndrome:
      choline acetyltransferase deficiency

2.3.5 Infantile neuroaxonal dystrophy
      (*PLA2G6* mutation)

2.4.1 Infantile neuronal ceroid
      lipofuscinosis

2.4.2 Pelizaeus–Merzbacher disease

2.5.1 Congenital cytomegalovirus
      infection

2.5.2 Menkes disease

2.5.3 Vertebral dissection

2.5.4 Moyamoya

2.5.5 Cerebroretinal microangiopathy
      with calcifications and cysts

2.5.6 L-2-hydroxyglutaric aciduria

2.5.7 Pontocerebellar hypoplasias 2

2.6.1 Occult neuroblastoma

2.6.2 GAMT (guanidinoacetate methyltransferase) deficiency

2.7.1 Glucose transporter 1 deficiency

2.7.2 Aicardi–Goutières syndrome

2.7.3 Alpers disease (*POLG1*)

2.7.4 Metachromatic leukodystrophy (late infantile)

2.8.1 Pompe disease

2.8.2 Vasovagal syncope

2.8.3 Guillain–Barré syndrome

2.9.1 Menkes disease

2.9.2 Glioblastoma multiforme

2.9.3 Cortical dysplasia

2.9.4 Juvenile metachromatic leukodystrophy

2.9.5 Congenital defect of the pyramidal tracts

2.10.1 Congenital cytomegalovirus infection

2.10.2 Congenital cytomegalovirus infection

2.10.3 Human herpesvirus 6 infection

2.10.4 Subacute sclerosing panencephalitis

2.11.1 Neonatal alloimmune thrombocytopenic purpura (NAITP)

2.11.2 NAITP

2.12.1 Hashimoto encephalopathy

2.12.2 Aicardi–Goutières syndrome

2.12.3 Occult ganglioneuroblastoma

2.12.4 Anti-NMDA (N-methyl-D-aspartic acid) receptor encephalitis

2.13.1 1p36 deletion

2.13.2 Pitt–Hopkins syndrome

2.14.1 Alpers (*POLG1*)

2.14.2 DBP (D-bifunctional protein) deficiency

2.14.3 Glutaric aciduria type 2

2.14.4 Cobalamin c deficiency

2.14.5 *PEX1* (peroxisome biogenesis factor 1) mutation

2.14.6 Pyruvate dehydrogenase deficiency

2.15.1 Benign neonatal sleep myoclonus

2.16.1 Late-onset pyridoxine-dependent epilepsy

2.16.2 Segawa disease

# Index

abdominal imaging 76
abetalipoproteinaemia, ERG 51
abscess, brain 319
   MRI 56
absence epilepsy/seizures 277, 284
   EEG 32, 277, 284
   myoclonic 277, 284
   with photoparoxysmal response 284
abstinence syndrome, neonatal 219
acanthocytes 112, 129
acetazolamide, diagnosis by therapeutic trial
   of 202
acetylcholine (ACh) receptors
   antibodies 136
   deficiency 217
acetylcholinesterase inhibitors, congenital
   myasthenic syndrome responses 216,
   217
acid maltase deficiency *see* Pompe disease
acquired immunity, disorders 134
acquired neurological deficits 310–17
ACTH unresponsiveness 357
activator protein deficiency 176
acute disseminated encephalomyelitis *see*
   encephalomyelitis
acute haemorrhagic leukoencephalitis 322
acute severe illness, ECG 107
acyl-CoA dehydrogenase deficiency, multiple
   *see* multiple acyl-CoA dehydrogenase
   deficiency

acylcarnitines
   blood 158
   urine 153
adaptive immunity, disorders 134
adenylosuccinate lyase (adenylosuccinase)
   deficiency 157, 174, 233, 261, 290
   epileptic seizures 290
adolescence
   epilepsy in 306
   progressive loss of skills and dementia 350
   *see also entries under juvenile*
adrenocorticotrophic hormone (ACTH)
   unresponsiveness 357
adrenoleukodystrophy 179, 348–9
   progressive loss of skills and dementia
   348–9
   speech/language impairment 267
age and progressive disorders 344
aggression 270
agitation, acute 272
agnosia, epileptic auditory *see*
   Landau–Kleffner syndrome
Aicardi, Jean 2, 48
Aicardi–Goutières syndrome 100–1, 123–4,
   219, 221, 248–9
   clinical vignettes 100–1, 137–9
   CT 69
   global developmental delay 226
   mistaken for cerebral palsy 248–9
airway obstruction, upper 300

ECG 106
albumin
    blood 158
    CSF 94–5, 169
alcin 352
*ALDH7A1* (antiquitin gene) mutation 191,
    205
Alexander disease 238
Allan–Herndon–Dudley syndrome 246
Allen Brain Atlas 145
alloimmune disorders (in general) 135
alloimmune thrombocytopenia/
    thrombocytopenic purpura, neonatal
    (NAITP) 131
    clinical vignette 131–2
Alpers disease (progressive neuronal
    degeneration of childhood) 176, 325
    clinical vignettes 101–2, 184–7
    EEG 28, 30, 32
alpha-amino-adipic semialdehyde
        dehydrogenase (AASA)
    blood 158
    urine 153
alpha-1-antitrypsin, blood 158
alpha-fetoprotein, blood 158
alpha-glucosidase deficiency *see* Pompe
    disease
alpha rhythm/wave 22
ambulatory EEG, digital 25, 35
amines, biogenic
    CSF levels 97, 171
    hypokinesia due to disorders of 220
amino acids
    blood/plasma 159
        in learning disability, child 262
        in learning disability, maternal 261
        in microcephaly 236, 237
    CSF 97, 169–70
        in microcephaly 237
    urine 153
        learning disability 261
ammonia, blood 159
amplitude-integrated EEG (aEEG) 25–6, 35
anaemia 265
    iron deficiency 129, 263
Angelman syndrome 224, 263, 266, 281, 309
    EEG 33, 224, 281
    mistaken for cerebral palsy 245
Angelman syndrome-like conditions 266
    mistaken for cerebral palsy 245

angiitis of CNS, primary 116, 322, 329
angiography
    catheter cerebral 72
    magnetic resonance 59
anoxic epileptic seizures 307
    clinical vignette 17–18
anoxic non-epileptic seizure 16
anterior horn cell lesions, floppiness 229
anterior opercular syndrome 266
antibodies (immunoglobulins)
    autoimmune
        ACh receptors 136
        aquaporin-4 314–15
        clinical vignette 136–7
        NMDA receptor *see* NMDA receptor
        voltage-gated potassium channel 135,
            319
    CSF 95
anticholinesterases (AChE inhibitors),
        congenital myasthenic syndrome
        responses 216, 217
antiepileptic drugs
    diagnosis by therapeutic trial of 201–7
    misinterpretation as effect of 90–1
    monitoring 198–200
antipsychotic (neuroleptic)-associated
        movement disorders 338
antiquitin gene (*ALDH7A1*) mutation 191,
    205
aphasia, epileptic *see* Landau–Kleffner
    syndrome
apnoea, neonatal 214–15
    severe, hyperekplexia with 43
apparent diffusion coefficient (ADC) map 60
apraxia, oculomotor, ataxia with 66, 255
*APTX* mutation 255
aquaporin-4 autoimmunity 314–15
arboviruses 319
arching in infancy 194–5
arginase deficiency 247
aromatic L-amino acid decarboxylase (AADC)
    deficiency 175
array comparative genomic hybridization 147
arrhythmias 105–7
arterial hypertension, systemic 328
arterial ischaemic stroke 131, 311–12, 338
arthrogryposis 220
    from anti-acetylcholine receptor
        antibodies 136
arthropod-borne viruses 319

*ARX* mutation 211, 263, 309, 342
arylsulphatase A (ARSA), lysosomal 103, 120, 175, 176, 348
asialotransferrin, CSF 96, 170, 336, 351, 352
aspartyl-tRNA synthetase deficiency, mitochondrial 89
asphyxia, birth, burst–suppression EEG 211
astatic seizure 35
    *see also* myoclonic–astatic epilepsy
asymbolic retardation, autistic spectrum disorder and 306
asystole, epileptic 106
asystolic syncope, reflex 299
ataxia 253–5, 255, 333–6
    acute 334–5
    cerebellar *see* cerebellar ataxia
    in eIF2B-related disorders 255, 336, 352
    episodic *see* episodic ataxia
    Friedreich *see* Friedreich ataxia
    gait abnormalities 253–5
    spinocerebellar *see* spinocerebellar ataxia
ataxia–telangiectasia 247, 254–5
'ataxic cerebral palsy' 228–9, 246
    clinical vignette of misdiagnosis of 54
*ATM* mutation 247, 255
'atonic' cerebral palsy 228
*ATP7A* mutation 118
ATRX syndrome 263
attention-deficit–hyperactivity disorder (ADHD) 270
audio and video, home *see* video and audio
auditory agnosia, epileptic *see* Landau–Kleffner syndrome
auditory unresponsiveness 226
    *see also* deafness
autism and autism spectrum disorder 226, 227, 269–70
    and asymbolic retardation 306
    clinical vignette 16–17
    EEG cautions 31
autoimmune disorders
    acquired 135
    innate 134
    *see also* antibodies
autonomic function tests 108–9
    clinical vignette 109–11
axial hypotonia 215–16

B-cell deficiency 135
band heterotopia, MRI 58

Bardet–Biedl syndrome, ERG 51
barium swallow, oesophagus 75
*Bartonella* 125
basal ganglia
    biotin-responsive disease of 357
    involvement
        in cerebellar atrophy 66
        in neonatal seizures 210
basilar impression (platybasia)
    gait abnormalities 254
    spasticity 256
Bassen–Kornzweig syndrome, ERG 51
bath-induced paroxysmal incidents in infancy 109
Becker muscular dystrophy, gait abnormalities 252
behavioural disorders 269–74
    clinical vignette 118–19
    paroxysmal 298
Behçet disease 136, 322
benign childhood epilepsy (benign rolandic epilepsy) with centrotemporal spikes 27, 28, 32, 284, 287–8
benign convulsions with mild gastroenteritis 282
benign familial alternating hemiplegia 301
benign familial infantile seizures 280
benign hereditary chorea 341
benign myoclonic epilepsy of infancy 280
benign myoclonus of early infancy (benign non-epileptic infantile spasms) 298, 338
    clinical vignette 18
benign neonatal–infantile seizures 279
benign neonatal sleep myoclonus 200, 209, 298
benign syncopes 299
benign tonic upgaze or downgaze 303
benzodiazepine ingestion/poisoning, EEG 32, 35
beta- (fatty acid) oxidation, assessment 181, 184
beta rhythm/wave 22
Bickerstaff encephalitis 136
bile acids 181
    blood 159
    urine 153
biochemical/metabolic disturbances/disorders *see* metabolic/biochemical disorders
biochemical/metabolic tests 151–98

clinical vignettes 184–95
CSF 152, 169–75
    protein *see* protein
    special 94–8
  global developmental delay 225
  learning disability 261
  microcephaly 236
  neonatal seizures 211–12
biopsies 112–22
  neurophysiological tests vs 43
biotin
  basal ganglia disease responsive to 357
  deficiency 257
  diagnosis by therapeutic trial of 202
biotinidase
  blood/plasma 160, 236
  deficiency 233, 236, 352, 357
birth asphyxia, burst-suppression EEG 211
birth trauma, brachial plexus injury 74
bleeding
  disorders 130–1
  general tests 130
  *see also* haemorrhage
blindness
  congenital retinal 241
  cortical *see* cortical visual impairment/
    blindness
  'hysterical' 271
blood biochemistry 152, 158–69
  global developmental delay 225
  learning disability 261–2
  neonatal seizures 211–212
blood (cell) tests *see* haematology
blood films/smear 129–30
  learning disability 263
blood oxygen level dependent fMRI 89
blood pressure, high 328
BOLD fMRI 89
bone(s), imaging 76
bone marrow sampling 115
borreliosis 125, 322, 360
bottom-shuffling 223–4
botulism, neonatal 216
brachial plexus imaging 74
brain
  abscess *see* abscess
  biopsy 116–17
  congenital muscular dystrophy with
    abnormalities of 230
  damage in very preterm neonate,

    predictive value of investigations 367
  floppiness related to lesions in 228–9
  function monitors 25–6
  infarction *see* infarction
  malformations *see* malformations
  prenatal destruction/lesions 220, 325–6
    global developmental delay 226
  trauma *see* trauma
  tumours 324, 355
    clinical vignette 118–19, 139–40
    gait abnormalities 254
    headache 327–8
  *see also* muscle–eye–brain disorders
brain death, mimic, clinical vignette 110–11
brain imaging 55–76
  functional *see* functional brain imaging
  global developmental delay 224
  learning disability 264
  microcephaly 236, 237
  neonatal abnormal neurology 221
  neonatal seizures 210
  unexplained, biopsy in 117
brainstem
  leukoencephalopathy with involvement of
    spinal cord and, and elevated white
    matter lactate, MRI 65
  malformations 215
brainstem auditory evoked potentials 52
  normal values 369
Bratton–Marshall test 152, 157
  learning disability 261
buffy coat, electronmicroscopy 113
burr cells (echinocytes) 112–13, 129
burst–suppression EEG *see* suppression burst

*CACNA1A* 335
caeruloplasmin, blood 160
calcifications and cysts, cerebroretinal
  microangiopathy with *see* cerebroretinal
  microangiopathy with calcifications and
  cysts
calcium, blood 160
  learning disability 261–2
*Campylobacter jejuni* 125
Canavan disease 238, 338
  macrocephaly 238
  mistaken for cerebral palsy 248
  progressive loss of skills and dementia 347
  proton MR spectroscopy 87
carbon monoxide poisoning 324

cardiology *see* heart
carnitine, blood 160
cat scratch fever 125
cataplexy 301–2
cataplexy–narcolepsy 135, 301
catheter cerebral angiography 72
*CDKL5* mutations 264, 279
cells 112–22
    CSF 94
central conduction studies 53
central hypoventilation 215
central nervous system, primary angiitis 116, 322, 329
centrotemporal spikes
    benign childhood epilepsy with (benign rolandic epilepsy) 27, 28, 32, 284, 287–8
    benign childhood epilepsy with 27, 28, 32
cerebellar ataxia 333
    clinical vignette 89–90
    *see also* spinocerebellar ataxia
cerebellar atrophy 66
    MRI 65
cerebellar atrophy plus 66
cerebellar hypoplasia
    gait abnormalities 254
    neonatal seizures and EEG 210
cerebellar leukoencephalopathy with presumed histiocytosis 116–17, 349
cerebellitis 315
cerebral function monitors 25–6
cerebral infarction *see* infarction
cerebral ischaemic attacks with induced hyperventilation for EEG 31
cerebral palsy (and so-called 'cerebral palsy') 243–50
    ataxic *see* ataxic cerebral palsy
    atonic 228
    EEG cautions 30–1
    floppiness 228–9
    misinterpretation as 243–50
    clinical vignettes 47–8, 54, 100–1
    neurodevelopmental impairment and 306
cerebral venous sinus thrombosis 131, 310, 312
cerebroretinal microangiopathy with calcifications and cysts (Coats plus; CRMCC) 81–2
    clinical vignette 81–2
    MRI 65

cerebrospinal fluid
    examination 93–104
        biochemical tests *see* biochemical tests
        clinical vignettes 100–4
        indications 98–9
        microcephaly 237
        proton magnetic resonance spectroscopy (H-MRS), global developmental delay 224, 225
        vaccine damage 44
    pressure *see* pressure
cerebrotendinous xanthomatosis 273, 358
ceroid lipofuscinosis, neuronal *see* neuronal ceroid lipofuscinosis
ceruloplasmin, blood 160
cervical cord
    trauma 218
    tumour
        clinical vignette 19–20
        spasticity 256
channelopathy, clinical vignettes 15–16, 46
    *see also specific ions*
Charcot–Marie–Tooth disease (hereditary motor and sensory neuropathy) 229, 254
    clinical vignette 45
    floppiness 229
    gait abnormalities 253
*CHAT* mutations *see* choline acetyltransferase
chest, imaging 75
Chiari I malformation 328
cholestanol, blood 161
cholesterol, blood 161
cholesterol ester trafficking 184
choline acetyltransferase (*CHAT*) mutations and deficiency 217
    clinical vignette 46–7
cholinesterase inhibitors (AChE inhibitors), congenital myasthenic syndrome responses 216, 217
chorea 341
    Sydenham *see* Sydenham chorea
chorea–encephalopathy 338
choriomeningitis, congenital lymphocytic 123
chromosome (karyotopic) abnormalities 146
    global developmental delay 224, 226
    learning disability 263
    microcephaly 236
    seizures 288
        neonatal 212

*see also* deletions; ring chromosome
chronic fatigue syndrome 331
clinical genetics services 147
clinically isolated syndrome (CIS) 314
clonic seizures 277
clotting (coagulation)
    disorders 130–1
    general tests 130
CMV *see* cytomegalovirus
coagulation *see* clotting
Coats plus *see* cerebroretinal microangiopathy
    with calcifications and cysts
cobalamin *see* vitamin B$_{12}$
coenzyme-A dehydrogenase deficiency,
    multiple *see* multiple acyl-CoA
    dehydrogenase deficiency
coenzyme Q10 (CoQ10; ubiquinone) 161,
    179
    deficiency 362
Coffin–Lowry syndrome 309, 342
collagen gene mutations, neonatal seizures
    213
collapsed neonate, clinical vignette 117–18
*COLQ* mutations 217
communication disorders 265–68
comparative genomic hybridization, array
    147
complex partial epileptic seizure, EEG 35
compound muscle action potentials
    apnoea/syncope of neonatal hyperekplexia
        8, 43, 215, 299
    exercise EMG 42
    slow channel congenital myasthenic
        syndrome (CMS) 217

compulsive Valsalva manoeuvre *see* Valsalva
    manoeuvre
computed tomography
    abdomen 76
    brain 68–9
        microcephaly 236, 237
    chest 75
    cytomegalovirus 76, 77
    spinal cord 71
    *see also* single photon emission computed
        tomography
conduct disorder 270
conduction studies 370–1
    central 53
    nerve *see* nerve conduction studies

normal values 368–70
confusion, acute 272
congenital defects of glycosylation *see*
    glycosylation
congenital dystrophies and myopathies *see*
    muscular dystrophy; myopathies
congenital hypomyelination *see*
    hypomyelination
congenital infections *see* infections
congenital malformations of brain *see*
    malformations
congenital myasthenic syndrome *see*
    myasthenic syndrome
congenital myopathy 231
    floppiness 231
    gait abnormalities 253
congenital retinal blindness 241
conjunctiva 113
contrast-enhanced MRI 56
conversion disorder
    gait disturbance 257
    headache 332
convulsions
    at age 3 signifying epilepsy, predictive
        value of investigations 366–7
    benign, with mild gastroenteritis 282
    infantile, paroxysmal dyskinesia with 308,
        340
convulsive syncope 108–9
copper
    blood 161
    urine 154
corpus callosum, agenesis 210
cortical dysplasia
    clinical vignette 119–20
    EEG 210
cortical visual impairment/blindness
    visual unresponsiveness 227
    wobbly eyes 241
cost of investigations 2–3
cramps 331
cranial ultrasound, *see also* ultrasound
craniocervical junction disorder 300
craniosynostosis, radiograph 69
creatine
    blood levels 262
    CSF levels 171
    deficiency syndromes 209
        proton magnetic resonance
        spectroscopy 87

synthesis disorders 97, 346
    progressive loss of skills and dementia 346
    speech/language disorders 265–6
    transporter deficiency 154
    speech/language disorders 265–6
creatine/creatinine ratio 154
creatine kinase, blood 162
    in learning disability 262
creatinine, blood 162
    see also creatine/creatinine ratio
Creutzfeldt–Jakob disease (CJD), variant 350
    brain biopsy 117
culture
    fibroblast 183–4
    virus, in microcephaly 236
cut-off point 366
cyanocobalamin see vitamin $B_{12}$
cyst(s)
    cerebroretinal microangiopathy with calcifications and see cerebroretinal microangiopathy with calcifications and cysts
    subcortical, megalencephalic leukoencephalopathy with, MRI 57
cystic encephalomalacia 210
cytochrome oxidase deficiency, MRS 88
cytomegalovirus (CMV) infection 124, 125–6
    clinical vignettes 77, 125–6
    CT 68, 77

D-bifunctional protein deficiency 226
    clinical vignette 187–9
dancing eye syndrome see opsoclonus–myoclonus syndrome
deafness 226
    speech difficulties 265
    and white matter lesions in congenital CMV infection 126
death in infancy, sudden unexplained 291
    see also brain death
7-dehydrocholesterol, blood 162
deletions
    1p36 148, 288
    22q– 267
    see also microdeletion
delirium, acute 272
delta rhythm/wave 22
dementia 344–54
demyelination (and demyelinating

neuropathies/disorders) 218, 313–15
    conduction studies 40–1
DEND syndrome (developmental delay, epilepsy and neonatal diabetes mellitus) 279, 358
dentato-olivary dysplasia 218
depression 271–2
dermatomyositis, juvenile, gait abnormalities 252
developmental delay/impairment 223–7
    cerebral palsy and 306
    clinical vignette 82–3
    global see global developmental delay
    see also DEND syndrome
DHAP-AT (dihydroxyacetone phosphate acyltransferase), blood 162
diffusion tensor imaging 6, 60
diffusion-weighted MRI 60
digital ambulatory EEG 25, 35
dihydrolipoamide acyltransferase, mutation 195
dihydroxyacetone phosphate acyltransferase (DHAP-AT) 181
    blood 162
diphtheria–tetanus–pertussis (DTP) vaccine 7, 325
    clinical vignette 3–6, 44–5
    febrile seizures and 296
diplegia, spastic 256
DLAT mutation 195
DNA repair disorders
    ataxia in 255
    ERG 51
DOK7 mutations 217
Doppler ultrasound, transcranial 68
Down syndrome (trisomy 21)
    epileptic seizures 288
    spasticity 256
downgaze, benign tonic 303
Dravet syndrome (severe myoclonic epilepsy in infancy) 7, 281, 325
    EEG 27, 33, 281
    genetic investigations 145
drugs
    diagnosis by therapeutic trial of 201–6
    toxic effects see toxic compounds
DTP vaccine see diphtheria–tetanus–pertussis vaccine
Duchenne muscular dystrophy
    creatine kinase 263

# Index

gait abnormalities 252
  mistaken for cerebral palsy 244–5
  speech/language disorders 265
*duranin* mutation 83
dyskinesias
  encephalitis with *see* encephalitis
  paroxysmal 302–3, 339
    with infantile convulsions 308, 340
dysmorphic neonate 221–2
dystonia 256–7, 341
  dopa-responsive 337, 341
    Segawa-type *see* Segawa-type dopa-
      responsive dystonia
  infancy, transient 339
  myoclonus and, clinical vignette 18–19
  paroxysmal kinesigenic, clinical vignette
    9–10
  stiffness and 331
dystonia–parkinsonism
  not rapid-onset 340
  rapid-onset 339, 340

ECG *see* electrocardiography
echinocytes 112–13, 129
echocardiography 75, 107
economics of investigations 2–3
edrophonium, diagnosis by therapeutic trial
  of 202
EEG *see* electroencephalography
EEG/ECG/EMG, in diagnosis of hyperekplexia
  8, 43, 299
eIF2B-related disorders 86, 232, 255, 296,
  336, 351, 352
  ataxia 255, 336, 352
  fever-related acute regression 296
  floppiness 232
  progressive loss of skills and dementia 351
electrocardiography (ECG) 65, 105–7
  EEG and, concurrent recording 24–5
electroencephalography (EEG) 22–39
  additional recordings with 24–6
  choice of 32–5
  electroclinical syndromes 27
  epileptic seizures 26–8, 32–4, 276, 277–9
    in distinction from non-epileptic events
      275
    neonates 210
  global developmental delay *see* global
    developmental delay
  hazards 30–1

hyperekplexia 8
indications 26–30
learning disability 264
microcephaly 236
paediatric intensive care unit 30
provocations 23–4
routine, request for 31
stroke-like episodes 313
electrolytes, blood 162
electromyography (EMG) 41–2
  clinical aspects 42–3
  clinical vignette 44–8
  EEG and, concurrent recording 25
  in fatigue 331
  ictal 276, 277–9
  practical aspects 42
electron microscopy, buffy coat 113
electroretinography (ERG) 49–50
EMG *see* electromyography
encephlitis
  anti-NMDA receptor *see* NMDA receptors
  Bickerstaff 136
  with dyskinesia 140–2
  limbic 135
  with psychiatric features/presentation 272
    and oral dyskinesia and autonomic
      dysfunction 135
  Rasmussen *see* Rasmussen syndrome
  toxoplasma 320
  viral 124, 319, 338
  *see also* leukoencephalitis; subacute
    sclerosing panencephalitis
encephalomalacia, cystic 210
encephalomyelitis
  acute disseminated (ADEM) 313, 314,
    315, 320–2
  monophasic 320–1
  MRI of brain 56, 313–14, 322
  MRI of spinal cord 70, 71
  multiphasic 321
  recurrent 321
  myalgic 331
encephalomyopathy of childhood, chronic
  177
encephalopathies 318–6
  acute 318–6
    febrile seizures and 295
  epileptic *see* Ohtahara syndrome
  glycine *see* glycine encephalopathy
  Hashimoto *see* Hashimoto

encephalopathy
  mitochondrial, with lactic acidosis and
    stroke-like episodes (MELAS) 177,
    329
  neonatal
    cranial ultrasound 67
    MRI 58
  *see also* chorea–encephalopathy;
    leukoencephalopathy
endocrine investigations 163
  learning disability 262
endoplasmic reticulum disorders 182–3
enteroviral infections 125
environment, impaired responsiveness 226–7
epilepsia partialis continua 289
  clinical vignettes 19–20, 101–2
epilepsy 275–93, 305–310
  coexisting with non-epileptic events
    305–10
  continuous/prolonged *see* epilepsia
    partialis continua; status epilepticus
  convulsions at age 3 signifying, predictive
    value of investigations 366–7
  drug effect in treatment of,
    misinterpretation as 90–1
  EEG in *see* electroencephalography
  explosive onset 325
  misdiagnosis of, clinical vignettes 15, 16,
    110
  polymorphous, diagnosis by therapeutic
    trial 201–6
  progressive loss of skills with 344, 345
  pyridoxine-dependent *see* pyridoxine-
    dependent epilepsy
  with regression, clinical vignette 16–17
  television-induced 24, 33
  temporal lobe, SPECT 86
  *see also* seizures
epileptic aphasia/auditory agnosia *see*
  Landau–Kleffner syndrome
epileptic ataxia 333
episodic ataxias 302, 309, 335
  diagnosis by therapeutic trial 202
episodic weakness 332
ERG (electroretinography) 49–50
erythrocytes (red cells) 112–13, 129–30
essential tremor 341
evoked potentials 49–54, 369
  clinical vignette 53–4
  normal values 369

examination 11–13
exercise
  cramps on 331
  EMG in 42
exertional dyskinesia, paroxysmal 303, 340
explosive onset of neurological disease 325
  clinical vignette 184–7
eyes
  benign tonic upgaze or downgaze 303
  closure, EEG on 23, 33
  compression, EEG on 24, 34
  congenital muscular dystrophy with
    abnormalities of 230–1
  'dancing' *see* opsoclonus–myoclonus
    syndrome
  examination, opsoclonus–myoclonus
    syndrome 12
  wobbly 240–2
  *see also* muscle–eye–brain disorders

face
  pain 79
  palsy 315–6
  weakness sparing the 216
failure to thrive, clinical vignette 193–4
fainting fit
  lethal 36
  simple 34–5
falling (clinical vignettes) 127–8
  from knees down 45
  with laughter, sleepy and sluggish and
    139–40
false negative proportion 366
false negative rate 365
false positive proportion 366
false positive rate 365
*FAM126A* 65
family history-taking 8
family members, genetic investigations 145
fat suppression on MRI 57
fatigue 330–1
  myopathy with 176
fatty acid (beta) oxidation, assessment 181,
  184
febrile seizures 286, 294–6
  differential diagnosis 294–5
febrile seizures plus 280
  genetic epilepsy with 287
febrile status epilepticus 280
ferritin, blood 163

fever, seizures with *see* febrile seizures
fibroblasts
    culture 183–4
    very
    chain fatty acids in 181
financial constraints on tests 2–3
FISH 146–7
fits *see* convulsions; fainting fit; seizures
fixation-off technique 23, 33
flaccid paralysis 315
FLAIR 57
flat ('lifeless') baby 214
floppy baby/infant 215–18, 228–4
    hoarse 45–6
    ill 215
    *see also* hypotonia
fluid attenuated inversion recovery (FLAIR)
    57
fluorescent in situ hybridization (FISH)
    146–7
fluorodeoxyglucose (FDG) in positron
    emission tomography 86
focal epilepsy/seizures *see* partial
    epilepsy/seizures
Foix–Chavany–Marie syndrome 266
folate deficiency 359
folinic acid-responsive seizures 289
    diagnosis by therapeutic trial 202
fragile X chromosome 263
Friedreich ataxia 351–2
    ECG 107
    echocardiography 107
    gait abnormalities 254
    misdiagnosis, clinical vignette 120–1
    skills loss 351–2
frontal lobe
    epilepsy, autosomal dominant nocturnal
        285
    MRI of lesions 56, 57, 58, 68
full blood count 130
    learning disability 263
functional brain imaging 85–92
    learning disability 264
functional disorders *see* psychogenic and
    functional disorders

G-banding 146
GABA, CSF levels 172
gadolinium-enhanced MRI 56
gait (walking) abnormalities 251–8

clinical vignettes 102–3, 191–3, 206–7
ganglioneuroblastoma, clinical vignette
    139–40
gangliosidosis *see* GM1 gangliosidosis; GM2
    gangliosidosis
Gastaut-type occipital epilepsy 33, 285
gastroenteritis, mild, benign convulsions with
    282
    *see also* neurogastrointestinal
        encephalomyopathy
GCH1 *see* GTP cyclohydrolase 1
gelastic–dacrystic seizures (from
    hypothalamic hamartoma) 15, 279
'generalized epilepsy'
    tonic–clonic seizures 277
    *see also* genetic epilepsy with febrile
        seizures plus
GeneTests website 144
genetic epilepsy with febrile seizures plus 8,
    287, 295
genetic (hereditary/inherited) disorders
    ataxias 336
    ECG findings 106
    epilepsy/seizures 288
    MRI diagnoses 65
    peripheral neuropathies 229
genetic epilepsy with febrile seizures plus 8,
    287, 295
genetic investigations 144–50
    avoidance of other tests 145
    'cerebral palsy' 243–50
    clinical vignette 149–50
    learning disability 263–4
    neonates
        with generalized weakness 216
        with seizures 212–13
    range 146–7
genomic hybridization, array comparative
    147
geographical constraints on tests 2–3
glioblastoma multiforme, clinical vignette
    118–19
glioma, cervical cord, clinical vignette 19–20
global developmental delay 224–5
    EEG 224
        in several delay 29
globoid cell in D-bifunctional protein
    deficiency 188
globoid cell leukodystrophy (Krabbe disease)
    346

*GLRA1* mutations 244
glucose
    blood/plasma 163
    CSF 96, 172
        in microcephaly 237
    in microcephaly 237
glucose transporter type 1 (GLUT1) deficiency
    2, 96, 100, 209, 219, 233, 237, 246, 280,
    291, 308, 340, 359
glucosidase deficiency *see* Pompe disease
GLUT1 (glucose transporter type 1) deficiency
    *see* glucose transporter type 1 (GLUT1)
    deficiency
glutamate *SLC25A22* mutation,
    mitochondrial 211
glutaric aciduria
    type 1 (GA1) 7, 337
        macrocephaly 238
        mistaken for cerebral palsy 247
        movement disorders 339
    type 2 *see* multiple acyl-CoA
        dehydrogenase deficiency
glycine encephalopathy (non-ketotic
    hyperglycinaemia) 212
    EEG 32, 211
    proton MR spectroscopy 87
glycine receptor (*GLRA1*) mutations 244
glycine transporter (*GlyT2*) mutation 9, 244
glycogenosis type 2, ECG 107
glycosaminoglycans, urine 154
glycosylation, congenital defects of (CDG)
    131, 182–3, 232
    floppiness 232
    global developmental delay 226
    mistaken for cerebral palsy 249
    type 1a 66
*GLYT2* (glycine transporter) mutation 9, 244
GM1 gangliosidosis, infantile 107, 346
GM2 gangliosidosis 107
    infantile 346
        ERG 50
    late onset 66
Golgi apparatus disorders 182–3
granular osmophilic deposits (GROD) 53–4,
    113, 350
gratification, infantile *see* masturbation/
    gratification
GTP cyclohydrolase 1 (GTP-CH1; GCH1)
    blood levels 163
    deficiency 245, 357

clinical vignette 206
    CSF pterins and monoamines 175
    mistaken for cerebral palsy 245
guanidinoacetate (guanidinoacetic acid; GAA)
    CSF 172
    urine 154
        learning disability 261
        speech/language disorders 265–6
guanidinoacetate methyltransferase (GAMT)
    deficiency 91, 261, 262, 265–6, 340, 359
    epileptic seizures 290
    progressive skills loss 352
guanosine triphosphate cyclohydrolase 1 *see*
    GTP cyclohydrolase 1
Guillain–Barré syndrome (acute
    inflammatory polyneuropathy) 135, 177
    clinical vignette 110–11
    echocardiography 108
Guthrie test 8, 36
    cytomegalovirus 8, 123, 126, 226, 236,
    259, 266
    long QT syndrome 36, 105, 291
    microcephaly 236

haematology (blood tests) 112–13, 129–33
    learning disability 263
haemoglobin 129
    *see also* methaemoglobinaemia type 2
haemolytic anaemia 129
haemolytic–uraemic syndrome 323
haemophagocytic lymphohistiocytosis 322,
    358
    bone marrow samples 115–16
    brain biopsy 116
haemorrhage (non-traumatic intracranial)
    310, 312–13
    intraventricular, cranial ultrasound 65
    *see also* bleeding
haemorrhagic disease of newborn, late 131
haemorrhagic leukoencephalitis, acute 322
haemostatic factor abnormality 131
hair 112
Hallervorden–Spatz disease (pantothenate
    kinase 2/PANK2 deficiency) 112, 349
    ERG 51
hallucinations 271
harlequin phenomenon 109
Hashimoto encephalopathy 135, 313, 319,
    359
    clinical vignette 136–7

head
    size abnormalities 235–39
    trauma *see* trauma
head-up tilt testing 108
    in clinical vignette 110
headache 327–29
hearing *see* auditory unresponsiveness;
        deafness
heart 105–7
    clinical vignette 109–11
    *see also* echocardiography;
            electrocardiography
hemiclonic seizures 277
hemifacial spasms 279
hemiplegia, alternating 301, 308, 339
heparan sulphate, learning disability 261
hereditary disorders *see* genetic disorders
herpes simplex encephalitis 124, 319, 338
herpes virus infections 124
heterotopia, neuronal 210
hexosaminidase A and B
    blood 163
    deficiency, mistaken for cerebral palsy 248
HHVs *see* human herpes viruses
hippocampal sclerosis, mesial temporal lobe
        epilepsy with 285
histiocytosis-related cerebellar
        leukoencephalopathy, presumed 116,
        349
history taking 7–9
HIV infection, congenital, mistaken for
        cerebral palsy 248
hoarse floppy infant 45–6
home video/audio *see* video and audio
homocysteine, blood 163–4
    elevated 192, 193
    in microcephaly 236
homocystinuria 261, 262
human herpes viruses (HHVs)
    HHV6 124
        clinical vignette 126–7
    HHV7 124
human immunodeficiency virus (HIV)
        infection, congenital, mistaken for
        cerebral palsy 248
Hunter syndrome, ERG 51
Huntington disease 350
hydrocephalus 237–38
    obstructive 254
4-hydroxybutyric aciduria 247, 261

5-hydroxyindole acetic acid (5HIAA), CSF
        175
4-hydroxy-methoxymandelic acid (HMA),
        urine 154–5
hyperekplexia (startle), neonatal 109, 208,
        215, 218, 299, 337, 359
    autonomic function tests 109
    clinical vignette 9
    mistaken for cerebral palsy 244
    with severe apnoea 8, 43
hyperekplexia plus 309
hyperglycinaemia, non-ketotic *see* glycine
        encephalopathy
hyperkalaemic periodic paralysis 332
hyperkinesia (increased movements) 219
hypertension
    idiopathic intracranial 328
    systemic arterial 328
hyperthyroidism 341
hypertonia, neonatal 218
hyperventilation
    induced for EEG 23–4, 32
        hazards 31
    learning disability with, clinical vignette
        148–9
    in various conditions 15
        Pitt–Hopkins syndrome 15, 149
hypocretin 135
hypogammaglobulinemia, chronic viral
        infection 124
hypokalaemic periodic paralysis 332
hypokinesia 219–21
hypomyelination, congenital 40, 229
    MRI 65
hypoparathyroidism 262, 341
hypothalamic hamartoma, gelastic–dacrystic
        seizures 15, 279
hypothalamic syndromes, paraneoplastic
        135, 302
hypothyroidism
    ataxia 255
    floppiness 232–3
    progressive loss of skills and dementia 346
hypotonia, axial 215–16
    *see also* floppy baby
hypoventilation, central 215
hypoxic–ischaemic encephalopathy 323
hypsarrhythmia 26
'hysterical' blindness 271

ictal EEG 276, 277–85
ictal EMG 276, 277–78
IgG index
    clinical vignette 141
    definition 95
    normal values 369

*IGHMBP2* mutation 218, 229
imaging 55–92
    functional 85–92
    neurophysiological tests vs 43
    structural 55–84
        brachial plexus 74
        brain *see* brain imaging
        clinical vignette 76–8
        muscle 73
        spinal cord 70–2
        other organs/tissues 74–6
immunoglobulin *see* antibodies;
    hypogammaglobulinemia
immunoglobulin μ-binding protein gene
    (*IGHMBP2*) mutation 217–18, 229
immunolabelling, muscle biopsies 115
immunological disorders 134–43
    clinical vignette 136–42
    of innate system 134
immunological tests, vaccine damage 44
infants
    arching 194–5
    bath-induced paroxysmal incidents 109
    benign myoclonus *see* benign myoclonus
        of early infancy
    benign seizures 279
        familial 280
        myoclonic 280
    desaturation 46–7
    developmental delay *see* developmental
        delay
    GM2 gangliosidosis, ERG 50
    hoarse floppy 45–6
    masturbation/gratification *see*
        masturbation/gratification
    microcephaly evolving over 236
    movement disorders 337–8
    myoclonic epilepsy, severe *see* Dravet
        syndrome
    myositis 231
    neuroaxonal dystrophy *see* neuroaxonal
        dystrophy
    neuronal ceroid lipofuscinosis *see*

        neuronal ceroid lipofuscinosis
    newborn *see* neonates
    paroxysmal non-epileptic events 298
        paroxysmal dyskinesia with
            convulsions 308, 340
    partial *see* partial epilepsy
    premature *see* premature infants
    progressive loss of skills and dementia
        346–8
    reflex myoclonic seizures 281
    spasms *see* spasms
    spinal muscular atrophy *see* spinal
        muscular atrophy
    spinocerebellar ataxia 177
    sudden unexplained death 291
infarction (neonates), localized 210
    hypokinesia 220
infections 123–8, 318–20
    ataxia due to 334
    clinical vignettes 76–8, 125–8
    congenital 123–4, 221
        devastating 76–8
        misdiagnosis as cerebral palsy 248
        misdiagnosis of 132
    febrile seizures due to 295
    *see also* microbiology
inflammatory myopathy *see* dermatomyositis;
    myositis
inflammatory polyneuropathy, acute *see*
    Guillain–Barré syndrome
inherited disorders *see* genetic disorders
injury *see* trauma
innate immunity, disorders 134
insertional electrical activity (in EMG) 41–2
intensive care unit, paediatric
    EEG 30
    EMG 43
interferon-alpha (IFN), CSF 96, 98
    clinical vignette 141
interictal EEG 276, 279–85
interventricular septal hypertrophy 107
intracranial haemorrhage *see* haemorrhage
intracranial hypertension, intracranial 328
intraventricular haemorrhage, cranial
    ultrasound 65
ion channels *see* channelopathy *and specific*
    *ions*
iron deficiency anaemia 129, 263
ischaemic attacks, cerebral, with induced
    hyperventilation for EEG 31

ischaemic forearm test 184
ischaemic stroke, arterial 131, 311–12, 338

jitteriness 219
Joubert syndrome 241
    ERG 50
    wobbly eyes 241, 242
juvenile dermatomyositis, gait abnormalities 252
juvenile late-onset spasms 282
juvenile myoclonic epilepsy, EEG 27, 33
juvenile neuronal ceroid lipofuscinosis see neuronal ceroid lipofuscinosis
juvenile parkinsonism 340

karyotypic abnormalities see chromosome abnormalities
KCNA1 mutations 244, 301, 335
KCNJ11 mutations 358
KCNQ2 mutations 309, 311
Kearns–Sayre syndrome 177
kidney, ultrasound 76
kinesigenic dyskinesia, paroxysmal 302, 339
kinesigenic dystonia, paroxysmal, clinical vignette 9–10
knees, falling from the 45
Krabbe disease 346

lactate
    blood 164
    CNS (incl. brain) 89
        CSF 97, 172
        elevated white matter, leukoencephalopathy with involvement of brainstem and spinal cord and, MRI 65
lactic acidosis and stroke-like episodes, mitochondrial encephalopathy with (MELAS) 177, 329
Lafora progressive myoclonic epilepsy (Lafora disease) 114, 351
    ERG 53
    progressive loss of skills and dementia 351
Lambert–Eaton myasthenic syndrome
    autonomic function tests 108
    ganglioneuroblastoma, clinical vignette 139–40
    repetitive nerve stimulation 41
laminin 2 deficiency 230
Landau–Kleffner syndrome (epileptic aphasia; epileptic auditory agnosia) 267, 283
    clinical vignette 37–8
    EEG 27, 28, 30, 33, 35, 283
    speech/language disorders 267
language disorders 226, 265–8
L-arginine:glycine amidinotransferase (AGAT) deficiency 261, 265
laughter
    seizures with crying and (from hypothalamic hamartoma) 15
    sleepy and sluggish and falling with 139–40
L1CAM mutation 246
L2HGDH mutation 83
lead intoxication 262, 263, 324
learning disability (mental retardation) 259–64
    aetiological clues 259–60
    asymbolic, autistic spectrum disorder and 306
    genetic evaluation 147, 148–9
    with hyperventilation, clinical vignette 148–9
    movement disorders with 342
Leber amaurosis complex, ERG 50
Leber hereditary optic neuropathy 177
Leigh disease 176–7, 242
    mistaken for cerebral palsy 249
Leigh-like syndrome 177
Lennox–Gastaut syndrome 282
    EEG 27, 282
leptospirosis 360
Lesch–Nyhan syndrome/disease
    mistaken for cerebral palsy 246
    movement disorders 338, 341
    urine urate 157, 167
leukocytes see white blood cells
leukodystrophy
    globoid cell (Krabbe disease) 346
    metachromatic see metachromatic leukodystrophy
    misdiagnosis 125–6
    progressive loss of skills and dementia in 351
    see also adrenoleukodystrophy
leukoencephalitis, acute haemorrhagic 322
leukoencephalopathy (white matter disorders)
    approaches to MRI interpretation 64

cerebellar, with presumed histiocytosis 116, 349
  deafness and, in congenital CMV infection 126
  neonatal seizures due to, imaging 210
  progressive loss of skills and dementia in 351
  with subcortical cysts, megalencephalic, MRI 57
  see also vanishing white matter disease
leukomalacia, periventricular 227
  cranial ultrasound 65
levodopa
  conditions responsive to
  dystonia see dystonia
  mistaken for cerebral palsy 245
  trial 162, 201, 203
    clinical vignette 206-7
L-2-hydroxyglutaric aciduria 329
  clinical vignette 82-3
'lifeless' (flat) baby 214
limbic encephalitis 135
lipofuscinosis, neuronal ceroid see neuronal ceroid lipofuscinosis
liver
  biopsy 116, 182
  ultrasound 75
local epilepsy/seizures see partial epilepsy/seizures
long QT syndrome 36, 105, 300, 349
Lowe syndrome 231
LQT mutation (= long QT syndrome) 36, 105, 300, 349
lumbar puncture 93
  contraindications 99
  see also cerebrospinal fluid
lupus erythematosus, systemic see systemic lupus erythematosus
Lyme disease (borreliosis) 125, 322, 360
lymphocytes
  B and T cell deficiencies 135
  vacuolated 113
lymphocytic choriomeningitis, congenital 123
lymphohistiocytosis, haemophagocytic see haemophagocytic lymphohistiocytosis
lysosomal arylsulphatase A (ARSA) 103, 120, 175, 176, 348
lysosomal enzymes (in general)
  blood levels 164

disorders 175-6

macrocephaly 237-8
macrocytosis 113
macrophage activation syndrome 322
MADD see multiple acyl-CoA dehydrogenase deficiency
magnesium, blood 165
magnetic resonance arteriography and venography 59
magnetic resonance imaging (MRI)
  abdomen 76
  brain 55-65
    in acute disseminated encephalomyelitis see encephalomyelitis
    approach to interpretation 63-4
    in headache 327
    in learning disability 264
    limitations 61
    in microcephaly 57, 236, 237
    in multiple sclerosis see multiple sclerosis
    in neurological diagnosis 64
    sequences 55-61
  chest 75
  muscle 73
  spinal cord 70-1
magnetic resonance perfusion imaging 89
magnetic resonance spectroscopy 86-9
  global developmental delay 224, 225
  learning disability 264
  neonatal seizures 210
magnetic stimulation 53
malaria 320
malformations of brain (congenital structural anomalies) 210, 216, 219, 221-2
  brainstem 215
  'cerebral palsy' 243
  global developmental delay 226
  metabolic disorders with 221-2
  movements related to
    decreased 220
    increased 219
  neonatal seizures due to 210
  pyramidal tract absence, clinical vignette 121
malignant migrating partial seizures 280
malignant syncopes 299-300
manganese, blood 165

manometry, CSF 93–4
maple syrup urine disease, intermittent 336
masturbation/gratification, infantile 298
    clinical vignette 15
maternal examination in myopathies 202
*MCT8* mutation 232, 241, 246, 247, 262, 267
measles, subacute sclerosing panencephalitis
    *see* subacute sclerosing panencephalitis
*MECP2* (methyl CpG binding protein 2 gene)
    duplication 245, 263, 265
    mutations 236, 237, 263, 352
megalencephalic leukoencephalopathy with
    subcortical cysts, MRI 57
MELAS (mitochondrial encephalopathy with
    lactic acidosis and stroke-like episodes)
    177, 329
meningitis
    pyogenic 318–19
    tuberculous 319
    *see also* choriomeningitis
Menkes disease 347
    burst–suppression EEG 211
    clinical vignette 77–8, 118–19
    epileptic seizures 290
    progressive loss of skills and dementia 347
mental retardation *see* learning disability
MERFF (myoclonic epilepsy with ragged red
    fibres) 177
merosin deficiency 230
mesial temporal lobe epilepsy with
    hippocampal sclerosis 285
metabolic/biochemical disorders 226, 325,
    355
    ataxia 255
    with brain malformations 221–2
    epilepsy/seizures 288, 289–91
    global developmental delay 226
    transient neonatal 219
metabolic/biochemical tests *see* biochemical/
    metabolic tests
metachromatic leukodystrophy (MLD) 103,
    120–1, 175, 176, 348
    ataxia 255
    clinical vignette 120–1
    progressive loss of skills and dementia 348
    urine sediment 113
meta-iodobenzylguanidine scanning 85–6
metal objects and MRI 61
methaemoglobinaemia type 2 337
methyl CpG binding protein 2 gene *see*

MECP2
5-methyltetrahydrofolate, CSF 172
MIBG (meta-iodobenzylguanidine) scanning
    85–6
microbiology 123–8
    clinical vignette 125–8
    CSF 98
    *see also* virology
microcephaly 235–7
    clinical vignette 12
    MRI 57, 236
    *see also* Aicardi–Goutières syndrome
microdeletions, learning disability 263
microscopy 112–22
migraine mimics 329
Miller–Fisher syndrome 136
mitochondrial disorders/cytopathies 176–9,
    185–8, 232
    ataxia 255
    biochemical tests 176–9, 185–8, 212
    clinical vignette 185–8
    diagnostic confusion 179
    dystonias 337
    ECG 107
    epileptic and non-epileptic events
        combined 308
    epileptic seizures 290
    ERG 51
    floppiness 232
    global developmental delay 226
    H-MRS 89
    mistaken for cerebral palsy 249
    mistaken for flaccid paralysis 315
    movement disorders 339, 340
    progressive loss of skills 345
    *see also specific disorders*
MLPA (multiplex ligation-dependent probe
    amplification) 147
molybdenum cofactor deficiency 212
    progressive loss of skills and dementia 347
    variant and atypical 261, 262
monoamine neurotransmitter disorders 152,
    337
monocarboxylate transporter 8 gene (*MCT8*)
    mutation 232, 241, 246, 247, 262, 267
monogenic disorders *see* single gene mutation
    analysis
morphological abnormalities, neonates
    221–2
mortality *see* brain death; death

motor and sensory neuropathy, hereditary *see* Charcot–Marie–Tooth disease
motor development, abnormalities 223–4
motor nerve conduction studies 40–1
 repetitive nerve stimulation 41
motor skills loss 344–54
 acute undiagnosed neurological illness with 28
 progressive 344–54
 subacute or chronic, EEG 29–30
movement(s)
 decreased 219–221
 increased 219
movement disorders 337–43
 CSF examination 99
 infancy 337–38
 mitochondrial 177
moyamoya disease 301, 308, 329
 clinical vignette 79–80
 EEG 32
mucolipidosis type 4, ERG 51
mucopolysaccharidoses 344
multiple acyl-CoA dehydrogenase deficiency (MADD; glutaric aciduria type 2)
 clinical vignette 189–91
 riboflavin-responsive 362
multiple sclerosis 313–14, 320
multiplex ligation-dependent probe amplification (MPLA) 147
mumps 320
Munchausen by proxy, poisoning in 233, 308
muscle
 biopsy 114
  EMG vs 43
  in mitochondrial disorders 179
 cramps 331
 imaging 73
 tone abnormalities *see* dystonia; hypertonia; hypotonia
 weakness *see* weakness
 *see also* electromyography *and entries under* myo-
muscle–eye–brain disorders 230, 231
muscular atrophy, spinal *see* spinal muscular atrophy
muscular dystrophy 216
 congenital, floppiness 230
 Duchenne *see* Duchenne muscular dystrophy
 ECG 106

gait abnormalities 252
mutism 266–7
 elective 37–8, 270
myalgic encephalomyelitis 331
myasthenia 230
 diagnosis by therapeutic trial 201, 202
 neonatal 215
myasthenia gravis 136, 330
 asymptomatic 136
myasthenic syndrome
 congenital 136, 216, 217, 230, 330, 360
  clinical vignettes 45–7
  EMG 42–3
  floppiness 230
  gait abnormalities 252–3
 Lambert–Eaton *see* Lambert–Eaton myasthenic syndrome
*Mycoplasma pneumoniae* 320
myelin basic protein, CSF levels 96, 173
myelination
 abnormalities *see* demyelination; hypomyelination
 normal for age, MRI 62–3
myelitis, transverse 135
 *see also* encephalomyelitis; poliomyelitis
myoclonic absences (myoclonic–absence seizures) 277, 284
myoclonic epilepsy (ME) 278
 EEG 278, 280
  juvenile ME 27, 33
 of infancy
  benign 280
  reflex 281
  severe *see* Dravet syndrome
 progressive 289, 351
  Lafora *see* Lafora progressive myoclonic epilepsy
 with ragged red fibres (MERFF) 177
 Unverricht–Lundborg progressive, ERG 53
myoclonic–astatic epilepsy 282
myoclonus 341
 benign infantile *see* benign myoclonus of early infancy
 benign neonatal sleep 200, 208, 298
 negative 278
 phenytoin monitoring 199–200
 *see also* opsoclonus–myoclonus syndrome
myoclonus–dystonia 257, 340, 341
 clinical vignette 18–19
myoglobin, urine 155

myokymia 43
  hereditary 244
myopathies 216, 220
  ECG 107
  with fatigue 176
  floppiness 230–1
  gait abnormalities 252–3
  hypokinesia 220
  microscopy 114–15
  *see also* encephalomyopathy
myositis, infantile 231
myotonic dystrophy 230
  ECG 106
  floppiness 230

N-acetylaspartate (NAA) in Canavan disease 87
narcolepsy–cataplexy 135, 301
natural (innate) immunity, disorders 134
necrosis, bilateral striatal 323
necrotizing encephalopathy, acute 323
necrotizing haemorrhagic leukoencephalitis, acute 322
negative likelihood ratio 365
negative myoclonus 278
negative predictive value 365
neonates (newborn babies) 208–22
  abnormal neurology 214–22
  alloimmune thrombocytopenia *see* alloimmune thrombocytopenia
  benign sleep myoclonus 200, 208, 298
  collapsed, clinical vignette 117–18
  congenital infections presenting at 123
  encephalopathy *see* encephalopathies
  haemorrhagic disease, late 131
  hyperekplexia *see* hyperekplexia
  peroxisomal disorder investigations 180–1
  preterm *see* preterm infants
  seizures 207–13, 279
  stiff *see* stiffness
neoplasms *see* tumours
neopterin, CSF 98, 173, 175
nerve conduction studies 40–1, 368
  biopsies 115
  clinical aspects 42–3
  clinical vignette 44–8
  normal values 368
  practical aspects 42
neuroaxonal dystrophy, infantile 232, 348
  clinical vignette 47–8

EEG 29, 32
floppiness 232
microscopy/biopsies 114
progressive loss of skills and dementia 348
neuroblastoma, paravertebral, clinical vignette 89–90
neurodegenerative disorders, EEG with suspicion of 29–30
neurogastrointestinal encephalomyopathy, mitochondrial (MNGIE) 177
neuroleptic-associated movement disorders 338
neuromuscular junction disorders 230
  floppiness 230
  repetitive nerve stimulation 41
neuronal ceroid lipofuscinosis
  buffy coat 113
  infantile (INCL) 113, 237, 347
    clinical vignette 53–4
    EEG 29, 32
    ERG 51, 52
    microcephaly 237
    progressive loss of skills and dementia 347
  juvenile (JNCL) 350
    ERG 51, 52
    progressive loss of skills and dementia 350
  late infantile (LINCL) 113, 348
    clinical vignette 17
    EEG 24, 29, 33
    ERG 51, 52
    progressive loss of skills and dementia 348
neuronal degeneration of childhood, progressive *see* Alpers disease
neuronal heterotopia 210
neuropathy
  Leber hereditary optic 177
  peripheral 218, 229–30
    demyelinating *see* demyelination
    floppiness due to 229
    hereditary motor and sensory *see* Charcot–Marie–Tooth disease
    *see also* polyneuropathy
neuroserpinopathy 117
  epileptic seizures 288
neurotransmitter disorders
  hypokinesia due to 220
  monoamine 152, 337
newborns *see* neonates

N-glycosylation disorders 182
Niemann–Pick type C disease 301, 349
   bone marrow samples 115
   cholesterol ester trafficking 184
   progressive loss of skills and dementia 349
night terrors 303
NMDA receptor, antibodies to 108, 135, 136,
   272, 338
   clinical vignette 140–2
nocturnal frontal lobe epilepsy, autosomal
   dominant 285
non-accidental injury
   self-administered 270–1
   skull radiograph 69
non-accidental poisoning 233, 308
non-epileptic events (incl. non-epileptic
   attack disorders/paroxysmal disorders)
   275–6, 297–309
   anoxic 15
   benign infantile, clinical vignette 18
   coexisting with epileptic disorders 305–9
   distinction from epileptic seizures 275,
     297
   EEG 34, 35
   movement disorders 339–40
   neonatal 208–9
non-ketotic hyperglycinaemia see glycine
   encephalopathy
non-kinesigenic dyskinesia, paroxysmal 303,
   339
nonspecific (innate) immunity, disorders 134
nuclear pore protein mutations 323

obsessive–compulsive disorder (OCD) 270
occipital epilepsy of Gastaut 33, 285
ocular investigations/problems, etc. see eyes
oculomotor apraxia, ataxia with 66, 255
oesophagus, barium swallow 75
O-glycosylation disorders 182
Ohtahara syndrome (infantile epileptic
   encephalopathy) 119–20, 226
   clinical vignette 119–20
   EEG 26, 27, 210, 211
   global developmental delay 226
   with suppression bursts 279
oligoclonal bands (of immunoglobulins),
   CSF 95
oligosaccharides, urine 155
3-O-methyldopa (3OMD), CSF 175
OMIM (Online Mendelian Inheritance in

Man) 144
Ondine's curse 215
1p36 deletion 148, 288
Online Mendelian Inheritance in Man
   (OMIM) 144
opercular syndrome, anterior 266
ophthalmological investigations/problems,
   etc. see eyes
opsoclonus, in GLUT1 deficiency 359
opsoclonus–myoclonus (dancing eye)
   syndrome 135, 242, 334
   ataxia 334
   clinical vignette 12–13
optic atrophy 241
optic nerve hypoplasia 240–1
   clinical vignette 131–2
optic neuropathy, Leber hereditary 177
organelle-related investigations 175–83
organic acids
   disorders
     floppiness 232
     progressive skills loss 352
   urine 155
     in learning disability 261
     in microcephaly 236
ornithine transcarbamylase (OTC) deficiency
   329
orotic acid, urine 156
osteopetrosis 238
   electroretinography 49, 50, 51
   macrocephaly 238
   wobbly eyes 241
ovary, ultrasound 76
oxalic acid, urine 156
oxidative phosphorylation disorders 177–8

paediatric intensive care unit see intensive
   care unit
pain see facial pain; headache; paroxysmal
   extreme pain disorder
palsy see cerebral palsy; paralysis
Panayiotopoulos syndrome 108, 283, 287,
   307, 328
   autonomic function tests 108
   ECG and rhythm disturbances 106
   EEG 32, 33, 283
   headache 328
PANDAS (paediatric autoimmune
   neuropsychiatric disorders associated
   with streptococcal infections) 135

panencephalitis, subacute sclerosing *see*
    subacute sclerosing panencephalitis
panic attacks 271
*PANK2* mutation *see* Hallervorden–Spatz
    disease
pantothenate kinase 2 deficiency *see*
    Hallervorden–Spatz disease
parainfectious disorders 320–2
    ataxia 334
paralysis (palsy)
    facial 316
    flaccid 315
    periodic 332
    *see also* cerebral palsy; diplegia;
        hemiplegia; paraplegia
paraneoplastic hypothalamic syndromes 135,
    302
paraparese, progressive spastic 352
paraplegia 315
    hereditary spastic, mistaken for cerebral
        palsy 246
paravertebral neuroblastoma, clinical vignette
    89–90
parkinsonism, juvenile 340
parkinsonism–dystonia *see* dystonia–
    parkinsonism
paroxysmal disorders (in general)
    history-taking 7
    non-epileptic *see* non-epileptic events
    non-epileptic and epileptic, combined
        305–09
paroxysmal extreme pain disorder (previously
    familial rectal pain) 208–9, 299, 360
    autonomic function tests 109
    clinical vignette 16, 38
paroxysmal gait disturbance 257
paroxysmal kinesigenic dystonia, clinical
    vignette 9–10
partial (focal/local) epilepsy/seizures 278
    benign
        of infancy 280
            with midline spike and wave during
                sleep, in infancy 282
    clinical vignette 17–18
    EEG 35, 278
    malignant migrating 280
pattern stimulation (EEG) 24, 33
Pearson syndrome 177
Pelizaeus–Merzbacher disease 241, 248, 346
    clinical vignette 54

mistaken for cerebral palsy 248
    MRI 64
    progressive loss of skills and dementia 346
    wobbly eyes 241
Pelizaeus–Merzbacher-like disease 241, 248,
    346
perfusion imaging, MR 89
periodic paralysis 332
periventricular leukomalacia *see* leukomalacia
peroxisomal disorders 179–82, 187–9
    biochemical tests 179–82, 187–9, 212
    clinical vignette 187–9
    ERG 50, 51
    global developmental delay 226
    history-taking 7
    mimic 189–91
pertussis vaccine *see* diphtheria–tetanus–
    pertussis
*PEX1* mutation, clinical vignette 193–4
phenylalanine load 184
phenylketonuria (PKU) 262
    epileptic seizures 290
    maternal 261
    progressive loss of skills and dementia
        346
phenytoin
    intoxication, gait abnormalities 254
    monitoring 198–199
        clinical vignette 199–200
philosophy of tests 2
phosphate
    blood 165
    urinary 156
phospholipase A2 (*PLA2G6*) mutation 48
phosphorus MR spectroscopy ($^{31}$P-MRS) 89
photic stimulation (stroboscopic activation),
    EEG 23, 32
    modifications 24
photon magnetic resonance spectroscopy 87
photoparoxysmal response 24
    absence epilepsy with 284
photophobia 240
photosensitive epilepsy, EEG 27
phytanic acid, blood 165
pigmentary retinopathy 193, 194
pipecolic acid, blood 165
    high 191
Pitt–Hopkins syndrome 264
    clinical vignette 148–9
    hyperventilation 15, 148–9

pituitary tumours, headache 328
*PLA2G6* mutation 48
plain films *see* radiography
platybasia *see* basilar impression
*PLP* mutation 54
pneumonia, Werdnig–Hoffmann-like
    syndrome with 109–10
poisoning *see* toxic compounds
*POLG1* mutations 145, 178, 179, 329
    clinical vignettes 3–6, 101–2, 184–7
    EEG 28, 29, 32
    skills loss 352
    sodium valproate and 199
poliomyelitis, vaccine-associated, clinical
    vignette 44–5
polygraphy 24–5, 34
polymerase gamma 1 mutations *see POLG1*
    mutations
polyneuropathy
    acute *see* Guillain–Barré syndrome
    chronic relapsing 253
polyols, CSF 173
polyspikes 23
Pompe disease (glycogenosis type 2; acid
    maltase/alpha-glucosidase deficiency )
    109–10, 231–2
    clinical vignette 109–10
    ECG 107
    floppiness 231–2
pontocerebellar hypoplasia 210
porencephaly 212
porphyrins, urinary 156
positive likelihood ratio 365
positive predictive value 365
positron emission tomography 86
posterior fossa
    surgery, mutism following 267
    tumour, gait abnormalities 254
posterior odds 364
Prader–Willi syndrome 215, 220, 337
    axial hypotonia 215
    hypokinesia 220
    mistaken for cerebral palsy 244
    neonatal 337
predictive value of investigation results
    364–67
prenatal brain lesions *see* brain
pressure, CSF
    high 328
    measurements 93–4

preterm infants
    cranial ultrasound 67
    retinopathy, ERG 49–50
    very, brain damage in, predictive value of
        investigations 366
prevalence 365
prior odds 365
probability 365
progressive disorders 344–54
    'cerebral palsy' 243
    febrile seizures and evidence of 296
    of movement 340
    of skill loss 344–54
    *see also* regression
progressive myoclonic epilepsy *see* myoclonic
    epilepsy
progressive neuronal degeneration of
    childhood *see* Alpers disease
prolactin, blood 165–6
prosaposin 176
protein(s), CSF 3, 94, 175
    normal values 369
protein palmitoyl thioesterase
    deficiency 54, 113
        progressive loss of skills and dementia
            347
    in microcephaly, assay 237
proteolipid protein 1 (*PLP*) mutation 54
proton MR spectroscopy (H-MRS) 87–9
    global developmental delay 224, 225
    learning disability 264
    neonatal seizures 210
pseudo-hypoparathyroidism 261
pseudo-peroxisomopathy 189–91
pseudo-Zellweger syndrome 189
psychiatric disorders 269–74
    encephalitis and *see* encephalitis
    *see also* PANDAS
psychogenic and functional disorders
    ataxia 333
    dyskinesia 303
    EMG and nerve stimulation 43
    movement disorders 339
'psychological' paroxysmal non-epileptic
    events 299
psychosis 271
*PTEN* mutations 238
pteridines, urinary 156
pterins, CSF 97–8, 173, 175
    *see also* neopterin; sepiapterin

purine nucleoside phosphorylase deficiency
135, 247
purine synthesis deficiency 211, 233
purpura, neonatal alloimmune
thrombocytopenic *see* alloimmune
thrombocytopenia
pyogenic meningitis or septicaemia 318–19
pyramidal tracts, congenital absence 121
pyridostigmine, diagnosis by therapeutic trial
of 203
pyridoxal phosphate (pyridoxal 5′-
phosphate)
CSF levels 97, 174
diagnosis by therapeutic trial of 204, 209
pyridoxal phosphate-responsive seizures 97,
289, 361
burst–suppression EEG 211
pyridox(am)ine phosphate oxidase deficiency
97, 209
pyridoxine-dependent epilepsy 201–6, 289,
361
AASA
blood 158
urinary 153
burst–suppression EEG 211
diagnosis by therapeutic trial of pyridoxine
204, 209
clinical vignette 201–6
pipecolic acid 191
pyruvate, blood 166
pyruvate dehydrogenase (PDH) deficiency
177–8, 183, 335–6, 362
ataxia 335–6
clinical vignette 194–5
mistaken for cerebral palsy 249
movement disorders 338
progressive skills loss 352

QT interval, long, (= long QT syndrome) 36,
105, 300, 360

radiography (plain films)
chest 75
skull *see* skull radiographs
rage 270
*RANBP2* mutations 323
*RAPSN* mutation 217
Rasmussen syndrome/encephalitis
brain biopsy 117
immunological tests 136

receiver operating characteristic 366
rectum
biopsy 116
pain, familial *see* paroxysmal extreme pain
disorder
red cells 112–13, 129–30
reference ranges, antiepileptic drug 198
reflex asystolic syncope 299
reflex myoclonic epilepsy of infancy 281
reflex seizures of early infancy, tonic 298
Refsum disease, ERG 51
regression (regressive disorders) 344, 345–6
CSF examination 99
EMG 43
epilepsy with, clinical vignette 16–17
fever-related 296
in peroxisomal disorders in school-age
child 181
speech/language impairment 267
*see also* progressive disorders
respiratory distress, spinal muscular atrophy
with *see* spinal muscular atrophy
restless legs syndrome 341
retina
electrical responses of various cell types
(electroretinography) 49–50
visual evoked potentials in disorders of 50
retinal blindness, congenital 241
retinopathy, pigmentary 193, 194
Rett syndrome 309, 347
clinical vignette of 12
clinical vignette of case mistaken for 53–4
hyperventilation 15
microcephaly 236, 237
mistaken for cerebral palsy 245
progressive loss of skills and dementia 347
rhabdomyomata 107
rhythm disturbances (cardiac) 105–7
riboflavin-responsive MADD 362
Riley–Day syndrome 108
floppiness 230
ring chromosome
chromosome 14, epileptic seizures 288
chromosome 20 283
clinical vignette 37–8
*RNASEH2B* mutations 101, 346
roast beef seizures 100
rolandic epilepsy, benign 27, 28, 32, 284,
287–8

saliva, antiepileptic drug monitoring 199
Sandhoff disease, infantile 346
Sandifer syndrome mistaken for cerebral
    palsy 244
Sanfilippo syndrome 261, 344, 348
sarcoglycan mutation 19
sclerosing panencephalitis, subacute *see*
    subacute sclerosing panencephalitis
*SCN1A* mutations 7, 145, 287, 325
*SCN2A* mutations 279
*SCN9A* mutations 109
screening test 2
Segawa-type dopa-responsive dystonia
    levodopa trial 201, 245, 255
        clinical vignette 206–7
    mistaken for cerebral palsy 245
    spasticity 256, 256–7
seizures (epileptic) 209–12, 275–93, 305–9
    anoxic–epileptic 15
    astatic 35
    cardiac rhythm disturbances 106
    coexisting with non-epileptic events 305–9
    CSF examination 99
    distinction from non-epileptic events 275,
        297
    EEG in *see* electroencephalography
    focal, clinical vignette 17–18
    gelastic–dacrystic, from hypothalamic
        hamartoma 15, 279
    neonatal 209–12
    pyridoxal phosphate-responsive *see*
        pyridoxal phosphate-responsive
        seizures
    roast beef 100
    *see also* convulsions; epilepsy
seizures (non-epileptic/in general/
    unspecified) *see* febrile seizures; non-
    epileptic events
self-injurious behaviour 270–1
senataxin gene (*SETX*) mutation 255
sensitivity (investigation results) 364
sensorimotor neuropathy, hereditary *see*
    Charcot–Marie–Tooth disease
sensory ataxia 333
sensory deficits 226–7
sensory nerve conduction studies 41, 368–69
    normal values 368–69
sepiapterin, CSF 174, 175
sepiapterin reductase deficiency 175, 206,
    245–6, 257, 266, 362

mistaken for cerebral palsy 245–6
    spasticity 257
    speech/language disorders 266
septal hypertrophy, interventricular 107
septicaemia, pyogenic 318–19
serine synthesis disorders 97, 209, 219, 362
    epileptic seizures 290
    learning disability 262
    microcephaly 236
serpinopathy, neural *see* neuroserpinopathy
*SETX* mutation 255
*SGCE* mutation 19
shuddering attacks 198, 338
    clinical vignette 17–18
sialic acid, urinary 156
sickle cell disease and traits 130
SimulConsult 1, 144, 259, 344, 345
single-fibre EMG, stimulation 42
single gene mutation analysis 147
    neonatal seizures 212
single photon emission computed
    tomography (SPECT) 85, 86
skeletal survey 75
skills *see* motor skills
skin biopsy 114
skull radiographs 69–70
    microcephaly 236
*SLC* mutations (and subsequent deficiency)
    *SLC2A1* (*GLUT1*; glucose transporter type
        1) 2, 96, 100, 209, 219, 233, 237,
        248, 280, 291, 308, 340, 359
    *SLC16A2* (*MCT8*) 232, 241, 246, 247,
        262, 267
    *SLC25A22* 211
sleep
    EEG in 24, 33
        spike-and-wave complexes *see* spike-
        and-wave complexes
    paroxysmal non-epileptic events 298
sleep deprivation, EEG 24, 34
sleep myoclonus, benign neonatal 200, 208,
    398
slow channel syndrome, clinical vignette 46
slow stroboscopic activation 24, 33
Smith–Lemli–Opitz syndrome 162
social unresponsiveness 227
sodium channel mutations *see* SCN
sodium valproate monitoring 199
solute carrier family *see* SLC
somatosensory evoked potentials 52–3

spasms 278
  benign myoclonus of early infancy
    (benign non-epileptic infantile
    spasms) 298
  hemifacial 279
  infantile
    benign *see* benign myoclonus of early
    infancy
    clinical vignettes 36
  juvenile late-onset 282
spastic parapareses, progressive 352
spastic paraplegia, hereditary, mistaken for
  cerebral palsy 246
spasticity 256–7
specific (acquired) immunity, disorders 134
specificity (investigation results) 364
speech disorders 265–68
*SPG11* mutation 246
spike(s) (EEG) 22–3, 28
  centrotemporal, benign childhood
    epilepsy with 27, 28, 32
  multiple closely spaced 23
spike-and-wave complexes 23
  frequent bilateral 26
  in sleep
    continuous (CSWS) 26, 30, 33, 36, 283
    midline, benign focal epilepsy in
    infants with 282
  slow, longs runs of 26
spinal cord
  floppiness due to lesions in 229
  imaging 70–2
  leukoencephalopathy with involvement of
    brainstem and, and elevated white
    matter lactate, MRI 65
  trauma 218
    autonomic function tests 108
  tumours
    clinical vignette 19–20
    mistaken for cerebral palsy 244
    spasticity 256
spinal dysraphism
  gait abnormalities 253
  ultrasound 71–2
spinal muscular atrophy 229
  distal 253
  infantile (Werdnig–Hoffmann disease)
    216–17
    ECG 106
    floppiness 229

intermediate, floppiness 229
with respiratory distress 217–18
  floppiness 229
spinocerebellar ataxia 352
  infantile 177
stains, muscle biopsy 114–15
startle *see* hyperekplexia
status epilepticus
  clinical vignette 126–7
  EEG 35, 281
  febrile 280
  minor, gait abnormalities 253
  in sleep (continuous spike–waves in sleep;
    CSWS) 26, 30, 33, 36, 283
stereotypies 298
stiffness 331
  baby/neonate 218–19
    clinical vignette 121
stimulation single-fibre EMG 42
storage diseases, lysosomal, disorders 175
striatal necrosis, bilateral 323
stroboscopic activation *see* photic stimulation
stroke 310–13
  arterial ischaemic 131, 311–12, 338
stroke-like episodes 313
  with antibodies, clinical vignette 136–7
  mitochondrial encephalopathy with lactic
    acidosis and (MELAS) 177, 329
structural anomalies *see* malformations
subacute sclerosing panencephalitis/SSPE,
    post-measles 124, 127–8, 349–50
  brain biopsy 116
  clinical vignette 127–8
  EEG 30, 32
  progressive loss of skills and dementia
    349–50
subcortical cysts, megalencephalic
    leukoencephalopathy with, MRI 57
succinic semialdehyde dehydrogenase
    deficiency (4-hydroxybutyric aciduria )
    247, 261
succinyl purines
  CSF 98, 174
  urinary 157
sudden unexplained death in infancy 291
sulphatides, urinary 157
sulphite oxidase deficiency
  burst–suppression EEG 211
  microcephaly 236
sulphite test 152, 157

learning disability 261
microcephaly 236
suppression burst pattern (on EEG)
epileptic encephalopathy with 279
neonatal seizures 210, 211
sural nerve biopsy 115
Swartz–Jampel syndrome 218
Sydenham chorea 125, 135, 338
valvular disease 107
syncopes
benign 299
convulsive 108–9
malignant 299–300
vasovagal/neurally mediated see vasovagal
syncope
see also fainting fit
systemic arterial hypertension 326
systemic lupus erythematosus 135, 136, 337
'congenital SLE', clinical vignette 137–9

T-cell deficiency 135
T1 inversion recovery 57
T1-weighted MRI sequences 55
T2-weighted MRI sequences 56
FLAIR 57
tache cérébrale 3
tau protein (asialotransferrin), CSF 96, 170,
336, 351, 352
Tay–Sachs disease 346
ERG 50
TCF4 mutation 149, 264
television-induced epilepsy 24, 33
temporal lobe epilepsy
mesial, with hippocampal sclerosis 285
SPECT 86
tendoskeletal disorders, floppiness 231
thalamic lesions, neonatal
hypokinesia 220
seizures, imaging 210
stiffness 218
therapeutic range, antiepileptics 198
therapeutic trial of drugs, diagnosis by 201–7
pyridoxal phosphate 204, 209
theta rhythm/wave 22
thiamine, blood 166
thrombocytopenia, neonatal alloimmune see
alloimmune thrombocytopenia
thrombophilias 131
thrombosis, cerebral venous sinus 131, 310,
312

thyroid function tests 166
global developmental delay 224
learning disability 262
see also hyperthyroidism; hypothyroidism
tics 270, 341
toe-walking 251–2
clinical vignette 102–3
tonic–clonic seizures
generalized 277
neonatal 279
tonic reflex seizures of early infancy 298
tonic seizures 278
tonic upgaze or downgaze, benign 303
tonsillar ectopia 328
torsion dystonia, idiopathic 257, 341
torticollis, paroxysmal 300
Tourette syndrome 270, 341
toxic compounds (drugs and poisoning) 326,
361
ataxia 334
deliberate (Munchausen by proxy) 233,
308
gait abnormalities 253–4
learning disability 262, 263
misinterpretation as 90–1
movement disorders 338
toxoplasma 320
transaminases, blood 167
transcranial Doppler ultrasound 68
transcription factor 4 gene (TCF4) mutation
149, 264
transferrin, blood 167
trauma/injury
brachial plexus 74
brain/head 324
neonatal seizures 212
non-accidental see non-accidental injury
spinal cord, autonomic function tests 108
tremors 341
tricyclic poisoning 308
tri-iodothyronine (T3), free 166
trisomy 21 see Down syndrome
Tropheryma whipplei 125
true negative proportion 366
true positive proportion 366
tuberculous meningitis 319
tuberous sclerosis
clinical vignette 36–7
echocardiography (for rhabdomyomata)
107

tumours/neoplasms
    brain *see* brain
    paravertebral, clinical vignette 89–90
    spinal cord *see* spinal cord
22q– deletion 267
*Twinkle* 177, 178
tyrosine hydroxylase deficiency 175, 207

*UBE3A* mutation 263
ubiquinone *see* coenzyme Q10
ultrasound
    cardiac (echocardiography) 74
    chest/abdominal/pelvic organs 75, 76
    cranial/brain 65–8
        microcephaly 236
    muscular 73
    spinal 71
Unverricht–Lundborg disease 351
    somatosensory evoked potentials 53
upgaze, benign tonic 303
uracil 157
urate
    blood 167–8
        in learning disability 262
    urinary 157
urea, blood 168
urea cycle defects 219
urine
    biochemistry 151–2, 153–8
        global developmental delay 225
        learning disability 261
        neonatal seizures 212
    sediment 113

vaccine-associated damage 7, 325
    clinical vignette 3–6, 44–5
    febrile seizures and 296
vacuolated lymphocytes 113
vagovagal reflex 108–9
Valsalva manoeuvre, compulsive 299
    clinical vignette 16–17
    ECG 106
    EEG 34
    home video/audio 15
valvular disease (cardiac) 107
vanillylmandelic acid (VMA), urine 154–5
vanishing white matter disease, floppiness
    232
varicella-zoster 125
vascular headaches 329

vascular stroke syndromes *see* stroke
vasculitis (angiitis) of CNS, primary 116, 322,
    329
vasovagal (neurally mediated) syncope 299
    clinical vignettes 35–6, 110
venography, MR 59
venous sinus thrombosis, cerebral 131, 310,
    312
ventricular septal hypertrophy 107
vertebra, neuroblastoma alongside, clinical
    vignette 89–90
vertebral artery dissection 79, 335
vertigo, paroxysmal 300
very long-chain fatty acids, blood/plasma
    168, 179, 181, 184
vestibular ataxia 333
video and audio (at home) 7, 12
    'cerebral palsy' 243
video-EEG 25, 34
video game epileptic seizures 289
video telemetry 25, 30, 35
viral infections 319, 338
    chronic 124
    *see also specific viral infections*
virology 123–4
    microcephaly 236
    vaccine damage 44
vision, low, late onset, ERG 51
visual evoked potentials (VEPs) 50–1
    normal values 369
visual impairment/defect
    congenital low vision, ERG 50
    cortical *see* cortical visual impairment
    late-onset low vision, ERG 51
    wobbly eyes and 240–1, 242
visual unresponsiveness 227
visuomotor ataxia 333
vitamin A, blood 168
vitamin B$_1$ (thiamine), blood 166
vitamin B$_{12}$ (cobalamin/cyanocobalamin)
    256
    blood 169
    deficiency (incl. malabsorption) 256, 341,
        363
    metabolic disorders 256, 358
        cobalamin C disorder, clinical vignette
            191–3
        progressive loss of skills and dementia
            346
vitamin E

blood 169
  deficiency 363
    ataxia 254

Walker–Warburg syndrome 231
  ERG 50
  floppiness 231
  muscle ultrasound 73
walking abnormalities *see* gait abnormalities
weakness, generalized 216–18, 330
  episodic 332
  gait abnormalities 252–3
Werdnig–Hoffmann disease *see* spinal
    muscular atrophy
Werdnig–Hoffmann-like syndrome with
    pneumonia 109–10
West Nile virus 125
West syndrome 280
  EEG 27, 280

Whipple disease 125
white blood cells (leukocytes)
  blood 113
  CSF, count 94
white matter disorders *see*
    leukoencephalopathy
whole-body MRI 61
Williams syndrome 262
Wilson disease 154, 161, 341, 350, 363
wobbly eyes 240–2
Worster-Drought syndrome 266

X chromosome, fragile site 263
xanthomatosis, cerebrotendinous 358

Zellweger syndrome (Zellweger-type
    generalized peroxisomal disorder) 193–4
  clinical vignette 193–4
  mimic 189

# Other titles from Mac Keith Press

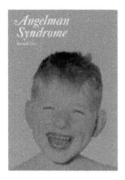

## Angelman Syndrome
Bernard Dan

Clinics in Developmental Medicine 177
2008 • £75.00 • €90.00 • $150.00 • Paperback • 256 pp
ISBN 978-1-898683-55-1

The diagnosis of Angelman syndrome has important implications for both medical management and counselling. Despite its severity and typical presentation, however, many physicians remain unfamiliar with the condition, first described by Harry Angelman in 1965. This comprehensive guide to the clinical management and basic science of Angelman syndrome will be of value to clinicians and researchers as well as parents and relatives.

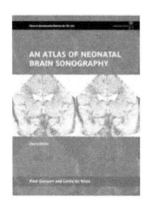

## An Atlas of Neonatal Brain Sonography
(2nd edn)
## Paul Govaert and Linda S de Vries

Clinics in Developmental Medicine 182-183
2009 • £125.00 • €150.00 • $225.00 • Hardback • 448 pp
ISBN 978-1-898683-56-8

This Atlas covers the entire spectrum of brain disease as studied with ultrasound, illustrated throughout with superb-quality images. Suggestions for differential diagnosis accompany all the sonographic findings, guiding the clinician in proceeding from an abnormal image to a diagnosis. This second edition of the Atlas has been brought up to date to include the many advances in technique and interpretation that have been made in the past decade.

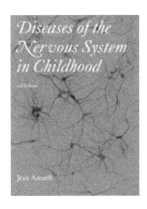

## Diseases of the Nervous System in Childhood (3rd edn)

Edited by Jean Aicardi with Martin Bax and Christopher Gillberg

2009 • £175.00 • €236.30 • $335 • Hardback • 956 pp
ISBN 978-1-898683-59-9

This is the essential resource for child neurologists, neurologists, paediatricians, and physicians in developmental medicine. The third edition has been extensively updated to incorporate the tremendous volume of new information since the previous edition, but remains as clinically oriented as its predecessors. Because of the enormous and wide-ranging amount of new material available, Aicardi and his co-editors have been joined by an eminent team of international experts who have contributed many of the chapters.

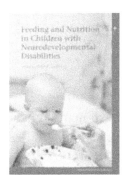

## Feeding and Nutrition in Children with Neurodevelopmental Disability

A practical guide from Mac Keith Press

Edited by Peter B. Sullivan

2009 • £20.00 • €24.00 • $40.00 • Paperback • 196 pp
ISBN 978-1-898683-60-5

This book is for all those who have responsibility for the nutritional and gastrointestinal care of children with neurodisability, providing an up-to-date account of the practicalities of assessment and management of feeding problems in these children. The emphasis throughout is on the importance of team-based care: it is written from a multidisciplinary perspective by a group of authors with considerable clinical and research experience in this area.

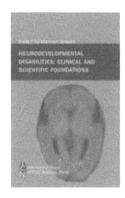

## Neurodevelopmental Disabilities: Clinical and Scientific Foundations

Edited by Michael Shevell

International Reviews in Child Neurology
2009 • £75.00 • €90.00 • $119.95 • Paperback • 504 pp
ISBN 978-1-898683-67-4

This comprehensive approach to addressing neurodevelopmental disabilities in childhood focuses in particular on the two most common childhood neurodevelopmental disabilities: global developmental delay and developmental language impairment. The book's attention to both clinical and scientific aspects is invaluable; it provides extensive information in a single source on often-overlooked areas such as medical management, rehabilitation, public policy, and ethics.

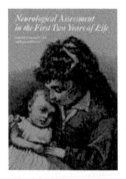

## Neurological Assessment in the First Two Years of Life

Edited by Giovanni Cioni and Eugenio Mercuri

Clinics in Developmental Medicine 176
2008 • £80.00 • €96.00 • $150.00 • Hardback • 256 pp
ISBN 978-1-898683-54-4

This book reviews the state of the art of neurological assessment in the first two years of life and identifies the most appropriate instruments for the follow-up of newborn children at risk of developing neurological abnormalities. It presents the various methods used, emphasizing how a combined approach of clinical and instrumental investigations can provide important diagnostic and prognostic information.

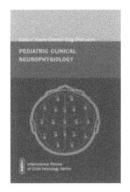

## Paediatric Clinical Neurophysiology

Edited by Karin Eeg-Olofsson

International Reviews in Child Neurology
2008 • £65.00 • €78.00 • $119.95 • Hardback • 254 pp
ISBN 978-1-898683-48-3

This book introduces clinical neurophysiology
and its applications to the paediatric neurologist.
The focus is on the methods applied in the setting
of a clinical neurophysiological laboratory. This
book will stimulate readers' interest in paediatric
clinical neurophysiology in their daily clinical work.
Particularly valuable are the examples and reference
values for nerve conduction studies, EMG, evoked
potentials, autonomic testing, EEG and transcranial
magnetic stimulation.

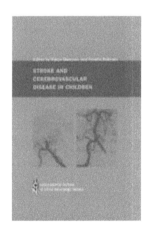

## Stroke and Cerebrovascular Disease in Children

Edited by Vijeya Ganesan and Fenella Kirkham

International Reviews in Child Neurology
2010 • £145.00 • €174.00 • $199.95 • Hardback • 448 pp
ISBN 978-1-898683-34-6

This major volume for the first time summarises
the state of the art in this field. A team of eminent
clinicians, neurologists and researchers provide an
up-to-the-minute account of all aspects of stroke and
cerebrovascular disease in children, ranging from a
historical perspective to future directions, through
epidemiology, the latest neuroimaging techniques,
neurodevelopment, co-morbidities, diagnosis and
treatment. The authors' practical approaches to the
clinical problems make this essential reading for
practising clinicians as well as researchers.